Ecosystem Effects on Avian Health and Disease

Ecosystem Effects on Avian Health and Disease

Julia Zaias

Department of Pathology & Laboratory Medicine
University of Miami
Miami, FL, USA

WILEY

Published by John Wiley & Sons, Inc., Hoboken, New Jersey.

Library of Congress Cataloging-in-Publication Data has been applied for:
Print ISBN: 9781394422012
ePDF ISBN: 9781394422036
ePub ISBN: 9781394422029
oBook ISBN: 9781394422043

Cover Design: Wiley
Cover Images: Thipwan/Getty Images, Robert Brook/Getty Images

Printed and bound by CPI Group (UK) Ltd, Croydon, CR0 4YY

C9781394422012_080926

I would like to dedicate this book to several people who inspired my love of birds! Dr Oscar T Owre and Dr Randall Breitwisch, who introduced me to birds. Harry & Darlene Kelton and Wendy Fox, who introduced me to pelicans and seabird rehabilitation. Dr Carolyn Cray, who taught me avian clinical pathology and always indulged my research ideas! THANK YOU!

Contents

Introduction

Driving home from work one day, there was a long line of cars stopped and not moving. After a few minutes, I saw three Muscovy ducks ambling across the street (see below)! This happened several times in the next few weeks. I saw the ducks literally walk to the sidewalk curb, turn their heads right and left, then jump down and start to cross the street! And the cars slowed and stopped to wait for these ducks to finish crossing the street! On a road that is a major egress point for the hospital, these ducks have made street crossing to a small stream, then back, part of their daily routines ... and our lives! They see no need to fly across the street or over the cars to avoid the risk of being run over. No need. They plod along in that rhythmic walking, kind of oscillating, motion ... at one speed ... the entire way across. I have never heard a car honk at them nor run over them (thankfully).

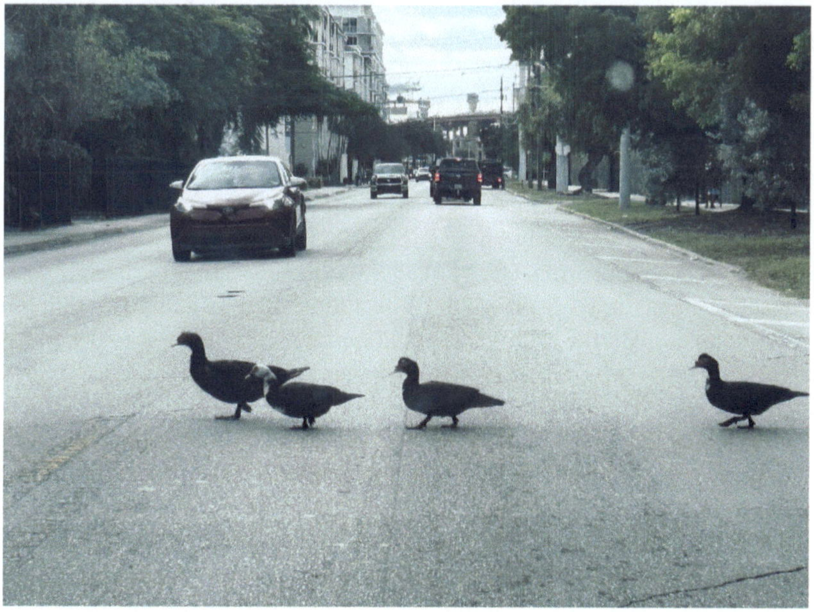

In South Florida, Muscovy ducks are considered "non-native" birds. This species thrives in urban and suburban areas and is often viewed as a pest. Muscovy ducks have learned to live, very comfortably, with humans in our world. It is but one example of a bird species that "embraces" and thrives in anthropogenic environments, not thwarted by a building or new road. Many other species common to urban areas (pigeons, crows, and starlings) also appear to do well in cities. Many other species, however, would not fare as well. Forest species need trees, tree canopies, and the insects that live there. How will they adjust to increasing urbanization, logging, and increased temperatures without the benefit of shade from the tree canopies?

The more I read and researched, the more I was astounded by how much environmental change and damage we humans have created. I cringed every time I read about seagulls foraging at garbage dumps (it's quite embarrassing). I was surprised by how much the sea surface and air temperatures have already increased. I was speechless when I read about the Hawaiian honeycreepers' demise from malaria! How can we have allowed all the damage and change to impact bird (or any) species around the world?

The general public is aware of temperatures rising, increased pollution in urban centers, elimination of farmland as people expand out to rural areas, etc. There is also general awareness of mitigation strategies and other actions we have initiated including carbon footprint reduction, increased use of electric vehicles, and changes in how we handle/use plastics. However, I was *not* aware of how extensive the damage and change were already! It is one thing to understand the *general concept* of carbon emissions affecting environmental temperatures, but it is an entirely different level of understanding to see in detail how increasing temperatures resulted in the expansion of the mosquito vector and introduced malaria (*Plasmodium*) to naïve avian species, causing near extinction-level losses.

How to help mitigate the negative consequences of these changes can also be hard to grasp. We can decrease our carbon footprint by driving an electric vehicle (and using solar panels to generate electricity), but reducing carbon effects is a huge problem which takes a long, long time to resolve. And my electric car in Florida is not directly mitigating the melting polar ice in the Arctic!

We need these types of actions, but there are also smaller scale actions to help save (or protect) some bird species. The more we learn about disease transmission for individual diseases and the entry points of contaminants into the environment, the better we can work with microbiologists, chemists, and others to find ways to prevent and/or mitigate their negative effects. We already know a lot of this information! We have lots of tools – medical, ecological, engineering, etc. – already! We just need an interdisciplinary approach to generate novel ideas and solutions. Specific solutions here and there for different smaller scale issues coupled with the large-scale goal to reduce carbon emissions and (try to) stall the increasing temperature trend. Not sure how realistic the latter is these days, but we must try.

What would it be like to not be able to show our grandchildren what a live toucan looks like? Will they only get to see one on the box of Fruit Loops cereal? Or will they only get to see it on social media? Every year I have a debate with my class about which interaction type (in-person interaction or video/social media) moved the students to want to work with and study animals (in their case, marine mammals). Consistently over the past 10 years, more than 95% have said "in-person interaction." We will only become invested in saving/studying what we learn to love and understand. This is most often solidified by seeing the animal in person. That's where zoos and captive breeding are integral and critical: integral to engendering love and interest in the animals and critical to the preservation of species that are on the brink of extinction.

Why this book? This book is an attempt to widen the exposure of health and welfare of birds in our changing environment. Avian health is not the realm of veterinarians only. Most other people who work and care for birds are critical to animal health. I feel it is important to understand the anatomy, physiology, and behavior of birds so that changes in behaviors or failing of physiological systems are recognized as soon as possible. If you do not know what is normal, then you do not know what is not normal.

The first section of the text covers some background in anatomy, physiology, immunology, and infectious agents in a (hopefully) easy but detailed way. The second section deals with managing health and reproduction primarily in managed care settings by introducing methods of sampling and testing, rationale and purpose of different types of blood tests, and reviewing management of breeding, egg laying, development (briefly), and the potential health impacts on the female. The last section of the text deals with various environmental factors that affect health and welfare of captive and wild birds. These include diseases known to cause epizootics, chemical contaminants, and physical contaminants (e.g., urbanization and associated problems). A chapter on stress touches on how to "diagnose" (or "verify") stress in birds and then what that means relative to welfare. After the summary chapter, I have a short chapter on the chicken and recognizing all the amazing and beneficial attributes and scientific knowledge we have learned from them (my indulgence if you don't mind). I hope you enjoy it.

Section 1

Basis of Health and Disease

1

Cells and Tissues in Health and Disease

Very simply, medicine is the study (and maintenance) of health – which requires appropriately functioning organ structure and function. Health that has gone awry or out of balance is *disease*. To understand how and why things go wrong in the body, we need to understand what is normal – normal anatomy, normal physiology, normal function. The starting point and basis for all health and disease is the cell. Cells form tissues, which form organs, which are responsible for an organism's life.

The eukaryotic cell is a remarkable creation! Self-sustaining, it contains all that is needed to survive and reproduce – mechanisms to replicate, create energy, create proteins and molecules to make substrates it needs, a storage depot, a way to import and export signals, and a way to remove and/or destroy waste. Each of these functions is mediated by specific organelles; that is, membrane-bound "factories" that carry out their specific tasks (Figure 1.1).

The cell and each organelle within it are surrounded by a membrane. The primary functions of the membrane are to enclose and protect the integrity of the cell and to mediate the movement of molecules and signals in and out of the cell. The membrane is composed of a lipid bilayer with proteins either located within the bilayer and/or protruding out either end. This structure supports the optimal function and flexibility of the cell.

The director of all activities in the cell (and body) lies within the genetic material, which resides in the nucleus. The eukaryotic nucleus houses DNA within genes tightly bound together in structures called chromosomes. When needed, these tightly bound structures will "unwind" to permit cell division or replication (mitosis) and/or protein formation.

Cell division, or mitosis, is simply the replication of the cell. DNA normally exists in a diploid state – two copies of the DNA per cell (i.e., two copies of each chromosome with all their genes within). In general, mitosis is preceded by the S phase of interphase (during which DNA replication occurs) and is often followed by metaphase, telophase (chromosomes split and spread apart), and ultimately cytokinesis. In cytokinesis, division of the cytoplasm, organelles, and cell membrane occurs, and two new cells are created, each containing roughly equal shares of these cellular components.

Gamete production occurs by meiosis, a process like mitosis but with distinct differences. In meiosis, the chromosomes duplicate (during interphase) and homologous chromosomes exchange genetic information (chromosomal crossover) during the first

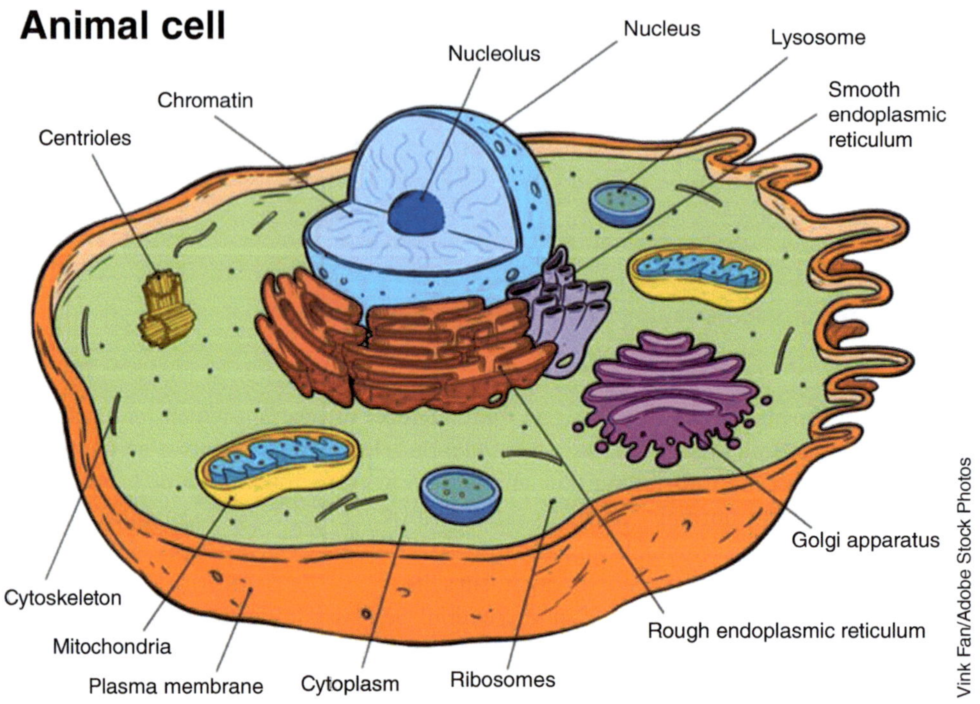

Figure 1.1 Diagram of a normal eukaryotic cell.

division, called meiosis I. The daughter cells divide again in meiosis II, splitting up sister chromatids to form haploid gametes. Gametes are haploid, i.e., they have only one copy of DNA, such that when the gametes from a male and female fuse to form a zygote, the diploid condition is restored. This process only occurs in the organs that produce gametes, the ovary and testicle.

Energy, in the form of Adenosine triphosphate (ATP), is created inside the mitochondria of cells. Energy is produced by oxidative phosphorylation (aka, aerobic respiration) which requires oxygen. Mitochondria have a double membrane system where there is an outer membrane surrounding the mitochondria and an inner membrane within the mitochondria that forms the substrate where ATP is produced. Mitochondria also have a function in cell cycle regulation and some other essential processes. Unique to this organelle is the presence of its own mitochondrial DNA (mtDNA), which is distinct from nuclear DNA (nDNA). Mitochondrial DNA is passed down via the females (matrilineal).

The endoplasmic reticulum, in concert with the Golgi apparatus, is involved with the production and movement of cellular products out of the cell. The rough endoplasmic reticulum (RER) contains ribosomes that are used to produce proteins targeted for release from the cell. The smooth endoplasmic reticulum (SER) has enzymes that metabolize steroids, lipids, some drugs, and glycogen. When the cellular products are ready to be released or excreted from the cell, they merge with the Golgi vesicles, which then fuse with the cell membrane and discharge the contents outside the cell (Figure 1.2).

Lysosomes are organelles that serve as waste receptacles for the cell. These organelles contain enzymes which can degrade molecules and other waste products. After degradation

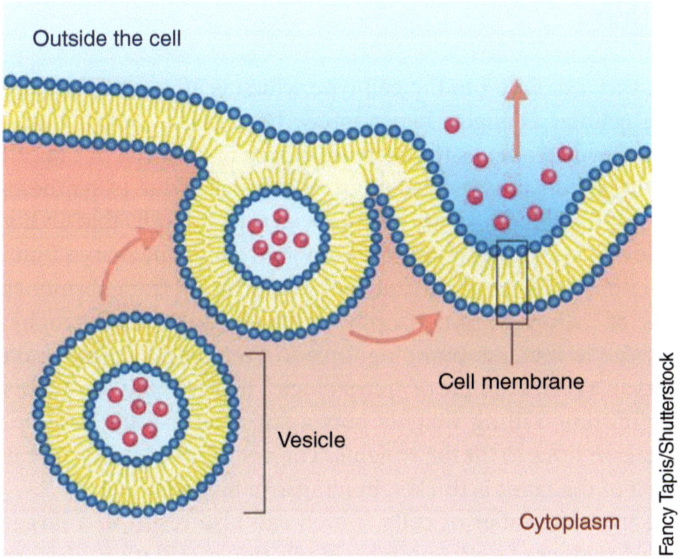

Figure 1.2 Diagram of an animal cell indicating the processes for excreting molecules and waste out of the cell. Molecules tagged for export out of the cell leave the Golgi vesicles, which merge with the membrane and expel their contents. Secondary lysosomes filled with waste also expel their contents after merging with the membrane.

of waste, they fuse with the membrane and discharge their contents (empty the garbage) out of the cell (Figure 1.2). Membrane integrity is critical for this organelle to prevent the enzymes within them from leaking out and degrading all other components of the cell.

The cell cytoskeleton is comprised of microfilaments, microtubules, and intermediate filaments. Each of these has a separate role in cell movement and shape. Microtubules are involved in mitosis when the cell divides in half and moves apart. Intermediate filaments help certain cell types move. For example, desmin is an intermediate filament involved in skeletal muscle contraction. In addition to proteins that reside on the outer surface, the cell may have "appendages" which stick out of the cell surface. These are small structures, such as cilia, which can help the cell sense the environment or move. Within the limits of the cell membrane is a watery, gel-like substrate (the cytoplasm) in which the filaments and organelles reside.

When the cell processes are all working well, the cell is in *homeostasis*. Homeostasis is the range of conditions wherein all cellular processes are functioning normally. Cells, tissues, organs, the organism, and the environment all have their own homeostatic parameters. When conditions change which challenge the organism's or the cells' homeostasis, it must respond to restore balance. It all starts with the cell.

The cell responds to challenges or stimuli by adapting and changing to restore homeostatic balance. These adaptations are often reversible, and the cell can change back once the imposing challenge/stimulus has resolved and/or ceases. In situations where the challenging stimulus does not immediately resolve, the cell can exist in this altered "homeostatic" state. Should the challenging stimulus persist, the cell may undergo irreversible changes which may ultimately lead to its death. In this latter situation, the greater number of cells that die, the more damage the tissue/organ will incur.

Reversible Cell Adaptations

Reversible changes of the cell vary according to the cell type which is affected. There are four basic types of reversible cellular changes: hypertrophy, hyperplasia, atrophy, and metaplasia (Cotran et al., 1999). Hypertrophy is the increase of size or function of the cell which results ultimately in enlarged organ size. The enlarged cell size is due to synthesis of more structural components of the cell. This type of response is seen in cells that do not regularly divide such as muscle and nerve. The stimulus for hypertrophy is increased functional demand (by pathologic or physiologic causes) and/or by stimulation from hormones or growth factors. An example of pathologic hypertrophy would be cardiac hypertrophy; the heart muscle increases in size to increase pumping force to overcome a downstream blockage (e.g., such as a faulty valve). An example of "physiologic" hypertrophy in humans would be subsequent to weightlifting. Lifting weights puts a stress on the arm muscles (e.g., biceps and triceps) to increase force to lift the weights. The net effect of the former is an enlarged heart; the net effect of the latter is thicker, bulging arm muscles.

Hyperplasia is the increase in the number of cells, which can also result in a larger organ size. The mechanism of increased cell numbers is via the stimulation of stem cells or the proliferation of mature cells. This adaptation is common in cell types which normally continually divide (e.g., epithelium of the gastrointestinal tract). As in hypertrophy, hyperplasia can be induced by physiologic or pathologic stressors. Physiologic hypertrophy occurs under hormonal influence in certain organs, such as the mammary gland during pregnancy. Near parturition (birth), mammary gland cells divide and increase in number resulting in mammary gland enlargement. Pathologic hyperplasia can be caused by excesses of hormones or growth factors resulting in pathologic conditions such as endometrial hyperplasia or prostatic hyperplasia.

Atrophy is the reduction in cell size or function (often due to underutilization), which results in a reduction in organ size. The decreased cell size can be due to decreased protein synthesis and/or increased protein degradation, as the cells are not in use and have much lower metabolic demand. As in the adaptations above, causes can be physiologic or pathologic, and atrophy is a common mechanism employed during embryo/fetal development. When a muscle has a reduced workload, such as when one has a cast over a broken bone, the decreased workload to the associated muscles results in disuse atrophy. When the bone mends and the arms/legs resume normal functioning, the muscle will undergo hypertrophy to return to normal size/function.

The last reversible adaptation is metaplasia. Metaplasia is a reversible change in the phenotype of a cell – one differentiated cell type is replaced by a different differentiated cell type. This is basically an adaptive substitution of cell type that will be more tolerant and less sensitive to the imposing stimulus. The new cell type originates from stem cells that receive a message to produce a different cell type. One example of this adaptation is in the respiratory tract. Normally the cells in the upper respiratory tract are columnar in shape and have cilia on their apical/luminal surface. In situations where the tract is chronically irritated from inhaling air with irritants, the columnar cells with cilia will be damaged easily. The body will respond by reprogramming the stem cells to produce squamous cells (instead of columnar cells), which are more robust and can handle the irritants. This must be a temporary change, as the squamous cell type cannot replace the cilia and the normal respiratory cell type's function.

Nonreversible Cell Injury and Cell Death

There are many causes of cell injury, but the ultimate mechanism of cell injury is the same. Depletion of ATP from decreased production in the mitochondria can be induced by many etiologies, all ultimately resulting from a decrease in oxygen (hypoxia). Even a slight 5–10% decrease in ATP from hypoxia can lead to decreased activity of membrane ion pumps, which results in a net gain of water into the cell and cell swelling. Altered metabolic pathways, calcium pump function, protein synthesis, and structural disruption also occur. If the extent of ATP decrease is very severe, the mitochondrial damage worsens. When this happens and the calcium pumps fail to keep calcium out of the cell, the injury becomes irreversible. Free radicals can build up inside the cell, intensify all the damage to the membranes, mitochondria, etc. that are already occurring leading to cell death.

If the injury or stimulus is very prolonged or severe, irreversible cellular changes will be observed, which ultimately lead to death of the cell (Cotran et al., 1999). If too many cells die, then organ function can be compromised. Cell death is a normal and essential process during embryogenesis, organ development, and the maintenance of homeostasis. There are two mechanisms by which cells can die, necrosis and apoptosis. The distinction between these two mechanisms has clinical relevance.

Let's start with necrosis. Cell death by necrosis involves cell membrane rupture and release of cellular contents and lysosomal enzymes out of the cell, which can digest adjacent cells/tissues (Figure 1.3, right side). The dying cells cannot maintain cellular

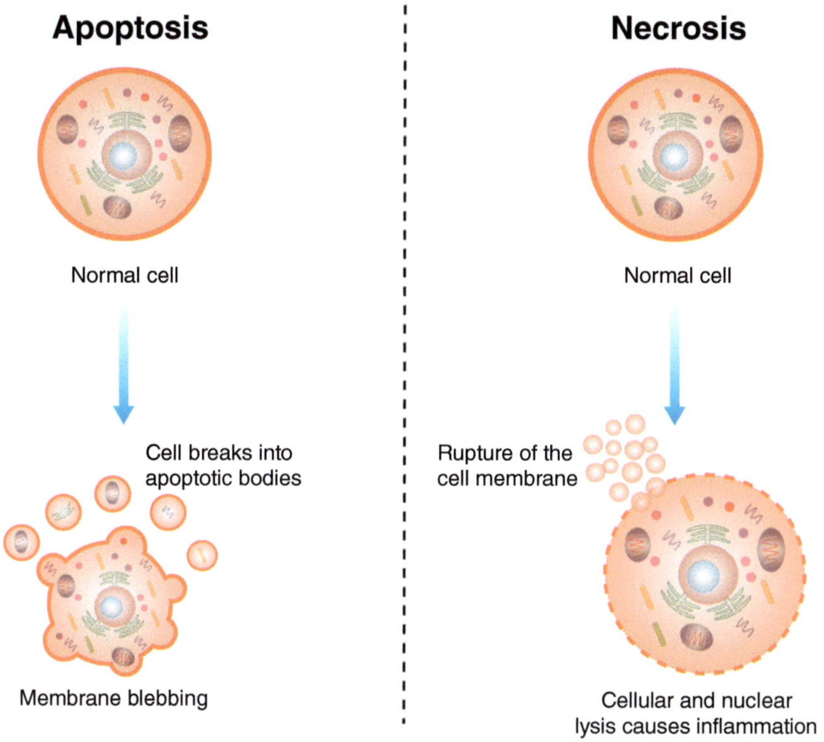

Figure 1.3 Pathways of cell death – necrosis and apoptosis. Details are discussed in the text.

membrane integrity, and contents leak out into the surrounding tissue. In necrosis, an inflammatory process is always incited. Necrosis is always a pathologic response to severe injury or pathology. Cellular necrosis can be seen via light microscopy as early as 4–12 hours after inception and earlier using electron microscopy. There are different patterns of necrosis depending on the etiologic agent and tissue affected, which can lead to its etiology. In coagulative necrosis (often bacterial in origin), the "ghosts" of cells can be seen under the microscope for a few days. In liquefactive necrosis (often viral or toxic in origin), all that is observed is a liquid mass of dead cells and debris. Caseous necrosis includes friable white tissue (grossly looks like cottage cheese) that is well circumscribed (encapsulated) by connective tissue and inflammation caused by acid fast bacteria. Finally, in affected blood vessels, fibrin and immune cell deposition occurs in the vessel walls and this is known as fibrinoid necrosis.

The other mechanism of cell death is called apoptosis (Figure 1.3, left side). In apoptosis, the cell membrane remains intact, and the dead cell fragments are formed into small, membrane-bound structures called "apoptotic bodies." Because the membranes remain intact, apoptotic cell death does *not* incite inflammation. Apoptosis is actually a very complex and tightly orchestrated process of "cell suicide." When damage is so severe to the cell proteins and DNA, the cell basically "signals" the process that results in death via apoptosis. This process is normal during fetal development but can also be induced by severe damage to the cell. The apoptotic bodies are visible under light and electron microscopy. However, the lack of cellular leakage and lack of an inflammatory process makes the diagnosis of this phenomenon *clinically* difficult.

From a clinical diagnostic perspective, necrotic cell death provides us with a mechanism to diagnose disease and the organs affected. When the cell membranes break open, all the enzymes within the cell come pouring out. They get absorbed into the blood circulation. Assaying the enzyme levels in the blood can identify the organ(s) affected. For example, when there is suspicion of a heart attack in people, the hospital will assay the blood for the appropriate cardiac enzyme. If the enzyme levels remain high, then this indicates heart muscle damage. Since the major mechanism of cell damage is lack of oxygen, this suggests a "heart attack" (cardiac infarct; reduced blood supply to the heart muscle). Additionally, when a sick individual presents to the clinic, blood work often shows evidence of inflammation. Combining evidence of inflammation with elevations of certain organ system enzymes can help narrow down the source of the inflammation (e.g., liver and kidney). Further details will be discussed later.

In summary, cell pathology underlies disease. Cell death by necrosis underlies our ability to clinically diagnose disease due to release of organ-specific enzymes into circulation and by inciting an inflammatory response – which is where we go next.

Literature Cited

Cotran, R. S., Kumar, V., and Collins, T. (1999). *Robbin's Pathologic Basis of Disease*, 6th Ed., pp. 3–42. W. B. Saunders Co.

2

Inflammation and the Immune Response

It is worthwhile discussing the inflammatory response, as this is not only one of the avenues to clinically identify when a disease process is underway, but inflammation is now known to underlie many diseases. We will discuss the basic processes here and then discuss the details of how to diagnose inflammation later when we discuss clinical pathology.

The goal of the immune response in the body is to go to, attack, and kill and/or sequester anything foreign. The immune system is composed of a barrier system (normal anatomic and physiologic functions), two main cellular arms (innate and adaptive systems), and specialized lymphoid tissue that all interact to protect the body from anything foreign. For our purposes, we won't go too deeply into detail regarding the cellular systems and their crosstalk, except maybe by example. However, this is a fascinating and multifaceted topic well worth further study! We will also touch on how biomedical research has/can take advantage of the immune system and the inflammatory response to treat and/or manage diseases, including developing cancer immunotherapies (using the host's immune cells to attack host cancer cells).

The body's first defenses to exclude pathogens or anything foreign are the natural body barriers. The main routes of entry of pathogens into the body are through the gastrointestinal system (beak and anus), respiratory route (nasal opening), across the skin/integument, and genitourinary route (via the cloaca). Little hairs and mucous line the internal surface of the nasal turbinates to catch any particulates that enter here during inhalation. Note that pathogens can attach to particulates and can enter the respiratory tract if the nasal barrier is successfully breached. Sneezing is one mechanism to remove from the nasal cavity what shouldn't be entering. In the nasal turbinates, the mucociliary system will be charged with catching the particulates, moving them up (backward) toward the nares. If the particulates make it past these respiratory barriers to the parabronchi, the alveolar macrophages located in the lower respiratory tract can engulf them.

The gastrointestinal tract (GIT) has many physiologic barriers that help keep particulates and pathogens from crossing through the GIT epithelium and into circulation. Saliva contains antimicrobial peptides and molecules including one type of antibody. The stomach is a highly acidic environment to which most pathogens succumb. The intestines have patches of lymphoid tissue which contain lymphocytes that survey ingesta to identify any pathogens attempting to gain access. The main physiologic barrier in the genitourinary system is urination which physically washes out any pathogens or agents.

As for the integument, any breach in the skin (epidermis and/or dermis) surface provides a route of entry into the body. Feathers can trap particles, keeping them away from the skin surface.

Once the pathogen penetrates the anatomic and physiologic barriers, the cellular immune system takes over. The innate arm of the immune system can be thought of as the first responder. Much like firefighters and police, innate immune cells are first on the scene to assess and attack anything foreign or any injury. This response, acute inflammation, follows a prescribed and predictable set of steps. Acute inflammation is accompanied by redness, heat, swelling, and pain at the injured site.

Inflammation is a main component of the immune response (Cotran et al., 1999). When tissues (i.e., cells in tissues) are injured, molecules (e.g., enzymes and proteins) are released from the cell (because the cell membrane is disrupted, and they leak out). These molecules stimulate inflammatory mediators, which cause the local blood vessels to dilate (*vasodilation*), resulting in an increase in blood flow (can be seen as redness in the area). Additionally, the widened blood vessels become "leakier" (pores open in the vessel walls). The opened "pores" serve as sites where circulating inflammatory cells can *see* receptors on the damaged tissue. If the circulating cells have binding sites that match receptors on the injured tissue, then binding occurs, and the immune cells leave the circulation and move into the injured area. Vessel dilation, membrane leakage, and cell migration are discrete and separate processes. The primary responders from the circulating pool of cells are heterophils (a type of white blood cell). Influx of inflammatory cells further enhances an already mounting cascade of actions designed to resolve or remove the injury/pathogen. This nonspecific, acute inflammatory response is only the first part of the process.

The inflammatory response first responds to the injury, but is then tasked to eradicate the pathogen, and finally to heal the injured tissue. The acute inflammatory response is the responder, and it begins the eradication of the pathogen. If extra immune support is needed to eradicate or contain the pathogen, the adaptive arm of the immune system is recruited. Much like human/animal patients are sent to medical specialists, the adaptive immune response responds in a specific way, targeting the pathogen/insult causing the harm. The cells that comprise the specific, adaptive response are called *lymphocytes*. There are various types of lymphocytes – B cells, T cells, and NK cells. Each type of lymphocyte responds to different pathogens in different ways.

Very simply, B cells produce antibodies which bind to and sequester the specific agents/antigens for which they have complementary receptors. (An *antigen* is any molecule/agent that is foreign and elicits an immune response.) T cells do not produce antibodies but will assist with an antibody response or directly "kill" the antigens for which they have specificity. Both cell types interact with and augment each other. When circulating, B lymphocytes are stimulated by successful binding to their antigen, the B cells divide, and the number of cells increases in an exponential manner. This huge increase in cell numbers and the antibodies that they produce attempt to eradicate or contain the offending agent. The method by which the B cells (and T cells for that matter) generate specific receptors for pathogens is way beyond the scope of this text. However, this cellular process is very specific.

So, here is where the immune system is so incredible! Young, naïve B and T cells are initially produced in the Bursa of Fabricius and bone marrow, respectively. Then the naïve T cells move to the thymus gland (which sits at the base of the heart) to be "educated" about what is "self." They learn that what is "self" is normal in the body and should not be attacked. Anything not learned as "self" is seen as "non-self" and will be targeted by the immune system for eradication/removal.

If a new or unknown pathogen enters and there is no previous antibody with the appropriate receptor, then it takes longer to generate the large antibody response needed to eradicate or control the agent. If the antigen has *never* been seen before by the body/cells, it takes 10–14 days for the immune system to mount a significant number of antibodies to successfully eradicate the antigen. However, if the body has seen the antigen before (and has created antibodies to it), then additional antibodies are produced much more rapidly and can reach effective levels within 3–5 days (Figure 2.1). This rapidity of response occurs because lymphocytes have what is termed "memory." The immune system has a head start because antibodies against this agent already exist, and lymphocyte replication proceeds quickly. This is the basis for successful immunization. Vaccines provide the "first" interaction with the antigen/agent. Then subsequent exposures (presumably natural exposures) stimulate a rapid antibody response that should mitigate the extent of the disease/illness. Without this "memory" function, vaccination would not work.

How does the body "know" when to mount an immune response? The answer lies within the lymphoid tissues and organs in the body. These are tissues that are well vascularized and contain lymphocytes. They are located near every orifice in the body and throughout the GIT so that if any pathogen enters, they will have the first opportunity to respond. If they recognize a pathogen (via specific receptors), pro-inflammatory chemical signals will be secreted into the bloodstream. Once the inflammatory cascade is triggered, it can progress exponentially and call in other cellular assistance to contain the pathogen.

To recap, once the body's barriers are breached, the innate arm responds immediately but in a generalized manner. An inflammatory response is triggered. Lymphocytes are

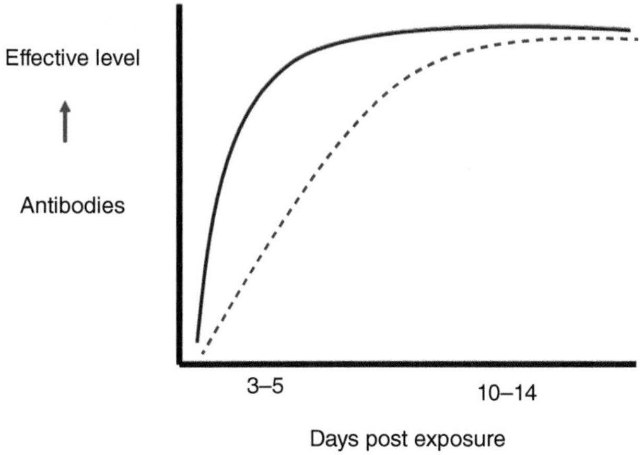

Figure 2.1 Diagrammatic illustration of the approximate timeline for the body to produce antibodies after first exposure (red) and repeat exposure (blue) to a pathogen. Note how much sooner the body can respond with antibodies on subsequent exposures. *Source:* Illustration by author.

called in for specific targeting of antigens. Chemical mediators (cytokines, chemokines, proteins, etc.) are recruited. These mediators serve to recruit other mediators and/or cells to stimulate different aspects of the inflammatory response. Acute phase proteins are an example. These proteins are signaled immediately and usually signal to continue the inflammatory response ("pro inflammatory"). They are short lived (hours up to two to three days) though. This short lifespan is useful in case the antigen is eradicated. Once eradication occurs, different noninflammatory acute phase proteins are stimulated which signal to "stop" the inflammatory process and pro-inflammatory signals are halted. Their short lifespan helps to regulate the inflammatory response more rapidly.

If the antigen is contained, then the inflammatory response changes to a reparative system, and different cells and signals come into play which direct healing (e.g., skin repair when cut). If the injury is not resolved (and not repaired), then the injury (and the inflammatory response) becomes chronic. Chronic inflammation can also result from repeated insult/injury.

Although intended for protection, sometimes the inflammatory response errs and the immune system attacks "self," i.e., host cells. These conditions are known as *immune-mediated diseases* and, in humans, include conditions such as Rheumatoid arthritis, Lupus, and Pemphigus. For unclear reasons (and many have been postulated), the immune system recognizes "self" tissues as foreign and attacks them... continually. These immune-mediated conditions in humans can be severely debilitating, difficult to treat, and can regress and recur due to various stressors. One issue managing these diseases is that treatment traditionally involves decreasing/lowering the body's immune response. However, in doing so, this may leave the person/animal unprotected and vulnerable against pathogens and/or infections. Biomedical research has led to the discovery of specific targeted medical treatments that focus on specific pathways in the inflammatory cascade to treat these conditions without nonspecifically decreasing the entire immune response.

Inflammation does not equal infection. The body can mount an inflammatory response in the absence of a bacterial/viral infection. For example, your ankle swells because you sprained and damaged it. Inflammation arises to rid the ankle of the damaged cells due to the sprain. As we discussed in last chapter, cell death by necrosis will result in an inflammatory response due to leakage of cell contents from destroyed cell membranes. Therefore, any damage to tissues or organs will also result in inflammation.

Specific Avian Immunologic Details

In general, the avian immune response is very similar to that of mammals. However, there are some unique differences. Bird lymphocytes include T and B cells. T cells develop and mature in the thymus as in mammals. However, B cells develop and mature in the Bursa of Fabricius, an organ unique to birds. The bursa produces a protein (bursapoietin) which stimulates B cell movement from the yolk to the bursa and then induces maturation of B cells (Doneley and Xie, 2025). The product of B cells are antibodies. In birds, IgG antibody is known as IgY. Developing embryos in the egg acquire immunity from passive absorption of antibodies (IgM and IgY) from the egg yolk and albumin (Doneley and Xie, 2025). After maturation, these cells then migrate from the bursa to secondary lymphoid tissue at approximately two to three weeks of incubation.

A fully active humoral response does not develop until about two weeks post hatch and is mature by four to six weeks (Doneley and Xie, 2025). Interestingly, glucocorticoids may be produced "locally" in the bursa and thymus and are involved in T and B cell regulation and development (Taves et al., 2017).

The respiratory system in birds, as discussed in the anatomy chapter, is susceptible to infection and/or damage due to its large surface area (15% greater than in terrestrial mammals), extent of the air sac system, and thinner blood gas barrier (56–67% thinner than in mammals; Maina, 2023; Mutua et al., 2016). To combat these features, birds have evolved a robust immune response in the respiratory tract. To start with, the multitiered air filtration system very efficiently filters particulates. As in mammals, portions of the bronchi contain a ciliated mucosal lining to trap and move undesired particulates out. There are resident immune cells in the airway epithelia and at other bifurcation points in the primary and secondary bronchi. Avian respiratory macrophages are not normally resident in the air capillaries. They will move into the lungs upon infection/stimulus. These macrophages have greater phagocytic and bactericidal activity than mammalian alveolar macrophages (Maina, 2023; Mutua et al., 2016). Avian erythrocytes (red blood cells) can phagocytize very small particles ($<0.2\ \mu m$ diameter; Maina, 2023; Mutua et al., 2016). The mechanism of how the erythrocytes literally engulf the particles is unclear – they do not have actin-myosin fibers to use. Very interesting!

How do we know when an inflammatory response is underway? And how do we know what is the target of the inflammatory response? There are several ways that we will go into in more detail in Chapter 5. For now, understanding the basics of inflammation and the immune response is the goal.

Literature Cited

Cotran, R. S., Kumar, V., and Collins, T. (1999). *Robbin's Pathologic Basis of Disease*, 6th Ed., pp. 43–78. W. B. Saunders Co.

Doneley, B. and Xie, S. (2025). *Avian Medicine and Surgery in Practice*, 3rd Ed. CRC Press.

Maina, J. N. (2023). A critical assessment of the cellular defences of the avian respiratory system: Are birds in general and poultry in particular relatively more susceptible to pulmonary infections/afflictions? *Biologic Reviews Cambridge Philosophical Society* 98(6):2152–2187. https://doi.org/10.1111/brv.13000.

Mutua, M. P., Muya, S., and Gicheru, M. M. (2016). Protective roles of free avian respiratory macrophages in captive birds. *Biological Research* 49(1):29. https://doi.org/10.1186/s40659-016-0090-7.

Taves, M. D., Hamden, J. E., and Soma, K. K. (2017). Local glucocorticoid production in lymphoid organs of mice and birds: Functions in lymphocyte development. *Hormones & Behavior* 88:4–14. https://doi.org/10.1016/j.yhbeh.2016.10.022.

3

Anatomy and Physiology

Normal anatomy and physiology are critical to understanding health and disease. When one understands "normal" form and function of any organ system, then it is easy to understand the downstream effects when there is an abnormality. As we go through the body by organ systems, we will highlight the adaptive changes that birds have compared to mammals.

Body Orientation

Describing the body, whether normal marks or lesions, requires specific language so that one can communicate an accurate location using only words. Standard terminology defines the body's orientation (Figure 3.1). Envision the normal posture of a tetrapod (four-legged) animal. *Dorsal* refers to "above" and *ventral* refers to "below" relative to a longitudinal (head to toe) midline through the animal. *Medial* refers to what is closer to the midline and *lateral* refers to what is away from the midline. For example, the wings are located laterally on the body.

When referring to or toward the head, one can use the words *cranial* or *anterior. Cranial* refers to the head. *Anterior* implies the forward direction of movement, which in animals is usually led by the head (but not in crabs!). *Caudal* or *posterior* refers to the tail/hind end or the direction from which one moved, respectively. For example, the avian ear opening is located caudal or posterior to the eyes.

For appendages (such as the wings), one can also indicate location by referencing the "insertion point" (the location where the wing connects to the body) or the "distal point," which would be any point lying farther away from the point of insertion. "Proximal" is a term that refers to near the insertion point, or more generally, the beginning part of any appendage or path (e.g., blood flow and food movement through the digestive tract). The insertion point of the appendage implies a more specific location than proximal, and the two words may not always be equivalent. An example of the above terms is "the nares are located at the proximal end of the beak."

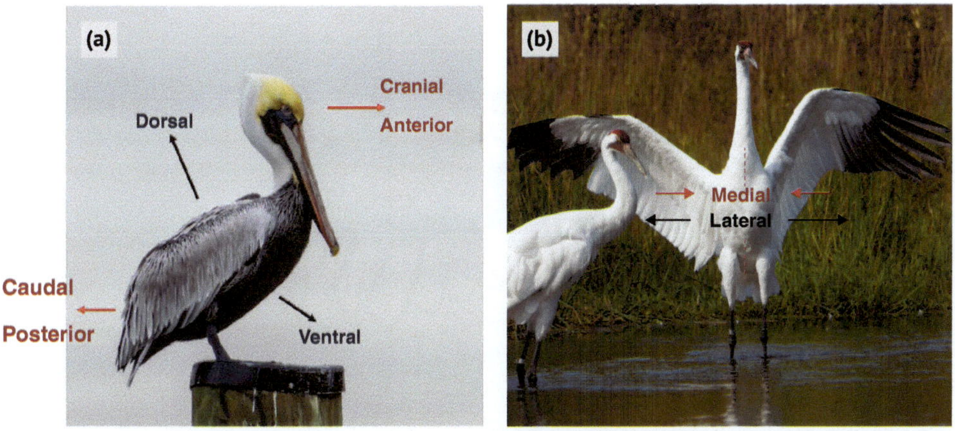

Jimkruger/Getty Images

Figure 3.1 Orientation terms. (a): Anterior is the forward direction; cranial is in the direction of the head. Posterior and caudal are terms for the "rear" direction/end. Dorsal is above the bird. Ventral is the underside of the bird. (b): Medial refers to body midline. Lateral refers to what is away from midline. (Photos: Left – Brown Pelican. Right – Sandhill Crane).

Skeletal System

The skeletal system of typical modern birds has undergone several modifications from the typical tetrapod (four legged) vertebrate to support flight and egg laying. Avian bones are structurally rigid but lightweight to permit flight (except in some nonflying birds such as penguins). Long bones of the leg are hollow, and the bone marrow is located only at the ends of each bone (contrary to mammals). The hollow bones are filled with air (*pneumatized*) and act as extensions of the lungs (this will be discussed in the "Respiratory System" section). In contrast, the leg bones of penguins are not hollow and are rather dense to permit diving (Wallace, 2015). Other skeletal modifications include fusion of various vertebrae and elongation of the neck from an increased number of vertebrae. The collar bones are fused together to form the *furcula* (which you may know as the "wish bone"). The keel (*sternum*) is the site of attachment of the pectoral (breast) muscles used in flight. In some flightless species, the keel is reduced or absent. The tail vertebrae are reduced and/or fused to create a short *pygostyle*. Teeth are absent in modern birds, likely in part because tooth enamel is relatively heavy and could hinder flight. The digits of the wings and legs are reduced in size, and other foot bones are fused (see below). There are additional modifications that are present only in some groups of birds. These can be found in any ornithology text.

As with mammals, the skeleton is formed by bone and cartilage, supports the body and internal organs, is the site for muscle attachment, and is the main reservoir for calcium, phosphorus, and various growth factors.

Limbs

Avian wings evolved from the anterior limbs. The wings function in flight and swimming (in certain species). The number of digits is reduced to three, the second of which is elongated for feather attachment (Figure 3.2). Primary feathers (or primary *remiges*) are used for flight and are located on the distal half of the wing. Secondary feathers (secondary remiges) are located proximal to the primaries. Bones of the wing, although pneumatized,

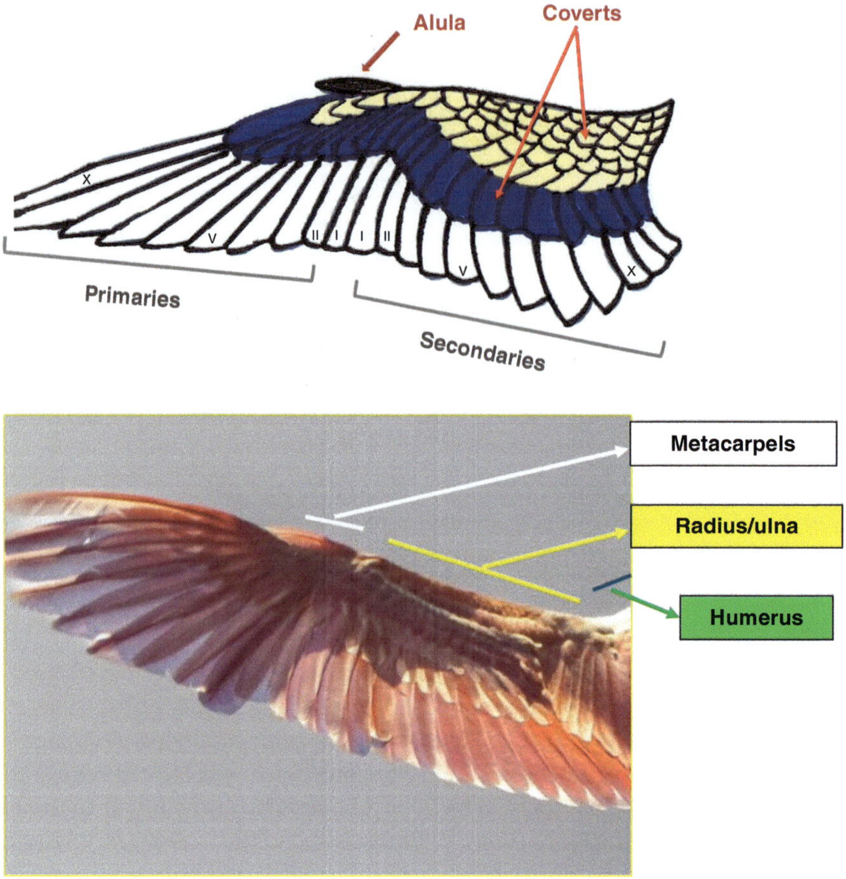

Figure 3.2 Wing detail showing feathers and bones of attachment. Top: Diagram indicating the primary, secondary, coverts (blue), secondary coverts (yellow), and alular feathers (black). Bottom: Underside of roseate spoonbill. Roman numerals indicate the feather number. *Source:* With permission of Jed Steiner, 2025.

are relatively heavy compared to other bones in the body due to stronger and denser outer walls. This is needed to support the muscles and other structures needed for flight.

The legs, or hind limbs, are generally similar to those of mammals, with a few modifications. The functions of the hind limbs are numerous – perching, walking, running, hopping, swimming, climbing, clinging, leaping, seizing and holding prey, holding food, preening, digging, carrying other objects, and fighting. The number of digits is reduced to four usually; however, some groups of birds have fewer. In some species, the first digit is rotated posteriorly. In species that rely on diving, the feet are webbed to various degrees.

The skull is similar to that of mammals. The eye sockets in birds are relatively large. Instead of teeth, birds have a *beak*, which is made from a thin layer of bone and keratin. The beak extends out anteriorly past the nostril openings (*nares*). The upper beak is mostly hollow and has openings for the *nares*. It is attached to the skull by a hinge permitting it to open its mouth very wide. The beak has tactile sensation (mechanoreceptors and neurovascular connections). This facilitates foraging especially in species that probe into substrate to catch small prey (du Toit et al., 2024). Additionally, in albatrosses and penguins, tactile contact of beaks is used in courtship. The lower bill is called the mandible. The openings of the ear canal are located caudal to the eye socket. Interestingly, the ear openings of owls are not located symmetrically on the right and left sides of the skull as in other birds. They are asymmetric, which allows them better acuity of sound to determine prey location (Faaborg, 2020).

Woodpeckers have a unique and interesting adaptation in the bones of the head. The hyoid bone (which is located just below the skull) is elongated and loops around the back of the head and to the forehead (Sykes, 2015). This arrangement helps absorb the vibration caused by pecking on wood/tress. The avian neck is relatively long and S-shaped. There are no intervertebral discs between the neck vertebrae. Instead, they have cartilage covering each end of the vertebrae permitting easier movement and sliding motion of the neck.

The *keel* is the structure to which the *pectoralis muscles* are attached. These are the primary muscles used to power flight. These muscles are called "fast twitch" muscles and are generally pale/white in color. This muscle type typically has many muscle fibers to permit rapid contraction and movement; however, it has relatively less blood supply, which results in it needing to operate via anaerobic respiration. This results in reduced efficiency, and the muscles tire easily. The muscles of the legs are known as "slow twitch" muscles and are redder in color (aka, "dark meat"). This muscle has fewer muscle fibers, but a much greater blood supply. It can support sustained movement using aerobic respiration.

Integument

The *integument* refers to the outer, protective layer of the body. The skin, composed of the *dermis* and *epidermis*, is protective because it provides a covering that is selective in what molecules are let in or out, is waterproof when intact, contains antimicrobial and immune surveillance cells, and is not uniform in thickness around the body. The outermost skin cells are the epidermal cells ("epi" means above, so "above the dermis"). These cells are produced by stem cells in the bottom (basal) epidermal layer. As these cells are produced, they move toward the outer surface, gradually changing shape from cuboidal (square shaped) to squamous (more flattened). In parts of the body, where there is constant high pressure applied (think bottom of feet), the thickness of the squamous epidermal layer increases, as does the total epidermal and skin thickness. This is an adaptation to provide a thick cushion to the areas that sustain this increased pressure. In addition, avian epidermis has a greater concentration of particular fats (cerebrosides) in the upper layers (stratum corneum), which act to decrease water loss.

In birds, feathers also serve a protective function by acting as a potential trap for particles, an additional "surface" outside the skin, and are used for communication (e.g., sexual displays). Similar to fur in mammals, feathers also function in thermoregulation. These functions are clearly enhanced when the feather is thicker with more "underfeathers."

The feather and hair are homologous dermal structures (Figure 3.3). The base of the follicle derives from the dermis and extends down into the subcutis (underneath the dermis). Adjacent to the feather follicle in the dermis are muscle bundles which contribute to stability and movement of the feathers. At the base of the follicle is the *dermal papilla*, which is well vascularized and supplies the developing feather with nutrients for growth and

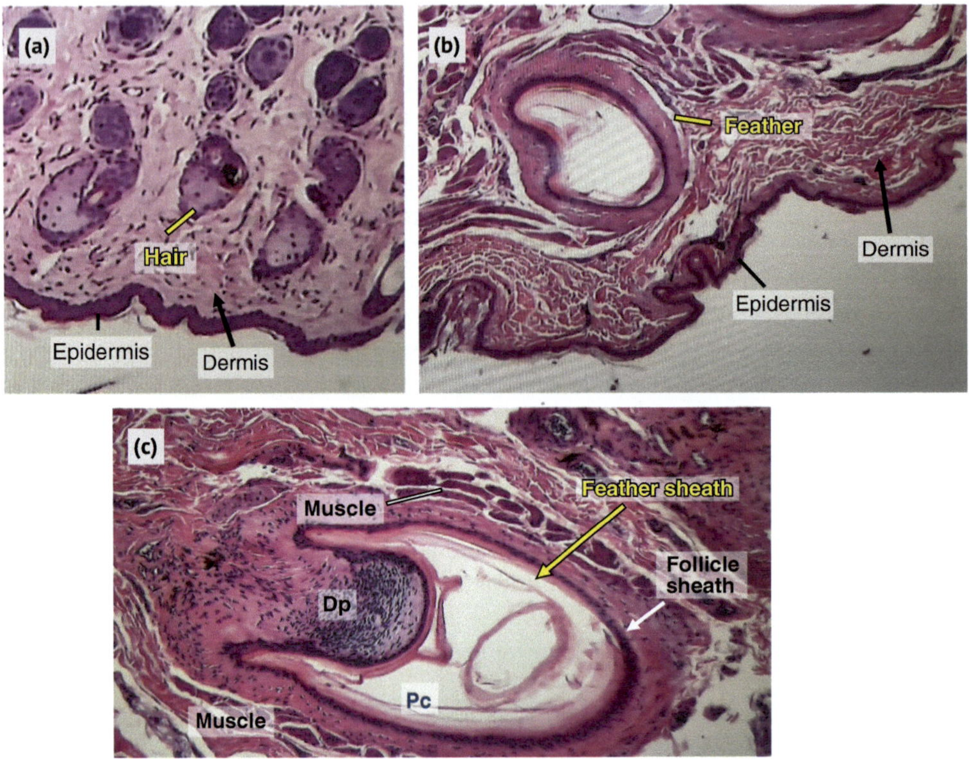

Figure 3.3 Homology of mammalian hair follicles (left, 40×) and avian feather follicles (right, 40×). Both follicles are located in the dermis layer. Muscle (maroon color) is obvious surrounding the feather follicle but too small to see surrounding the hair follicle. Bottom is a close-up (100×) of the feather follicle. Dp = dermal papillae. Pc = pulp cavity. This is a later stage feather; thus, the pulp cavity has minimal pulp.

development. Unlike haired mammals, in birds, there are no dermal glands associated with feathers. The few exceptions to the presence of skin glands include the uropygial gland, the auricular gland (near the ear), and vent glands near the cloaca. In general, the avian skin is much less innervated than mammalian skin *except* immediately adjacent to follicles and in many nonfeathered areas (e.g., the beak).

Birds have integument adaptations to maintain as smooth a surface as possible, especially the species that swim. The feathers lay flat on the body, and while they can puff up a bit, they cannot elevate off their skin in the same way mammalian hair can (think goose bumps in humans). The feather follicle is more rigidly embedded in the skin and cannot move as much as mammalian hair can. The relative decrease in movement of the feather follicles helps maintain the feather structure and configuration that optimally benefits thermoregulation and flight. If the feathers were able to move perpendicular to the skin, that would create drag during flight.

The feather shape itself tapers toward the distal end, as does the body shape. If you look at a cross section of a wing, the cross section would be larger cranially and taper caudally (Figure 3.4). This shape optimizes aerodynamics and reduces drag as the bird flies.

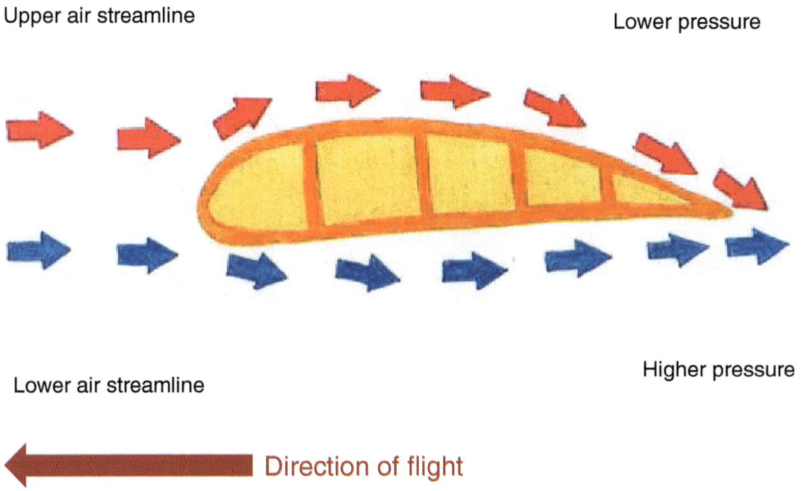

Figure 3.4 Wing cross-section. Note the larger, rounded, leading edge, and the thinner trailing edge. This shape provides smooth streamlining flowing over the wing with minimal turbulence. Airplane wings have the same structure. In addition, under the trailing edge, the air pressure is greater than above it is resulting in "lift" (air moves from higher to lower pressure), which enables birds and planes to take flight. *Source:* With permission of S. Mannone.

Feathers

There are several types of feathers in birds (Figure 3.5). Wing feathers, also called *remiges*, are divided into primary and secondary remiges (Figure 3.3). The 10 primary feathers are the feathers primarily involved in flight. They arise from the fused carpometacarpal bones. Because of the stress imposed by the wing movements during flight, the base of the feathers is securely seated in the skin and has desmosomal connections to the underlying bone. Secondary feathers arise from the ulna, which is located closer to the body. Both the primary and secondary feathers are covered at their proximal ends by *covert* feathers. Finally, on the wing are *alular remiges*, which are located near the alular bone (Figure 3.2). These feathers become important for maneuverability in some birds. Under the remiges are smaller feathers known as *plumules* (down feathers), powder down feathers, and filoplumes. These are small feathers with a central calamus, but they have many thin tufts of keratinized filaments (Figure 3.5). They function in thermoregulation and/or water proofing. Tail feathers, also known as *rectrices*, arise from the rump.

Birds molt (shed their feathers) annually either one or few at a time or all at once during one or more short, defined periods. Molting comes with a physiological cost – it takes energy to regrow new feathers. In a sequential or continual molt, losing one or few feathers over a long period of time, the energy cost can be redistributed over time. If molting occurs all at once (called a catastrophic molt), all feathers regrow in a short period of time and there are also other costs. Molting needs to be completed before migration. Thus, the timing of migration involves, in part, feather replacement.

Consider this scenario. If you live in a cold environment, molting can reduce your ability to thermoregulate. For species that molt all their feathers in one short period of time, this can be a drastic event! This will prevent them from foraging in (or even entering) the water. Without feathers to thermoregulate, they will not be able to swim in cold waters to forage.

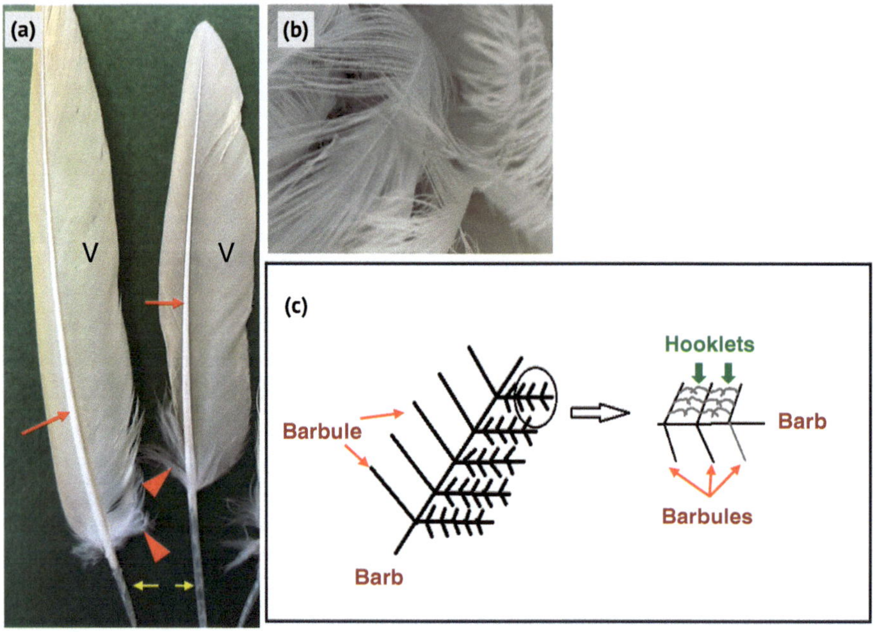

Figure 3.5 Feather detail and feather types. (a) primary flight feather of a cockatiel. Red arrows point to the *rachis* running down the feather midline. Yellow arrows indicate the hollow shaft, the *calamus*. Red arrowheads indicate *downy barbs* at the base of the feather. V = the *vane*. (b) close-up view of light wispy *underfeathers*. (c) detailed anatomy of the *barbs*, which emanate from the rachus. *Barbules* emanate from the barb and have *hooklets* at their tips. These *hooklets* keep adjacent feathers in alignment.

Some penguins molt feathers all at once and are stranded on land until the feathers regrow. So, hairless, cold, out on land, and without food, these birds are also now more susceptible to terrestrial predators and pathogens from the land.

How do feathers prevent body heat loss? The structure of feathers and how they interlock with each other provides a barrier to air. In addition, the downy feathers underneath the larger feathers trap air bubbles within and underneath them. This creates a layer that traps heat preventing heat loss. If the bird loses its ability to trap that air layer, then they will not be able to prevent heat loss. This is exactly what happens when animals (birds and mammals) get oiled in an oil spill. The oil does not allow the downy feathers (or under hairs in mammals) to trap the air, and the animal cannot insulate itself.

Maintaining this type of insulation system requires a lot of feather management and grooming. Birds are frequently seen preening their feathers with their beaks (or sometimes feet). This grooming behavior ensures the barbs and barbules of the feathers are correctly positioned and overlapping. In addition, birds have an oil-producing gland, called the *uropygial* gland, which is located on the rump. With their beak, they will get some oil from this gland and then preen the feathers with it. This provides water resistance to the feathers and ensures a smooth outer surface. The uropygial secretions also contain antimicrobial compounds active against bacteria and/or fungi (Mora-Rubio et al., 2025).

Let us move across the integument and into the body cavity to go through the organ systems.

Cardiovascular System

Birds have a four-chambered heart – right atrium, right ventricle, left atrium, and left ventricle. These chambers are connected in sequence to each other through valves. Valves are unidirectional thin leaflets designed to open only in a single direction (i.e., in the direction of blood flow). The valves are named logically as to what chambers they connect and the blood flow direction. Blood flows from the right atrium to the right ventricle through the right atrioventricular valve (RAV). Blood moves from the left atrium through the left atrioventricular valve (LAV) to the left ventricle. (Human medical terminology has alternate names for these valves; however, because the intent is to understand the blood flow path, we will not worry about the alternate names.

Let us follow the path of blood flow. The heart is a large muscle. From the body, the blood (returning from the organs, low in oxygen, high in carbon dioxide) flows from the vena cava into the right atrium. From here, the blood moves down to the right ventricle through the RAV. The blood is then pumped into the lungs and air sacs through the pulmonary valve to get reoxygenated and to offload the carbon dioxide, which will be exhaled. After oxygenation in the lungs, the blood returns to the left atrium, which then shuttles the blood down to the left ventricle through the LAV. Now, fresh oxygenated blood is ready to supply the body. It is pumped to the aorta through the aortic valve and then out to the body.

The aorta is the largest artery in the body. It has the thickest walls that are composed of elastin fibers and smooth muscle. These fibers provide flexibility, elasticity, and strength to withstand the great pressure under which the blood is expelled when the left ventricle contracts. The elastic recoil then pushes the blood on its way to circulate through the body. Arteries have thicker walls than veins throughout the body. The thickness comes from smooth muscle and elastin, which function to keep the blood moving.

If you were to hold the heart in your hand, you could easily differentiate between the right and left side of the heart. The thickness of the left ventricular wall muscle is greater than that of the right ventricular wall. It is easy to feel the differential thickness. Cutting into the heart (like you would during a necropsy) or evaluating the heart by echocardiography (ultrasound), you can measure the wall thickness. The left ventricular wall is thicker because the heart muscle needs to apply more force to pump the blood out and throughout the entire body. It takes less force to pump blood to the lungs nearby; therefore, the right ventricular muscle wall is thinner.

How do you tell if something is wrong with the heart? What are the resulting effects of some pathology or injury to the heart? It is easiest to think of the heart as a plumbing system. The heart pumps blood through a series of pipes (the vessels). As in plumbing, if there is a blockage in a pipe, it affects (slows or stops) the flow downstream of the blockage and affects the heart muscle preceding the blockage point. If the blockage does not completely stop the flow of blood (i.e., it lets some through as the vessel injury/pathology makes the lumen smaller), the heart muscle immediately preceding (in front of) the blockage will need to pump harder and stronger to get the same amount of blood through the now-narrowed lumen of the vessel. This increased need to pump harder and stronger causes the heart muscle to *hypertrophy*. The muscle cells enlarge to provide more force to the muscle. As a result, the thickness of that part of the heart will increase. The same effect can occur if the valves do not open fully or if cholesterol builds up in the arteries. Buildup of cholesterol in arteries is known as atherosclerosis. If the buildup of cholesterol is large enough, it can significantly narrow the vessel lumen and impair blood flow. Parrots (order Psittaciformes) and ducks (order Anseriformes) appear to be susceptible to atherosclerosis. Risk factors include older age (parrots >15 years old), sex (females more prone to disease), lack of exercise, and, of course, high fat diet (Doneley and Xie, 2025).

What if the blockage was complete? Now, no blood can pass that blockage and down through the vessel. The heart will continue to hypertrophy and enlarge to try and keep pumping the blood through this blockade. Downstream, though, no blood will flow, and the body will not receive the blood or the nutrients it provides. Full blockage is rare, but I mention it for illustrative purposes.

The longer the blockage persists, the heart muscle immediately preceding it will continue to thicken, and then this pathologic change will progress backward. Consider this example: the valve that lets blood flow into the lungs/air sacs from the right ventricle is thickened and opens only 50% of normal. The right ventricle (immediately preceding the affected valve) will thicken first. If this blockage persists, the right atrium may become thickened because still more pressure is required to get the correct amount of blood moving along. So, now both the right atrium and ventricle are thicker than normal. Over time, if the blockage persists or progresses, the blood will back up and eventually accumulate in the liver (hepatic congestion) and fluid in the body will accumulate (aka, ascites). This hepatic congestion is one sign of heart failure – the problem is just too much to overcome. Just by determining which wall thickness is abnormally enlarged, one can narrow down the location of the heart problem. It will be downstream (in the path of the blood) of the location of the thickened heart wall. Once the location of the problem is determined, the veterinarians can determine the etiology (cause) of the problem.

The above deals with the heart's role in pumping blood through the body. The heart also has its own blood supply to provide it with oxygen and nutrients. These vessels are *coronary* vessels and are visible on the outside of the heart (Figure 3.6). If the coronary vessels

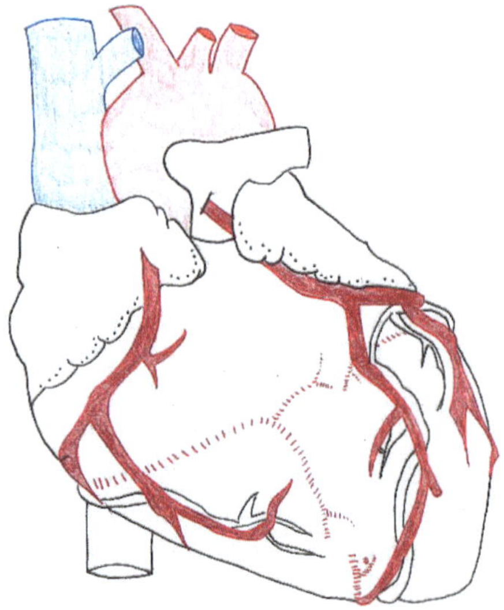

Figure 3.6 Coronary arteries (red) bring oxygen and nutrients for the heart tissue itself. Blockage and/or failure of flow in these vessels can result in death of the heart muscle. *Source:* With permission of S. Mannone.

become obstructed (like they can in humans with high cholesterol, which can form cholesterol plaques), then the amount of blood feeding the heart muscle decreases or ceases if the blockage is complete. When this occurs, the heart muscle that is fed by these vessels will die. This is called a myocardial infarct (*myo* = muscle; *cardia* = heart; *infarct* = death of tissue from lack of oxygen) commonly referred to as a "heart attack." Fortunately (for humans), medical science has angiography – a radiologic method using contrast agents to examine the patency of the vessels. The flow rate, wall thickness, and any blockages can be diagnosed before the blockage is complete and treated before an infarct occurs. The treatment usually involves placing a stent in the vessel to increase the lumen diameter, so blood flow resumes smoothly. (Cholesterol-reducing medicines are also prescribed in humans!). If the lumen is so reduced in size and stenting is not possible, then a coronary artery bypass surgery may be required. This procedure involves replacing the portion of blocked coronary artery with a segment of new vessel usually obtained from the leg. This new vessel segment is sutured in to provide an alternative route for the blood to flow around the blocked portion. With blood flow restored, the heart will receive oxygen and nutrients. Birds have unique and impressive cardiovascular parameters as compared to mammals.

Respiratory System

Upper Respiratory Tract

Air enters through the nares on the dorsal aspect of the beak. From there, air enters the nasal cavity which is divided by a nasal septum. Within the nasal cavity are highly vascularized and folded *nasal conchae* or *turbinates*. Turbinates have three parts which are differentiated by the type of epithelium and innervation. The function of the turbinates is to modulate water and heat loss from the body. It also helps modulate the temperature of the air entering the nasal cavity.

There are various sinuses in the head (Figure 3.7) which contribute to the functions of the upper respiratory tract. These functions are regulation of water loss and evaporation,

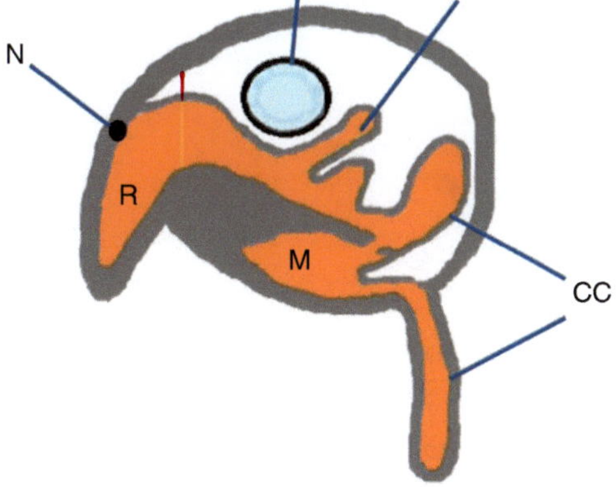

Figure 3.7 Cranial sinuses in birds are comprised of many sinus diverticula. Orange color represents the sinuses. Note, they are all connected. Blue area is the orbital socket. N = nares; R = rostral diverticulum; M = mandibular diverticulum; CC = cervicocephalic diverticulum with cranial and ventral lobes; PO = posterior infraorbital diverticulum; IO = infraorbital diverticulum.

insulation for heat retention, buoyancy control, filtering out particulates, and support of the head during sleep. In fish eating birds, the sinuses also help dampen the force of impact of the water.

Lower Respiratory Tract

The lower respiratory track of birds differs from mammals in various ways. The avian trachea has cartilaginous rings that are fully circular (vs. partially circumferential in most mammals). These rings frequently ossify. The last two rings fuse to form the *syrinx*, the structure responsible for vocalizations (see below). Avian lungs are not lobed. The lungs and air sacs are attached to the dorsal body wall which provides structural support and prevents collapse. Finally, the site of gas exchange is in the tertiary bronchi aka. *parabronchi*, not alveoli as in mammals.

Air is inspired through the nares and/or mouth. The air enters the trachea, then the primary bronchi, and ultimately goes to the caudal air sacs (Figure 3.8). From here, the still fresh air moves into the parabronchi for gas exchange. On expiration, the air moves into the cranial air sacs, again passing through the parabronchi, primary bronchi, then out via the trachea. The parabronchi have a unique structure which results in a much larger (approx. 10 x larger) area of gas exchange than alveoli surface area in mammals.

Inspiration and exhalation involve muscle contraction. There is no diaphragm as in mammals. Various muscles contract to permit breathing. In addition, wing muscle movement during flight can also provide the muscular force needed to breathe. During the downward stroke of the wings, the muscles contract resulting in inhalation. Exhalation occurs during the upward stroke of the wings. The air sacs function as 'bellows' and move the air. Air exchange does not occur within the air sacs.

Figure 3.9 shows the arrangement of air flow, air capillaries, and blood capillaries within the parabronchi. This arrangement results in a counter current system where the air flow and blood flow run perpendicular to each other. The parabronchus is fully perfused along its entire length. Parabronchi are of uniform lengths and have simple squamous epithelium lining their lumina. There are areas in them called atria that have openings leading

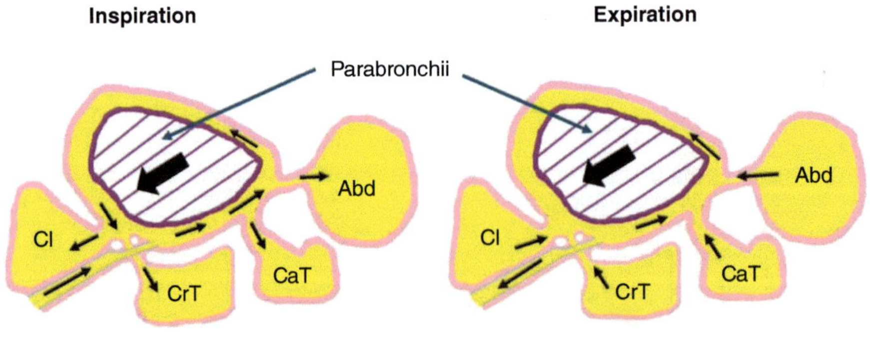

Figure 3.8 Pathway of the flow of air (yellow) on inspiration and expiration in birds. Arrows indicate direction of air flow. Air enters and exits via the trachea (lower left vessel). Note how the air proceeds far caudally on inhalation, then returns cranially on expiration. The air passes through the parabronchi during each phase of respiration resulting in double the opportunity to exchange oxygen/carbon dioxide. Cl = clavicular air sac; CrT = cranial thoracic air sac; CaT = caudal thoracic air sac; Abd = abdominal air sac.

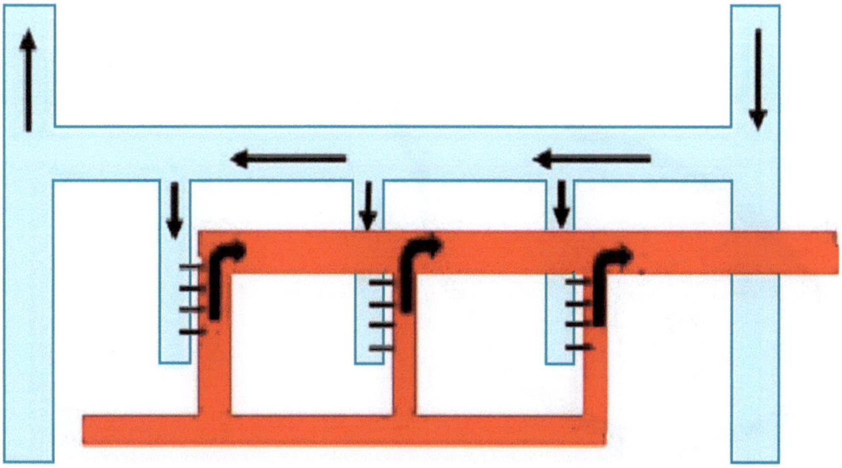

Figure 3.9 Detail (enlarged) of oxygen exchange in the parabronchi. Blue signifies air flow in air capillaries. Red signifies blood flow in blood capillaries. Arrows indicate direction of air or blood movement. The vertical series of dashes demonstrate where oxygen and carbon dioxide are exchanged. This arrangement provides a huge surface area for gas exchange.

to air capillaries at their base. These air capillaries intertwine with blood capillaries which increases the surface area for gas exchange. The walls of capillaries are one cell thick which permits diffusion.

Gas molecules can move in or out of air and/or blood capillaries by diffusion. Oxygen will move from the inhaled air across capillary walls into the blood (which is oxygen depleted) and replenish the oxygen in the red blood cells (RBCs). Oxygen moves from higher concentration in air to lower concentration in the RBCs. Conversely, carbon dioxide will move out of the blood in the capillary and into the air capillaries ultimately to be expelled from the body via exhalation. With the RBC replenished with oxygen, the blood returns to the heart through arteries of increasing diameter and then back into the left ventricle of the heart ready to supply the body with oxygenated blood.

The are typically nine air sacs in birds (Figure 3.10). Air sacs are thin-walled cavities that connect to the lungs. Their functions include acting as bellows to move air, several connect to and enter various bones (called *pneumatic* bones), and they contribute to the lighter body weight. The air sacs span the entire body and therefore drastically increase the surface area of the entire respiratory system. This makes birds more vulnerable to respiratory diseases because of the increased area. Air sacs can be used to optimize inhalation anesthesia (Doneley and Xie, 2025).

The *syrinx* is the structure responsible for vocalizations and song. The syrinx lies just cranial to the primary bronchus through which air enters and then leaves the respiratory tract. There is a membrane (*internal tympaniform membrane*) that, in conjunction with distention of the interclavicular air sac, protrudes into the bronchus. When air flows past, the internal tympaniform membrane and the associated muscles vibrate, and sound is produced. Sound characteristics depend on the tension of the membrane and air sac. Interestingly, puncturing the interclavicular air sac will prevent sound generation.

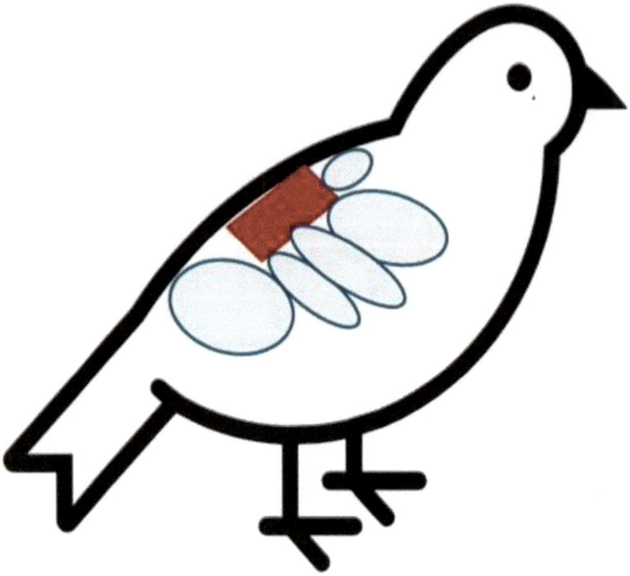

Figure 3.10 Diagram of orientation of the air sacs in birds. From the top clockwise: cervical, clavicular, cranial thoracic, caudal thoracic, and abdominal air sacs flank the parabronchi (red).

GI System

The gastrointestinal (GI or GIT) system is the system that encompasses ingestion, digestion, nutrient and water absorption, and then excretion. GI systems have evolved based on the type of food consumed (e.g., strict carnivore, strict herbivore, or omnivore). Beginning with intake, food is taken into the beak. Modern birds have no teeth; thus, beak shape has evolved to handle particular food items. For example, seed eaters (granivores) have short, thick, and conical beaks. Birds that eat smaller insects (insectivores) have small, thin, pointy beaks for precise manipulation of the insect. Nectar-feeding species have generally longer beaks that may be curved to get into the flowers far enough for it or the tongue to reach the nectar.

From the beak, the food is swallowed and passes into the esophagus, down to the stomach, then into the small intestine, cecum, and rectum, then out of the body via the cloaca. Seems like an easy, quick system! But there is so much variety and adaptation involved. There are additional organs that play a big role in the GI system. These organs are salivary glands (which produce and deliver saliva into the mouth; much more developed in granivores), pancreas (produces digestive enzymes that are delivered to the upper small intestine), liver, and gall bladder (in those species that have them), which provide bile to aid in fat emulsification and store bile, respectively. More on these organs will be discussed later.

The *esophagus* is a muscular tube. The function of the esophagus is just that, a conduit for food to pass through on its way toward the stomach. It is composed of skeletal and smooth muscles and has a lumen lined by squamous epithelium. The squamous cells that comprise the inner epithelium are flattened cells that contain no glands within them. They are sturdy cells that can withstand rough food scratching against them, like fish with scales. The *crop* is an outpouching of the esophagus. It is used to hold, store food, and to moisten and predigest food.

The esophagus connects to the stomach. The functions of the stomach are to hold food, begin the process of mechanically and chemically reducing the foodstuff to small and smaller bits. There are two parts or chambers of the stomach in birds. The first is the *proventriculus*. This is the glandular stomach, which produces digestive enzymes. The second is the *ventriculus*. This stomach is used for the mechanical breakdown of food. In granivorous species, the walls of this stomach are very, very thick to generate the power to crush seeds. In general, a bird's stomach shape varies with diet. A carnivore's stomach is a large, single sac. In granivores, there are two distinct sections. Nectar and fruit eaters' stomachs are intermediate in configuration between these two.

Why does the stomach begin the process of mechanically breaking the food into smaller and smaller bits? Because the goal of consuming food is to absorb its nutrients across the cells and into the bloodstream. An intact 10 inch fish with scales or a large nut cannot be absorbed across the lining of the small intestine. So, the first task of the stomach is reducing the size of the food item. This is done mechanically by muscle contraction and "crushing," if you will. There are mucus glands and digestive glands in the proventriculus. Secretion of mucus into the stomach lumen helps to soften the food items, basically by immersion in a mucous fluid, which can help with mechanical breakdown. The now moistened foodstuffs begin breaking down further by the digestive enzymes. As smaller and smaller food bits are generated, they move down through the pylorus to the small intestine for absorption.

The *small intestine* is composed of three regions: the *duodenum*, *jejunum*, and *ileum*. Along its path, the intestine continues chemical digestion and absorbs the nutrients within. The liver produces bile, which emulsifies fatty molecules, and the pancreas, which produces various types of digestive enzymes, deposit their contents into the duodenum via ducts from their respective organs. The small intestine mucosal surface is lined by small finger-like protrusions called *villi*. The presence of villi effectively increases the surface area across which absorption can occur. Overall, the avian intestine is shorter in length than comparably sized mammals. Similar to patterns in other animals, the granivores and herbivores have longer intestinal tracts than the carnivorous and fruit-eating birds.

The *cecum* is next in the path. With nutrient absorption complete, the cecum's main function is to break down cellulose (from plant materials) and for bacterial fermentation. The *rectum* and *cloaca* are then charged with absorbing excess water. Then feces exit through the opening of the cloaca, the *vent*. This makes sense, right? Food comes in whole, is broken down to very small units for absorption, and then we (humans) excrete it (usually) as more solid fecal material. So, the fluid digesta in the stomach becomes firmer feces by virtue of water reclamation in the rectum. That is true for humans and carnivorous mammals. However, depending on the environment and species, the excreted fecal product is not always firm. In birds, the feces are not solid and are excreted simultaneously with urine. In the cloaca, there are two openings (Figure 3.11). The *coprodeum* is the opening through which feces pass into the cloaca. The *urodeum* is the pathway through which urine passes into the cloaca. They combine to exit through a common opening, the vent.

How does food actually move through the GI tract from beak to anus? The GI organs all contain smooth muscle layers. Smooth muscle is an autonomic or involuntary muscle; that is, it contracts and relaxes without oversight by our wishes or commands. The rhythmic movement through the GI system, which moves food items down to the cloaca is called *peristalsis*. Peristalsis keeps things moving in the GI tract.

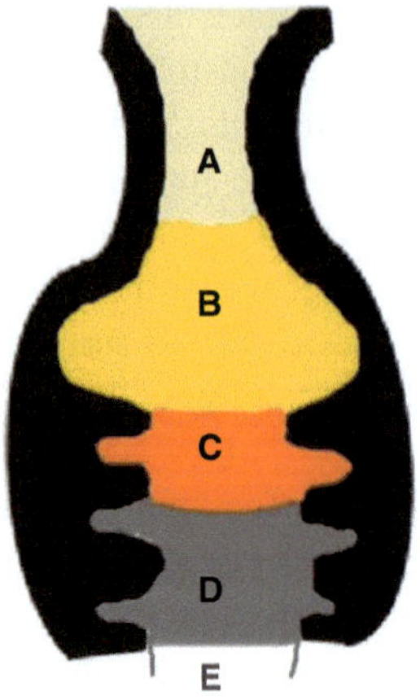

Figure 3.11 Anatomy of the lower urinary structures, cloaca, and vent of birds. A = rectum; B = coprodeum; C = urodeum; D = proctodeum; E = vent.

Understanding how the GI system normally functions allows us to understand why and how things go wrong in the body regarding this system. Let us run through an example of how understanding normal function can direct you to clarifying where to look to find the answers if the GIT is impaired. This is somewhat of a simplification as there may be interacting factors; however, knowing where to look to find a problem greatly hastens the diagnostic exercise.

Example The feces of your animal are harder and firmer than normal. Knowing the different parts of the GI system, where would you investigate first?

I would go to the rectum first because that is the main site of water reabsorption leading up to the final fecal product. In order to have harder than normal feces, too much water must be drawn out of the fecal material in the rectum and retained into the body. How can this happen in the rectum? It must be either spending too much time in there (in the rectum) or the water resorption function is not working correctly (for whatever reason). If the feces are moving through the rectum too slowly (i.e., peristalsis rate is decreased below normal), then there is more time to remove water from the fecal matter, yielding a harder fecal product. If the peristaltic rate is normal, then maybe the water resorption function is absorbing too aggressively, leaving a harder fecal product. So, now you have two processes to investigate – peristaltic rate and water resorption activity in the rectum, and you can develop a list of potential etiologies which may well be different for those two dysfunctions.

In the case of diarrhea (watery feces), the opposite problems would be observed. The general reasons for watery feces are increased peristalsis (moving through the rectum too fast for full water resorption) or increased water in the tract (either added in the small intestine or not enough removed in the rectum due to decreased resorption function). Now one can proceed to investigate etiologies.

Liver

The *liver* is a large, bi-lobed organ that is responsible for many processes. A few of its main roles include detoxification of toxic and/or foreign substances, production of proteins, production of bile, and glucose storage. Detoxification reactions usually render toxic substances nontoxic or reduce their toxicity. These reactions are mediated by a variety of different enzymes. This detoxification process is discussed in more detail in the contaminants chapter.

The liver produces many proteins that participate in endocrine, osmoregulatory, and inflammatory processes. The liver produces the protein *albumin*, which is the main protein responsible for maintaining the osmotic pressure of circulating blood (more on that in Chapter 5). Many proteins that carry hormones through the bloodstream are made in the liver. Other liver-derived proteins include acute phase proteins and others that are integrally involved in increasing and decreasing the inflammatory response (discussed in Chapter 2). Bile is produced in the liver and is stored in the gall bladder (if present). When needed to emulsify fatty food items, bile is released from the gall bladder to the intestines via the bile duct. In species that do not have gallbladders, the bile duct extends from the liver directly to the intestine.

Urinary System

Osmoregulation refers to the management of water and salt balance (aka fluid balance) in the body. The urinary system functions to remove body waste via the urine and to assist in fluid balance in the body. The urinary tract includes the kidneys (where water and salts are actively regulated and urine is produced), the ureters (through which the urine travels), and the urethra (which carries the urine to its point of exit in the cloaca). Birds do not have a urinary bladder (too weighty). The kidney is critical to osmoregulation in mammals; however, in birds, this function is shared between the kidney, rectum, and cloaca.

The avian kidney has three lobes which are connected. They are embedded in the synsacrum in the dorsal body cavity. The kidney has three regions – cortex, medulla, and pelvis. The glomerulus resides in the outer cortex and contains many capillaries through which the waste products and "good" nutrients are filtered out of the blood into the kidney tubules. In the proximal tubules, the desirable nutrients are reabsorbed back into the blood. The kidney medulla has numerous tubules that manage the body's water balance by pumping sodium and chloride (along with water) in or out of the body depending on the body's needs. If an animal is dehydrated, the kidney tubules will retain water in the body resulting in a more concentrated urine.

The urine is an excellent biological sample to analyze. In birds, however, there may be fecal contamination since they are excreted together. There is a "normal" range of specific gravity (think of this as the urine's concentration), amount of protein, glucose, pH, blood cells, etc. If these parameters are abnormal, you can tell which part of the kidney is likely to be poorly functioning and then search for the etiology. The specific gravity or urine concentration can indicate the body's hydration status. If red or white blood cells are found in the urine, it may indicate there is inflammation somewhere along the urinary tract. Glucose should be absent from urine; therefore, if glucose is present in the urine, this suggests that the tubules are not reabsorbing it. Alternatively, the tubules may be functioning correctly, but the amount of glucose is so high that some spills over into the urine. In this latter case, the first disease to check is if the animal has diabetes.

Hormones act on, and are produced in, the kidney. The kidney produces the hormone erythropoietin that regulates RBC production. If the kidney fails (as in chronic renal failure), the production of this hormone will be reduced, or it won't be produced at all, resulting in a decrease in RBC production and ultimately anemia. Vasopressin and renin are two hormones that act on the kidney tubules to help regulate osmotic and water homeostasis. Vasopressin, in the presence of hyperosmotic plasma, will act to reabsorb more water resulting in more concentrated urine. Renin has the opposite effect. The renal pelvis (or distal collecting area) is the third region of the kidney. In this area, the urine collects and then moves into the ureters on its way to the urodeum in the cloaca.

Reproductive Systems

Male reproductive organs in birds are similar to those of other species. Male birds have a *penis, paired testes, epididymis* (in which the sperm is stored), and the *vas (or ductus) deferens* (which connects to the urethra). Male birds may have a protrusive or non-protrusive penis which, when stimulated, is extruded via lymph fluid. Testes are located internally in the body cavity. Since body temperature in birds is higher than the optimal temperature for sperm generation and maturation, they have an adaptation to prevent the testes from becoming overheated from the internal body temperature. This adaptation is an *arteriovenous anastomosis* (called *rete venosus*), which detours heat from entering the testis. (Arteriovenous anastomoses are discussed more below).

Sperm production occurs in the seminiferous tubules of the testis under the influence of testosterone, which is produced by Leydig cells in the testis (Figure 3.12). When mature, the sperm will then be held in the epididymis. The ductus deferens carries the sperm down to the cloaca entering at the level of the coprodeum. In seasonally breeding species, the testes will regress (become smaller in size) from involution of seminiferous tubules in the nonbreeding season. In the breeding season, as the amount of daylight (photoperiod) increases, the pineal

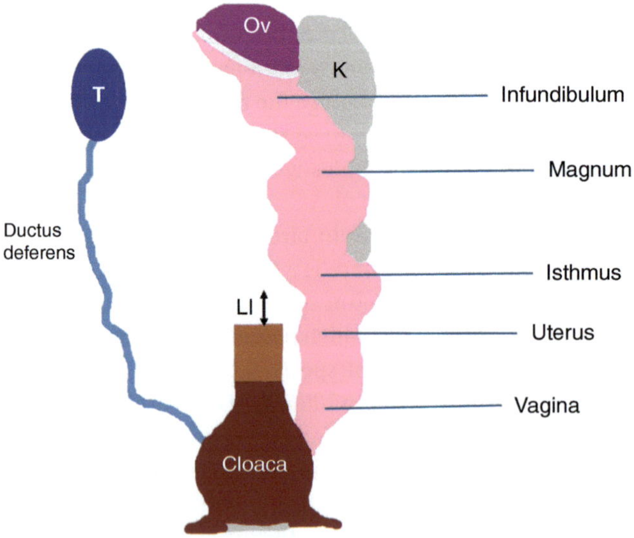

Figure 3.12 Anatomy of the reproductive and urinary tract in birds. T = testis; LI = large intestine; Ov = ovary; K = kidney (bilateral, but only one side pictured); light gray line under the ovary is the ostium.

gland signals melatonin to be released, which stimulates hormones (GnRH: gonadotropin-releasing hormone) to start reproductive processes. The testicular mass increases, and testosterone concentration increases in circulation stimulating spermatogenesis.

Female reproductive organs include the *ovary*, *uterus*, and *uterine horns* (Figure 3.12). As with mammals, females are born with the maximum number of eggs already in the ovary. At the age of sexual maturation and increased photoperiod, the ovarian follicles will begin enlarging, and the largest egg follicle will begin developing into the stage where it will ovulate. In most birds (except birds of prey), the left ovary is dominant, and the right ovary and tubules regress leaving only a single functioning ovary. The uterine horn connects the ovary to the body of the uterus, and it is within the horns that the embryo will begin embryogenesis. The developing egg is discussed further in the reproductive chapter. In seasonal species, as in males, the females will be triggered by melatonin during increasing photoperiod and begin activation and growth (hyperplasia) of reproductive organs under the influence of hormones.

Lymphoid Organs and Other Glands

The lymphoid organs are generally similar to those of terrestrial mammals with notable exceptions. Birds have a *spleen*, *thymus*, *bone marrow*, and various *lymphoid tonsils/aggregations*. They generally lack lymph nodes (except in some birds), and they have a unique organ called the *Bursa of Fabricius*. This bursa is located on the dorsal side of the cloaca. The *thymus* is responsible for the generation and education of T lymphocytes, while the bursa is responsible for the generation and education of B lymphocytes. In addition to its immunologic/lymphoid role, the spleen is the site of clearance of senescent or damaged RBC.

The aggregates of lymphoid tissues in the GIT and other locations serve as sentinel sites where the lymphocytes survey the incoming air or food for pathogens, harmful, or foreign agents. When the cells encounter something foreign or pathogenic, the lymphocytes signal the immune system to proliferate and attack the intruding agent (as described in Chapter 2).

Typical mammalian glands are present in birds. There are two types of glands: endocrine and exocrine. *Endocrine* glands secrete their hormone product directly into the bloodstream or lymphatic vessels. *Exocrine* glands secrete their product into an adjacent location but not into the bloodstream. Endocrine glands include the *thyroid, adrenal*, and the *pancreas*. Exocrine glands include the *salivary gland* and the pancreas. Notice that the pancreas acts as both an endocrine and exocrine organ.

The thyroid gland is located along the trachea cranial to the heart. Its function is to regulate metabolism in the body via thyroid hormones. The adrenal gland is located at the cranial pole of the kidneys (bilaterally). Its function is to regulate glucose homeostasis, but it also serves a critical role in stress response and other processes. Its primary products are glucocorticoids (cortisol or corticosterone), noradrenaline, and aldosterone. The salivary gland is an exocrine gland that secretes saliva into the oral cavity. Along with saliva are bacteriostatic agents and antibodies.

The pancreas has a dual function as an endocrine and exocrine gland. The endocrine portion of the pancreas is responsible for the production of insulin, glucagon, and a few other hormones in the islets of Langerhans. These islets comprise less than 5% of the entire gland. Insulin and glucagon have a primary role in regulating blood sugar levels and are the primary players in diabetes disease. The exocrine portion of the pancreas (comprising ≥95% of the organ) produces digestive enzymes to break down food to aid in the absorption of nutrients. These enzymes are deposited (through ducts) into the distal part of the proventriculus and the anterior portion of the duodenum.

The master endocrine gland is the pituitary gland, which is located at the base of the brain. On signal from the hypothalamus (located anterior to the pituitary), the pituitary releases hormones that activate target organs such as the ovary, testes, and adrenal glands. The activation is regulated by a negative feedback loop to the hypothalamus such that when sufficient target hormone is produced, it acts to decrease the signal from the hypothalamus, thus halting the signal emitted from the pituitary. We will return to hormonal regulation and feedback loops later in the stress chapter.

Central Nervous System

The central nervous system (CNS) includes the brain (*cerebrum* and *cerebellum*), *spinal cord*, and *cranial nerves* (which emanate from the brain). The peripheral nervous system includes the nerves that radiate from the spinal cord and innervate the organs/tissues in the body. As in mammals, sensory signals from the body make their way to the brain. The midbrain and the cerebellum receive visual, vestibular, and auditory input, then coordinate motor function, posture, and locomotion. The hindbrain continues posteriorly to become the spinal cord. There are 12 cranial nerves that derive from the brain, similar to mammals.

The areas of the brain are similar to those of mammals, but there are some notable differences in the avian brain. First, and most obviously, the cerebrum (*telencephalon*) is smooth (not convoluted as are human brains). There are no gyri nor sulci, as is characteristic of mammals. Avian intelligence shatters the myth of "the bigger and more convoluted the brain (cerebral cortex), the smarter one is." Second, the anterior-most aspect of the cerebrum, the olfactory lobe, is much reduced compared to terrestrial mammals (see senses section). Third, there is no corpus callosum in avian brains. The corpus callosum connects the right and left hemispheres of the brain of mammals, but in birds, other tracts connect the sides. Fourth, the spinal cord in birds continues all the way down to the last vertebrae compared to down to the pelvic girdle in mammals. Lastly, many functions that are regulated by the brain in mammals are regulated by the spinal cord as reflex arcs in birds.

Senses

The vast majority of avian species have a reduced olfactory sense. They rely mainly on vision and hearing. The anatomy of the visual system in birds is similar to that of mammals. Birds see in the range between ultraviolet and infrared. They employ rods and/or cones depending on if they are diurnal, nocturnal, or crepuscular (active at dawn and/or dusk). Birds, however, have an extensive visual field and binocular vision.

Hearing is a primary sense in birds. Vocalizations are commonly used and function in parent–offspring interactions, intraspecific communication, and mate choice. Most birds lack a pinna (outer ear) except for owls. The auditory signal is transferred to neurons by hairs on the cochlea, like in mammals. Unique to birds, however, is the ability to regenerate those auditory hairs if damaged! (If only humans could regenerate auditory hairs, we wouldn't need hearing aids!) Owls have an additional adaptation (in addition to the pinna) to optimize location of prey. Their ears are not symmetrically placed on the left and right sides of the head. One ear is lower than the ear on the other side of the head. This allows them additional information to localize prey because sound will arrive at each ear at different times.

Some birds actually echolocate! The Neotropical oil bird (*Steatornis caripensis*) and swiflets in the genera *Aerodramus* and *Collocolia* live and roost in dark caves. The ability to echolocate apparently evolved independently in these two groups. The echolocation is not exactly similar to that of bats, as these birds do not hear ultrasonic frequencies. However, they use clicks in the typical avian hearing range and listen for return echoes (Koppl, 2022).

While olfaction is poor, birds do taste all the major categories of taste sensation. They have taste buds in the oral cavity. Additionally, birds can use magnetoreception to orient themselves and for navigation purposes. There is a lot that is still unknown about the details of avian taste and magnetoreception.

Unique Avian Physiology and Systems

Oxygen Extraction and Uptake

In birds, oxygen extraction from the air is much more (10 times more) efficient than in other vertebrates. In addition to the unique anatomy of parabronchi in the lungs, the avian system has evolved to minimize the distance for diffusion of oxygen. This is made possible by an increased number of capillaries per cross-sectional area of flight muscle (3–6 times that in rats; Powell, 2022). The blood capillaries are also very tortuous and have a lot of folds, thereby increasing the surface area that contacts the air capillaries. This feature and the fact that the capillary walls are very thin increase the rate of transfer of oxygen into the muscles' mitochondria. In addition, birds are relatively tolerant of a low oxygen atmosphere (Powell, 2022). High-altitude flying birds carry on efficient oxygen exchange during flight.

How is oxygen carried in the blood? Oxygen is attached to a hemoglobin molecule inside the RBCs. Oxygen is also stored in a related protein called myoglobin ("myo" refers to muscle). Myoglobin is present in all animal muscles; however, some species, such as diving birds, high altitude flying birds, and hummingbirds, have a much greater density of myoglobin in their muscles because of the increased need for oxygen, either because of very high muscle activity and/or oxygen storage. Additional storage is needed if there is not continuous access to getting more oxygen as in diving birds, for example. The myoglobin is what makes the muscles look very dark, dark red. (Think about eating chicken for dinner – there is "white" meat, which is breast muscle and "dark" meat, which includes the thigh and legs/drumsticks. The "dark" meat is darker in color due to more myoglobin because of the sustained activity needed in those parts of the body.) Similar to deep-diving marine mammals, the concentration of myoglobin is greater in species that dive deeper (Powell, 2022). Box 3.1 has more unique avian physiology facts!

Box 3.1 The unique physiology of birds

The avian heart is relatively larger than the heart of similar-sized mammals. A bird's heart rate (HR) is also faster, usually 200 beats per minute (bpm), compared with an average small adult dog whose HR = 100–140 bpm. (At rest, human HR = 72 bpm. Hummingbird HRs range from 500 to 1,200 bpm!) The higher HR is due to a larger number of myocytes with a smaller diameter, which allows depolarization more rapidly. A larger heart and a higher HR lead to a greater cardiac output (Dzialowski and Crossley, 2022). To manage these features, the average arterial blood pressure is high (140–250 mm Hg vs. 100 in humans). This is quite remarkable and requires a lot of energy!

Other bizarre bird facts! The gastrointestinal tract of birds is shorter than that of mammals of comparable size. Obviously, this helps reduce weight for flying. But now the intestine must be more efficient at nutrient absorption because there is less area for this function. In an experiment, Rufous and Anna's hummingbirds (*Selasphorus rufus* and *Calypte anna*, respectively) absorbed 97% of a glucose–water solution in 15 min (Karasov et al., 1986)!! How is this for rapid absorption? Their intestines also appear to have greater plasticity and passive nutrient absorption than terrestrial animals (Hawkes, 2025). Birds also have "two-way" peristalsis. That is, they can move food down toward the cloaca (usual direction) and move ingesta back toward the small intestine (Faaborg, 2020)! This permits more absorption of nutrients as the ingesta has a second pass across the intestines. (This is similar in concept to cows regurgitating some food (cud), chewing it, and then swallowing it again.)

Birds are also able to tolerate very high levels of glucose in their blood, often double or more than the levels in mammals, and diabetes does not develop (Hawkes, 2025). It is suggested that this appears to be due to resistance to the effects of insulin, thus leaving glucose for metabolism. Hyperglycemia does not appear to cause physiological pathology (e.g., oxidative damage to tissues) as it does in mammals (Hawkes, 2025).

Finally, birds do not seem to develop loss of lean muscle mass (sarcopenia) with age as do mammals, at least humans (Hawkes, 2025)! So they do not lose body condition with age! This makes sense in light of the need to migrate annually. Maintenance of body condition and reduction of oxidative damage (above) contribute to long-living animals. Examples of aged birds (which can be found at https://euring.org/data-and-codes/longevity-list) include Laysan albatross – 73 years old; Manx shearwater – 51 years old; and Puffin – 45 years old.

Heat Conservation and Loss

Like all animals, birds are faced with the need to thermoregulate; that is, conserve heat when cold and release heat when hot. As birds have a higher basal body temperature than vertebrates (relative to size), they have continual pressure to conserve heat. Since water transduces 25× more heat loss from the body than does air, sea birds and diving birds have greater pressure to retain heat. Heat loss in birds occurs across the nonfeathered skin areas, across the beak (vasodilation favors heat release), and from the respiratory tract due to high ventilatory rates and/or panting (and/or gular fluttering). Heat loss can also occur across the cornea (eye) and cloaca. Some birds that live at higher latitudes have feathers all the way down to their toes to reduce heat loss across the legs. However, there are other novel ways to manage heat loss. They have to do with adaptations of the vasculature – the blood vessels in the body.

In some areas of the body where it is critical to avoid heat loss or avoid an organ from getting too hot, the vessels come to the rescue! Arteriovenous anastomoses (aka AVA, also known as countercurrent heat exchangers) are structures whereby arteries and veins that lie in close proximity have interconnecting capillaries that run between them (similar concept as in the parabronchi). These "capillary bridges" shunt the heat of the blood in arteries (hot and coming from the heart) to the veins for return to the body core *before* the blood reaches the skin, where it would radiate away. This prevents heat from being lost across the skin. This same mechanism can prevent an organ from becoming overheated. Let us run through an example to understand.

The testes produce sperm. This process is optimized to function best at certain body temperatures. In species with externally located testes (e.g., humans and dogs), temperature control can be managed by moving the scrotal sac (and the testes within) closer to the body if more warmth is needed or farther away if they need cooling. However, in species that have internal testes (all bird species), males need a way to avoid the testes from overheating and destroying the sperm and/or preventing spermatogenesis. There is an AVA system adjacent to the spermatic arteries. The warmer blood coming from the body's core needs to dump some of its heat before entering the testes. The heat diffuses across the capillaries via osmosis to the cooler veins within these AVAs. This results in the blood continuing into the testes, but the heat associated with the core blood is wicked away across the capillaries of the AVA and then heads back to the heart in the veins.

Other areas of the body are also in critical need of mechanisms to prevent heat (and water) loss. The brain functions optimally at a lower temperature than body temperature. There is an AVA (*rete opthalmicum*) at the brain base to prevent overheating (Wild, 2022). Another area is the nasal turbinates. Here, the presence of AVA helps recover heat (and water lost via evaporation) in expired air due to the increase surface area of the turbinates. In addition, the turbinates can increase the temperature and moisten inspired air. Another mechanism to prevent heat loss is to constrict the peripheral vessels. Constriction (temporarily) effectively closes the vessel so no blood flows beyond the constriction. This process is reserved for diving and when the environment is very cold. In fact, in some penguins, the body becomes *heterothermic* – the body is at different temperatures in different areas simultaneously. In this example, the penguin would have high internal body temperature and colder extremity temperatures during vasoconstriction.

There are several behavioral mechanisms to cool down if temperatures increase in the environment. Birds can go down into burrows, sit in shady areas, roost or sit in groups (communal roosting), stay out of windy areas (which would stimulate heat loss), or sit in positions where their surface area for heat loss is maximized. In addition, some species have evolved to have darker plumage, which minimizes heat gain.

Adaptations of Sea Birds and Diving

The species of birds which we refer to as seabirds vary greatly. So this discussion is general. All birds that regularly visit the water (swim, dive, and feed) have some degree of webbing between their toes. Many seabird species also either lack or have "closed" or non-perforate nares, so water does not enter the nasal cavity and respiratory tract. Several birds that float on the water (vs. dive down) have subcutaneous air sacs to facilitate floating.

Diving birds, especially penguins, have several additional adaptations. On land, the atmospheric pressure is 1 Atmosphere (ATM). For every 10 m (approximately 30 ft) you descend from the water surface, the pressure increases 1 ATM. So, the deeper you dive, the more physical pressure from the water is imposed on your body (internally and externally). In order for diving into the depths to be a successful foraging strategy, diving birds evolved several adaptations to overcome, or at least mitigate, the negative effects of increasing pressure. Similar to diving marine mammals, diving birds have an increased concentration of myoglobin in their muscles. Some of the long bones are dense rather than hollow, allowing them to descend underwater. These birds also tend to have broader wings (although there is variation). To help mitigate tracheal and pulmonary collapse, the trachea has complete cartilaginous, often ossified rings, and the lungs are embedded/wrapped within the ribs, which provide some support.

Flight

Flight has evolved four times in four different types of animals – insects, bats, birds, and pterosaurs. And why not? Flight in the air is much less energetically expensive overall than terrestrial locomotion. In addition, there are ways to maximize energy savings while flying, such as soaring, gliding (both non-flapping flight), and/or using thermals. Thermals are rising heat currents that will lift birds into the air without effort. In birds, the primary flight muscles are the pectoralis (pec) muscles. These muscles attach to the keel and move the wing for flapping or positional adjustment for maximal aerodynamics during flight. Aerodynamics is an important factor in body and wing design to minimize drag forces (which act against forward flight). The shape of the wing viewed from its leading edge is optimal for smooth air flow over it (recall Figure 3.4). It is so adaptive that marine mammal flippers have the same cross-sectional shape as they move through water and humans have copied it to use in aircraft!

Birds have a wide array of anatomical and physiological adaptations for efficient flight. Penguins have optimized these adaptations to swim/fly underwater. For starters, the avian body, looked at head-on, is shaped like a torpedo and tapers to the rear. In addition, the shape of feathers themselves follows the same pattern. Feathers have a very limited ability to change orientation like mammal hair can do when we get goose bumps. (In goose bumps, the hair stands up because of the contraction of a tiny muscle attached to each hair.) Inability to change the orientation of the feather ensures there is a smooth outer surface that minimizes drag. Preening, in addition to maintaining waterproofing, removes particulate debris from the feather surface. And of course, hollow pneumatized bones and dispensing with some organs contribute to lighter body weight.

Flapping flight consumes a lot of oxygen to generate ATP energy. There are several physiologic adaptations birds have evolved to augment oxygen retrieval and storage (McWilliams et al., 2022). The system for oxygen removal from air in the parabronchi is very efficient, as we discussed earlier in this chapter. Enzymes critical to *aerobic* metabolism are abundant, especially in migratory species, particularly those that fly at high altitude. The capacity for *anaerobic* metabolism is similarly enhanced. The number of blood capillaries in flight muscles is increased, mitochondrial density in flight muscles is increased, and muscle fiber diameter is decreased (increasing the density of muscle fibers), which favors oxygen retrieval into the blood and then passing oxygen to the muscle cells (Bishop and Guglielmo, 2022). Myoglobin is also present in higher concentrations, especially in birds that fly at high altitudes where oxygen partial pressure is low.

The most expensive part of a flight is taking off and slow speed flight. Depending on the bird type, the energy to take flight can be derived anaerobically since it is needed for only a short period of time. To get "lift" and rise into the air, the bird needs to be facing into the wind. The differential pressure above and below the wing (Figure 3.4) provides the initial lift off the ground. Then wing flapping keeps it going. The pectoral muscles contract for the downstroke (it is actually down and forward). The opposing supracoracoid muscle then flexes causing the upstroke.

Approximately 20% of all avian species migrate. Migration distances vary widely; the farthest migration distance annually is 71,000 km by the Arctic tern (see Box 3.2). Before migration, the bird needs to increase its energy stores and the flight muscles need to have sufficient aerobic "fitness" (Bishop and Guglielmo, 2022). In fact, the heart muscle hypertrophies. All the feathers have to be in (i.e., molting completed) and intact. Energy is stored as fats since fats have the highest energy density. Enzymes efficient at catabolizing fat to usable energy are abundant. Oxygen is stored in myoglobin in the muscles and in hemoglobin in RBC. Breathing continues during flight, so oxygen is easily obtainable. Perhaps the most interesting detail is that the type of muscle fiber can vary between four types (Halevy and Velleman, 2022). Each of those types *specializes* in aerobic or anaerobic respiration, can vary in diameter, and can have different capillary arrangements. They are used preferentially in different circumstances.

Box 3.2 Migration

Migration is the seasonal movement from nonbreeding to breeding area and back again annually. Some species will stop along the way to forage and refuel; others will fly straight through nonstop to their destination. Migration evolved to maximize reproduction and overwintering in optimal habitats. That makes sense as the arctic birds (for example) certainly cannot survive the polar winters! But do they really need to fly to the other side of the world? Apparently, some do!

Below are the five species that fly the farthest annually on their migration. (For reference, the distance from Miami to Los Angeles = 3,700 km or 2,300 miles. Faaborg, 2020.)

- Arctic tern (*Sterna paradisaea*) – annual round trip = 71,000 km (44,000 miles); Arctic to Antarctic and back; they will stop to eat along the way.
- Sooty shearwater (*Ardenna grisea*) – annual round trip = 64,000 km (40,000 miles); New Zealand to the Northern Pacific Ocean and back; they fly nonstop.
- Swainson's Hawk (*Buteo swainsoni*) – annual round trip = 14,000 km (8,700 miles); North America to Argentina and back; they will stop to feed opportunistically.

(Continued)

Box 3.2 (Continued)

- Bar-tailed godwit (*Limosa lapponica*) – annual round trip = 12,200 km (7,500 miles); Alaska to New Zealand/Australia and back; they fly nonstop.
- Blackpoll warbler (*Setophaga striata*) – annual round trip = 4,800 km (3,000 miles); NW Canada/Alaska to South America and back; they will fly nonstop over the ocean but may stop to eat when flying over land.

Preparation for migration is a substantial undertaking! Birds need to add lots of fat stores to derive energy. Their rate of fat deposition is due to a 40–50% increase in feeding rate (Hawkes, 2025). The Blackpoll warbler actually doubles its body weight before migrating! The pectoral muscles and heart hypertrophy and the stomach, intestines, and liver will atrophy a bit to get ready for the flight. While in flight, many birds use gliding or soaring, fly in V-formation, and use other ways to minimize energy. Some species can even sleep during the migration flight by shutting down half of their brain to "sleep" while the other side keeps functioning. During migration, the HR and oxygen uptake increases 6–10× more than when at rest (McWilliams et al., 2022).

How does this relate to health? Marshalling energy reserves for a long migration takes energy away from other body functions, including the immune response. If the species flies to an area that is being degraded or severely affected by humans and/or climate change, they may not be able to find sufficient nutrients to raise young or fly back in the nonbreeding season. High concentrations of birds at stopover locations or destinations due to decreased habitats put all those individuals at risk of contracting an infectious disease. All these factors potentially put the bird's survival and reproduction at risk. And if they successfully make the flights, they may be inadvertent carriers of infectious agent or contaminants to and from their destinations. Some species have "site fidelity" to their destinations. That is, they fly to the same exact places every year. Can birds be flexible and find alternate stopover sites, feeding, or nesting grounds? Human-induced environmental changes, pollution loads, and temperature increases are occurring at very rapid rates! Let's hope that they will be able to adjust quickly if needed.

There are downsides to flight. Flapping flight requires a lot of energy, as we discussed. Flapping flight also generates a lot of body heat, elevating the birds' core body temperature. There is an ultimate maximum temperature above which would be disastrous. The options then are to stop flying, change the type of flight to soar, rising on thermals, etc., which don't require flapping, or increase the mechanisms for dispelling heat. Wings that are longer, thinner, and pointier are adapted for long-distance flying and soaring (Figure 3.13). Wings with more rounded (less thin and pointy) ends are the more average-shaped wing. Increased ventilatory rate is one of the main mechanisms to dispel heat during flight. However, increased ventilation also causes more water loss, so the bird needs to balance that into the equation. Amazingly, however, evolution has worked out sufficient solutions to permit very long migrations without stopping and even "allowing" sleeping while in flight!

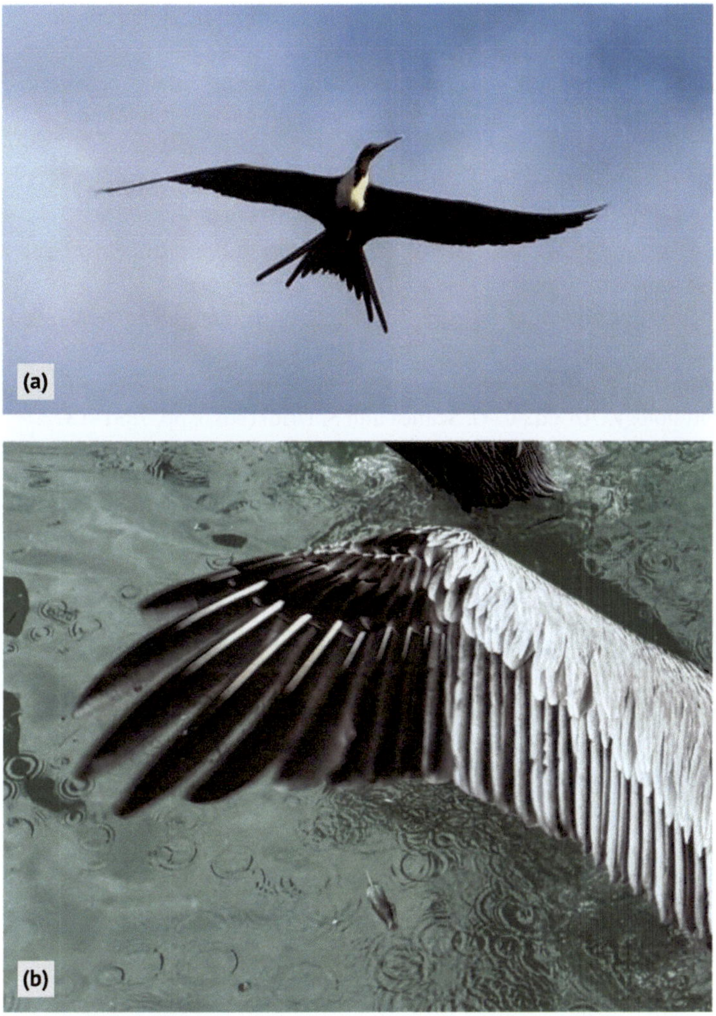

Photographs by author

Figure 3.13 Wing shapes and associated flight types. (a) Frigatebird viewed from below. Note the extreme pointiness and thinness of the long wing. This wing shape is adapted for soaring high up. (b) Close-up of a pelican wing. Note the rounded shape of the distal edge of the wing. This rounded shape is seen with most birds.

Literature Cited

Bishop, C. M. and Guglielmo, C. G. (2022). Flight. In: *Avian Physiology*, 7th Ed., C. G. Scanes and S. Dridi (eds.). pp. 1265–1330. Academic Press.

Doneley, B. and Xie, S. (2025). *Avian Medicine and Surgery in Practice*, 3rd Ed. CRC Press.

du Toit, C. J., Chinsamy, A. and Cunningham, S. J. (2024). Good vibrations: remote-tactile foraging success of wading birds is positively affected by the water content of substrates they forage in. *Journal of Avian Biology* 2024:e03243. https://doi.org/10.1111/jav.03243

Dzialowski, E. M. and Crossley, D. A. (2022). The cardiovascular system. In: *Avian Physiology*, 7th Ed., C. G. Scanes and S. Dridi (eds.). pp. 327–410. Academic Press.

Faaborg, J. (2020). *Book of Birds. Introduction to Ornithology*. Texas A&M University Press.

Halevy, O. and Velleman, S. G. (2022). Skeletal muscle. In: *Avian Physiology*, 7th Ed., C. G. Scanes and S. Dridi (eds.). pp. 565–590. Academic Press.

Hawkes, L. A. (2025). Why the superb physiological capacity of birds matter. *Journal of Experimental Biology* 228:jeb247986. https://doi.org/10.1242/jeb.247986.

Karasov, W. H., Phan, D., Diamond, J. M., et al. (1986). Food passage and intestinal nutrient absorption in hummingbirds. *Auk* 103(3):453–464.

Koppl, C. (2022). Avian hearing In: *Avian Physiology*, 7th Ed., C. G. Scanes and S. Dridi (eds.). pp. 159–178. Academic Press.

McWilliams, S. R., Ramenofsky, M., and Pierce, B. J. (2022). Physiological challenges of migration. In: *Avian Physiology*, 7th Ed., C. G. Scanes and S. Dridi (eds.). pp. 1331–1372. Academic Press.

McWilliams, S. R., Ramenofsky, M., and Pierce, B. J. (2022). Respiration. In: *Avian Physiology*, 7th Ed., C. G. Scanes and S. Dridi (eds.). pp. 445–484. Academic Press.

Mora-Rubio, C., García-Longoria, L., and Marzal, A. (2025). Preening for protection: A systematic review of the antimicrobial properties of uropygial secretions. *Journal of Avian Biology* 2025:e03425. https://doi.org/10.1111/jav.03425.

Powell, F. L. (2022). Respiration. In: *Avian Physiology*, 7th Ed., C. G. Scanes and S. Dridi (eds.). pp. 445–484. Academic Press.

Sykes, IV., J. M. (2015). Piciformes (Honeyguides, Barbets, Woodpeckers, Toucans). In: *Zoo and Wild Animal Medicine*, R. E. Miller and M. E. Fowler (eds.). vol. 8, pp. 230–235. Elsevier.

Wallace, R. S. (2015). Sphenisciformes (Penguins). In: *Zoo and Wild Animal Medicine*, R. E. Miller and M. E. Fowler (eds.). vol. 8, pp. 82–88. Elsevier.

Wild, J. M. (2022). The avian somatosensory system: A comparative view. In: *Avian Physiology*, 7th Ed., C. G. Scanes and S. Dridi (eds.). pp. 123–138. Academic Press.

4

Etiologic Agents of Infectious Disease

The approach to managing infectious disease in birds living in managed care/zoos and free-ranging/wild can be vastly different. Understanding the biology of microbes is critically important for managing an infectious disease in a managed care population. Can the agent be medically treated and eradicated? How can the environment be sanitized or disinfected to remove the agent in question? Where does the agent live, where can it live, and when and in what circumstances does it reproduce? How can the agent be spread around the facility or from animal to animal? The answers to these questions vary with the type of microbe. In wild bird populations, it is important to understand the etiology of infectious diseases to understand the relationship between the agent, the environment, and the host. In wild populations, the approach to managing infectious diseases includes understanding the mechanisms of how the etiologic agent spreads to other animals, other species, and far from the source, especially if the bird is a migratory species. Human and veterinary epidemiologists and medical practitioners are integral to working out the possible impact on humans and other species. We touch on those issues in the last section of the book. This chapter will focus on the infectious agent itself.

There are several types of infectious agents that cause disease. Understanding the basic biology and life cycles of infectious agents helps us understand how and why the agents spread and how to manage and treat them. The major agents we will review are bacteria, viruses, fungi, protozoans, and parasites.

Let us review some terms. There are three major types of organisms – *prokaryotes*, *eukaryotes*, and *archaea*. *Prokaryotes* are single-cell organisms that lack membrane-bound organelles. The components of the cells are present freely in the cells. The genetic material is not within a separate entity (i.e., no nucleus), nor is there a mitochondrion (to make energy). Typical prokaryotes include bacteria, viruses, and cyanobacteria. *Eukaryotes* include single and multicellular organisms whose cells have organelles that are encased within cell membranes. They are evolutionarily younger than prokaryotes and include plants, animals, fungi, protozoans, and other single-celled organisms. *Archaea* are the most primitive type of organism. Like prokaryotes, they lack organelles and nuclei. However, they have unique properties that prokaryotes lack and can use more diverse energy sources, including oxygen, ammonia, and hydrogen sulfide. Archaea can live in eukaryotes (e.g., in gut and oral microbiomes); however, none have yet been discovered to be directly pathogenic (Borrel et al., 2020).

Viruses

Viruses are small, obligate, intracellular parasites that depend on the host cell's metabolic machinery (e.g., production of sugars and nutrients) to survive and replicate. They can live outside of a cell, but they cannot replicate unless within the appropriate cell. They have a nucleic acid genome (either RNA or DNA) surrounded by a protein coat (called a capsid) and may or may not have a lipid membrane surrounding the capsid. Viruses are classified in various ways: by type of nucleic acid genome (RNA or DNA), shape of capsid (icosahedral or helical), presence or absence of lipid membrane, mode of replication, tropism (preferred cell type), and type of pathology they cause (cell rupture [aka cytolysis] or no rupture; Cotran et al., 1999). The presence of an outer lipid membrane is a key factor in virus eradication. Lipids are susceptible to detergents, and therefore, detergents used in cleaning will degrade and destroy the lipid membrane and kill these enveloped viruses. Viruses in the environment that lack a lipid membrane are far more difficult to eradicate by cleaning procedures.

Viruses are very small in size (20–300 nm; Figure 4.1). As such, they are not directly visible using the naked eye nor by using a light microscope. Visualization of actual viruses requires electron microscopy. However, one can often see the effects of certain viruses using light microscopy. For example, certain pathologic changes or "signatures" are produced by some viruses, such as inclusion bodies or multinucleated syncytial cells (paramyxoviruses). Detection of a virus relies upon molecular techniques, such as polymerase chain reaction (PCR), gene sequencing, or electron microscopy.

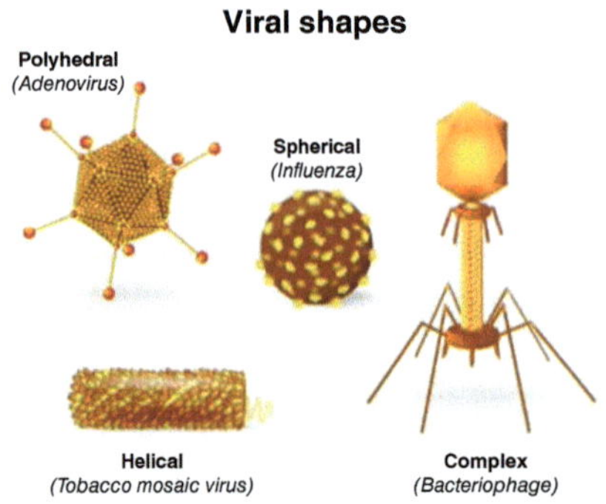

Designua/Adobe Stock Photos

(a)

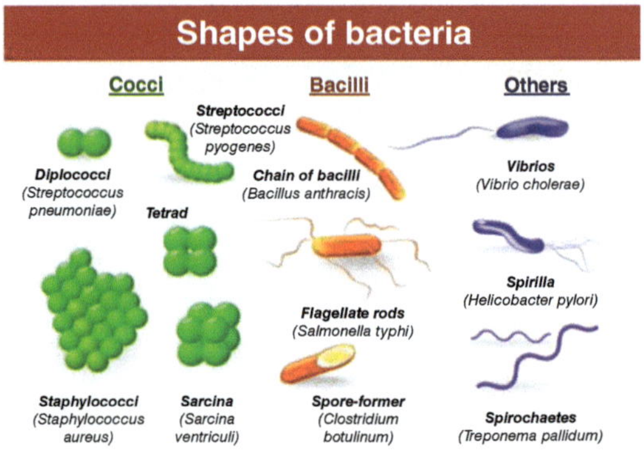

Designua/Shutterstock.com

(b)

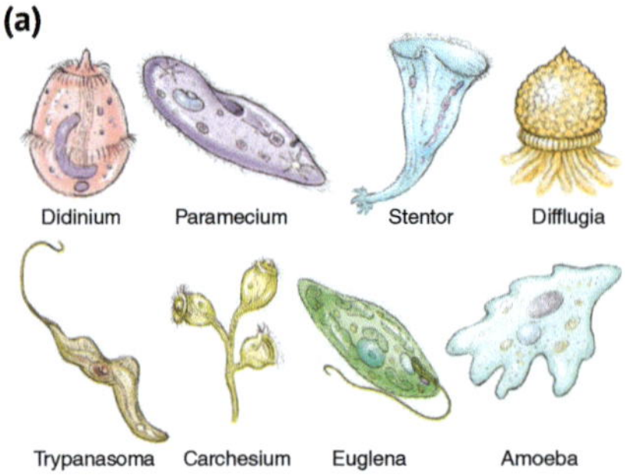

(c)

Figure 4.1 Bacteria and virus characteristics and shapes.

Viruses can cause diseases that are transient and clear by themselves, or they can cause long-standing diseases. Viruses can remain in the body and persist in host cells for years, be asymptomatic and dormant, and then potentially recur; that is, they begin multiplying and become active again. Examples of this phenomenon in humans include herpes zoster virus, the cause of chicken pox, which can reside latent in some dorsal ganglia and be reactivated later in life causing the disease shingles. A latent infection means that the virus is persisting in a nonreplicating form but is alive. Some viruses are *oncogenic* (cause cancer), producing either benign or malignant tumors. For example, there are various strains of human papillomavirus, some of which are benign, while others cause malignant cervical cancer.

The severity of disease (*virulence*) caused by some viruses depends on the exact strain of the virus and the condition of the host (e.g., immune competent or deficient). Vaccines for humans and many domestic species exist for many viruses. In fact, some diseases have been putatively eradicated by widespread vaccination (e.g., smallpox). However, contrary to bacteria, viruses cannot be eradicated and cleared from the body using medications. This has been dogma for many years. However, in recent years, new medications (antiretroviral therapies) have reduced the incidence of disease in people with certain viral infections and reduced the risk of transmission by drastically reducing viral reproduction (reduced viral load, such as in HIV).

Bacteria

Bacteria are prokaryotes (have an outer cell membrane but lack membrane-bound nuclei and organelles), and most have a "cell wall" around the cell membrane. Some bacteria have a thick wall surrounding the cell membrane; others have a thin wall sandwiched between two phospholipid membranes. The former type can absorb crystal violet (purple) stain and is known as gram-positive bacteria. The latter type cannot retain the stain and are referred to as gram-negative bacteria.

Bacteria have quite diverse lifestyles. Most can synthesize their own nutrients and proteins (in contrast to viruses), but they depend on the host for favorable growth conditions. Some bacteria require oxygen to live (*obligate aerobes*), some cannot tolerate oxygen (*obligate anaerobes*), and others can tolerate both *(facultative aerobes*). Many have flagella (long helical filaments) for movement. Some have pili, which are appendages on the cell surface used for attachment. Some bacteria reside outside of the cell (*obligate extracellular*); others must live inside cells (*obligate intracellular*), and some can live either in or outside of the cell (*facultative intracellular*). An example of an obligatory intracellular bacteria is *Chlamydia*. *Chlamydia* organisms need to obtain adenosine triphosphate from their host for biologic functions and to replicate inside membrane-bound vacuoles (Elwell et al., 2016).

Normally, all people and animals have millions of bacteria colonizing them daily (microbiome) in different parts of the body. For example, 10^{12} bacteria on skin, 10^{10} in mouth, and 10^{14} in the gastrointestinal tract (GIT). Usually, the microbiome contains one to a few species at each location. In normal intestinal flora, there may be many species, but only a few predominate in numbers. What we have learned in the recent past is that these normal microbiomes are also critical barriers to prevent disease.

Fungi

Fungi are multicellular eukaryotes. They have thick, chitin cell walls and ergosterol-containing cell membranes. Fungi can grow as yeast cells or as slender filamentous hyphae. Hyphae can be distinguished as septate (cell walls dividing individual cells) or nonseptate. They show thermal dimorphism; that is, they can grow into different forms depending on the temperature (yeast at higher body temperatures and hyphae at lower temperatures). Reproduction can be sexual (through spores) or asexual (through conidia), which is more common (Cotran et al., 1999).

Many fungi are ubiquitous in the environment and are opportunistic pathogens. Fungi usually cause superficial skin diseases involving hair, nails, or skin (e.g., ringworm). However, if the host and other conditions are favorable, deep, systemic infections can occur, usually in immunocompromised hosts. Example species of fungi in birds include *Aspergillus* and *Candida*.

Protozoa

Protozoans are single-celled eukaryotes, as their organelles are all membrane-bound. They can replicate intracellularly (e.g., inside red blood cells – such as *Plasmodium* in the disease malaria or *Leishmania* living inside white blood cells in the disease leishmaniasis). They can also replicate extracellularly, for example, in the urogenital system or intestine. In developing countries, protozoans are a major cause of human disease.

Protozoans are known for their complex life cycles, which often include multiple life stages and vectors. The most prevalent gastrointestinal (GI) protozoans in humans are *Entamoeba* and *Giardia*, which can exist in two forms: mobile trophozoites that attach to the intestinal wall and invade across the mucosa or immobile cysts that are resistant to stomach acids and are infectious when ingested. Cysts can be found in contaminated water and food sources and are the main form of disease transmission. Blood-borne protozoans include *Plasmodium, Trypanosoma*, and *Leishmania*, which are transmitted by mosquito vectors within whom they replicate before being passed to new humans or animals through bites.

One of the most familiar protozoans is *Toxoplasma* (Figure 4.2). *Toxoplasma* has a complex life cycle and can be acquired by contact with fecal oocysts (shed by cats) or by eating cyst-ridden, undercooked meat. The cyst wall is broken down by enzymes releasing the motile form, which can then invade the intestinal epithelial cells and begin multiplying. In humans, clinical disease is often a mild flu-like disease but can also include neuropsychiatric and behavioral changes. *Toxoplasma* infects warm-blooded animals, and birds are not immune to infection. It has been found to cause encephalitis and blindness in poultry, pet, and wild birds (Darwich et al., 2012; Buschang et al., 2025).

Parasites

Helminths (the "worms") are probably the most common type of internal parasite – parasitic worms are highly differentiated, multicellular eukaryotes. They can have complex life cycles alternating between sexual reproduction in the definitive host and asexual multiplication in the intermediary host or vector species. Usually when adult worms are in

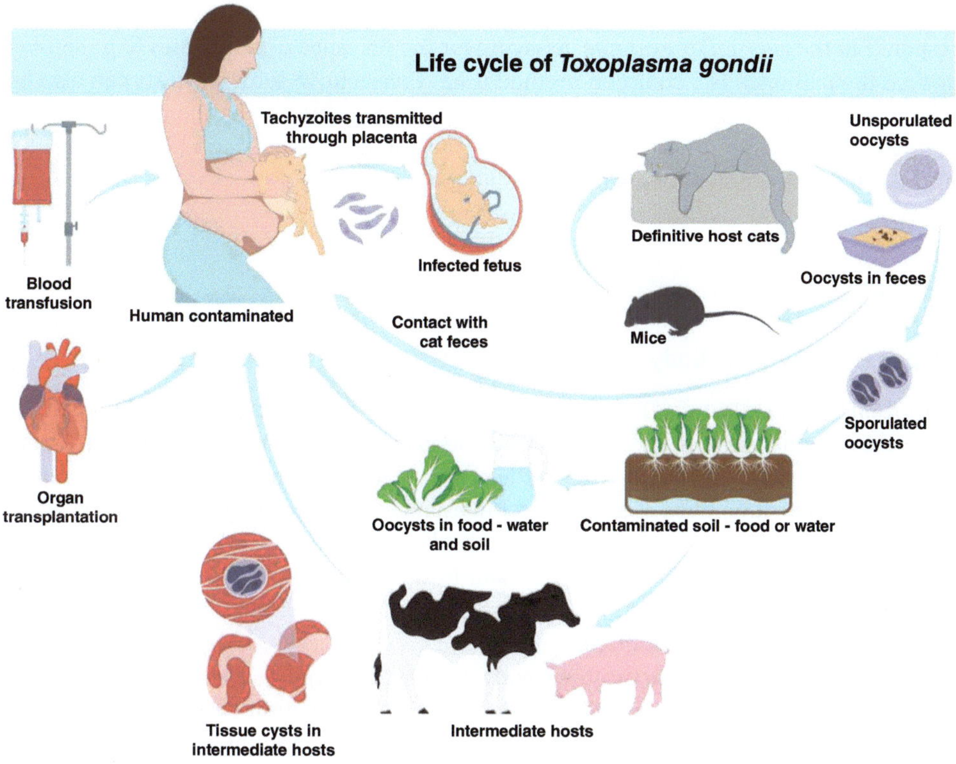

Figure 4.2 Toxoplasmosis life cycle.

the GIT, they produce eggs that can then pass out into the environment through feces and can infect other hosts. Common types of helminths include roundworms and hookworms. Treatment of these parasites is usually successful if the life cycle details are known.

Ectoparasites can also be seen in birds. Arthropods (e.g., insects and arachnids) that attach to or live on skin or feathers are the most common type of ectoparasites. They may produce local disease or insult to the skin (dermatitis) and/or transmit bacterial pathogens (e.g., Lyme disease is carried by ticks.). Parasites, by definition, have a negative consequence for the host. Mites are common ectoparasites in birds (Doneley and Xie, 2025). Blood-sucking species can cause anemia, especially in weak or young individuals.

Diagnosing Infectious Agents

Infectious agents can be diagnosed by a variety of methods. Some can be seen grossly – by the eyes without a microscope. Others require high magnification, such as with a light microscope. Standard stains can highlight the pathogen and any associated disease or lesion. Special stains can be used to highlight different aspects of the agent (such as the type of cell wall) to narrow down the species. In the case of viruses, an electron microscope must be used to visualize the agent because they are so small. Molecular diagnostics, such as PCR, in situ hybridization, and Northern and Southern blots, apply small segments of DNA or RNA to tissues to detect complementary binding and thus defining the pathogenic organism.

Detection of infectious agents may be better accomplished by assessing the body's response to the agent. For example, assaying for the presence of antibodies (e.g., serology) against the pathogen is a common method used. Consecutive serologic tests can also help define whether the infection is actively increasing, decreasing, or possibly reflecting a prior and resolved exposure. Indirect evidence of infection can also be found by looking at the host tissues for the potential effects of the pathogen.

How Pathogens Invade the Body

Step 1: Entry into the Body

Pathogenic (disease causing) microorganisms need to pass through the body's defenses, enter the body, and disseminate through the bloodstream to their preferred organ/tissue in the body. Once they arrive there, they settle in and begin to reproduce. From the organisms' perspective, they then need to get the host to excrete their new progeny out of the body to continue infecting new hosts. From a host bird's perspective, clinical symptoms appear once the organism reaches its preferred site in the body and begins reproducing. Thus, reducing the load of the invading organism (through medications, vaccination, etc.) can lead to fewer clinical signs of disease.

The methods/routes of entry into the body include inhalation (nares and beak), ingestion (beak), sexual transmission, and/or crossing the skin or mucosal barrier (cuts, scratches, and bites). The latter route can be breached by insect bites, animal bites, scratches, or, in seabirds, by spines penetrating through the body. If the bird resides in managed care/zoo, we need to include injections by syringe as another way to cross the skin or mucosal barrier. Let us review the body's defenses (physical, chemical, and functional) in relation to each of these routes.

The first defenses are physical barriers – intact skin and structures protruding from the skin (think fur and scales on fish). The integument is composed of the skin (epidermis and dermis), subcutis, and any structures protruding into the environment from the skin surface like feathers. In intact skin, there are normally no routes available for the pathogen to cross the skin and enter the body. The skin has a normal resident bacterial flora, which can deter the entry of pathogenic bacteria. The keratinized outer epidermis is also a formidable barrier. In addition, throughout the dermis, the acidic environment (low pH), the presence of certain fatty acids that can inhibit the growth of nonresident microbes, cerebroside fats, and the tight intercellular junctions between epidermal cells can all inhibit penetration.

In the GIT, consumption and ingestion of contaminated food or water is the most common mechanism of microbe entry. Saliva in the mouth contains antibodies and antimicrobial peptides. The acidic environment of the stomach is often an effective mechanism to deter (by killing or decreasing function) some microbes; however, we do see microbes (e.g., *Shigella* and *Giardia* in humans) that are resistant to, and can withstand, the acidic environment. Other defenses in GIT include a layer of viscous mucus covering epithelial surfaces, lytic pancreatic enzymes, bile detergents, mucosal antimicrobial peptides called defensins, normal GI flora, and secreted IgA antibodies in mucosal-associated lymphoid tissue. These foci of lymphoid tissue contain specialized "M" cells that are important for transport of the microbe to the lymphoid foci and for binding and uptake of gut pathogens.

In the respiratory tract, particles gain entry by inhalation through the nares and beak/oral cavities. Inhaled pathogens gain entry on dust, aerosolized particles, or water droplets. Larger, heavier particles settle out in the upper tract – from the nasal cavity down to the trachea and the larger primary bronchi. If the nasal cavity is stimulated by too many particles or irritating stimulus, the animal may sneeze expelling the irritants. The mucus in the upper tract traps microbes, and cilia move the trapped microbes to the back of the throat by ciliary action, where they may be swallowed. Small, lighter particles ($<5\ \mu m$) will be able to go further down into the lower airway – to the parabronchi and air sacs. In the lower airways, alveolar macrophages (immune cells that reside in the parabronchi) can engulf the microbes.

The main defense against invading pathogens in the urogenital and reproductive tract is by urination/defecation. The entry point to both systems is through the cloaca and then up the urethra. Urination effectively flushes out the urethra, taking with it any invaders. If pathogens are not washed out by the urine (e.g., if they evolved a way to attach to the urethral cells), then they can spread into the genital and/or urinary system.

Given the body's defense tactics, how do pathogens get through this first line of defense and cause disease in the body? Assuming the host is normally healthy, the body's defense mechanisms work very well! When the host immune system is compromised – either by stress, illness, or immunosuppressive disease – these local defenses may weaken. For example, the host may have an altered GI flora because they are taking an antibiotic. In this case, other pathogens (e.g., fungi) may be able to penetrate past this altered microflora and into the bloodstream when normally they would not.

Pathogens, especially bacteria and viruses, have evolved several mechanisms to overcome these primary defenses and enter the host. Microbes that invade the normal respiratory tract have evolved specific mechanisms to overcome the mucociliary defense or avoid destruction by alveolar macrophages. Some viruses have evolved ways to attach to lower respiratory epithelial cells, which then induce the host to engulf the virus. Now engulfed, the virus is inside a cell where it can hide. The influenza virus is a terrific example of a virus finding ways to avoid the normal respiratory defense system (see Chapter 10). Other pathogens impair ciliary activity (e.g., toxins paralyze cilia or act as ciliostatic agents), thereby failing to remove the pathogen from the respiratory tract. Still, other pathogens have evolved mechanisms to escape phagocytosis and killing by alveolar macrophages. In the GIT, some pathogens can withstand the acidic environment of the stomach. Enveloped viruses can be inactivated by bile and some digestive enzymes; however, non-enveloped viruses are very resistant to this defense.

Step 2: Dissemination and Cell Injury

Once past the first line of defenses and successful entry into the host, the pathogen must spread and disseminate within the body. Some pathogens will proliferate locally at the site of infection. Others have evolved ways to penetrate epithelial barriers and spread throughout the body via lymphatics, blood, or nerves. In these situations, manifestations of an infectious disease can appear at sites distant from the point of entry. Many pathogens are invasive by virtue of their motility or ability to secrete lytic enzymes destroying deterrents in their path. Some sporadic bloodstream invasions by low-virulent or nonvirulent microbes occur (e.g., in tooth brushing), but they are quickly controlled by normal host defenses. However, if invasion is by a virulent pathogen or the host is immunocompromised, the normal host defenses fail, and the infection may become systemic (throughout the organ systems).

Which system is affected depends on where the pathogen can bind. Some pathogens have a propensity for certain tissues or cells. This preferential binding is called *tropism*. The pathogen preferentially binds to a particular cell type in a particular organ because those cells have the appropriate receptors that the pathogens' binding sites recognize. Similar to a lock and key system where only a particular key can open the lock, the pathogen's binding depends on a match between its binding sites and the target cell's receptor sites. This specificity is critical. From a different perspective, this specificity (the virus binds only to respiratory tract cells) is why the influenza virus generally causes primarily respiratory symptoms but not usually GI symptoms.

Microbes, especially bacteria and viruses, have an amazing "war chest" of ways to fight more than the host's primary defense response, cause damage, and invade cells within the host! Once an infection is established, there are three general ways to damage host tissues. The first is that contact or entry into host cells directly causes cell death. Second, the pathogen can stimulate the release of toxins that may kill cells at a distance away from the infection site and release enzymes that degrade tissues, and/or damage blood vessels, which can result in tissue death. These can induce a host immune response targeted to the invader, but which also could cause damage to the host itself in the process. Finally, some can induce the cell to transform into a neoplastic (cancer) cell (Cotran et al., 1999).

Once inside the host (past innate defenses), microbes have various approaches to evade the host immune system. They can grow in niches that are inaccessible to the host immune system, for example, in the lumina of the intestine or gallbladder. They can multiply quickly before the host's immune system kicks in, thereby overwhelming the immune response. The formation of cysts (which have an outer capsule) provides protection from antibodies. Finally, viral latency is the ultimate strategy whereby the pathogen takes residence in a cell or tissue and "lays low" (does not stimulate clinical symptoms nor replicates). It just "hangs out" until the immune system falters and then the pathogen can recrudesce (replicate and cause disease).

The pathogen can also fool or "antagonize" the host's immune response. It can undergo antigenic variation, which means that the pathogen's antigens change/mutate resulting in variation of their outer membrane. This variation can fool the immune system into thinking that it has not seen this pathogen before, so it takes longer to mount a full immune response. The pathogen can resist the immune defenses by escaping the phagocytic cells, using capsules that are protective, killing, or weakening the phagocytes themselves, covering themselves with host proteins so that they are not seen as "foreign," and finally by producing/secreting molecules that inhibit or impair the immune system.

Other bacteria can survive and increase their virulence by living within cells. These are known as "intracellular bacteria," and they can be further classified as *facultative* (can live either inside or outside of the cell) or *obligatory* (must live inside the cell to survive). Once inside the cell, the pathogen is relatively safe and hidden from many immune effector mechanisms, and it is free to grow, replicate, and spread directly from cell to cell. To do this, these bacteria have evolved mechanisms to enter cells, often by manipulating the host immune phagocytic response to gain entry. Other species can manipulate the cell cytoskeleton to gain entry. For example, some gram-negative bacteria use needle-like structures on their surface to bind the host, cause pore formation in the host cell membrane, and then inject proteins that mediate rearrangement of the cell cytoskeleton opening new entry points. Once inside the cytoplasm, the bacteria can inhibit host protein synthesis, replicate quickly, lyse the host cell, and/or block the fusion with the lysosome, which normally would kill it.

Bacteria do not stop there! Many bacteria can produce and secrete toxins. A toxin is any bacterial substance that contributes to illness. There are two basic types of toxins, endo and exotoxins. *Endotoxins*, also known as lipopolysaccharides (LPS), are components of the gram-negative cell wall. LPS stimulates a protective host response. However, as part of this host response, cytokines are produced. If levels of LPS are very high, this can cause septic shock due to the high levels of cytokines produced.

Exotoxins are chemicals produced and secreted by bacteria. They can cause cellular injury and/or death. Exotoxins are classified by their mechanism of action. One type of exotoxin is enzymes. An enzyme is designated by the "...ase" ending of its name. For example, proteases degrade proteins, while coagulases damage coagulation molecules. The enzyme is effective because of its binding specificity to the active subunit of the target (e.g., proteases target only proteins). Generally, these types of enzymes alter intracellular signaling or interfere with regulatory pathways. Neurotoxins are another type of exotoxin. Neurotoxins inhibit the release of neurotransmitters, which results in muscle paralysis. They do not kill neurons, rather they cause death of the organism by paralyzing the diaphragm or other muscles leading to respiratory failure. The last general category of exotoxin is "superantigens." These toxins stimulate a large number of T cells leading to massive T-cell proliferation and cytokine release. Shock and death may result. One example of this phenomenon in women is toxic shock syndrome.

Some of the most "famous" bacterial exotoxins are secreted by enteropathogenic bacteria (bacteria that attack the GIT). Some strains of *Staphylococcus* release enterotoxins (toxins in the intestines) that result in symptoms of food poisoning. *Vibrio cholera* and toxigenic *Escherichia coli* strains release exotoxins that cause gut epithelium to secrete large volumes of fluid resulting in diarrhea. Some strains of *Shigella, Salmonella*, and *Campylobacter* go one step further. They damage the intestinal mucosa and lamina propria causing ulceration, inflammation, and hemorrhage, which results in clinical dysentery (bloody diarrhea). Finally, *Salmonella typhi* has been known to invade and damage mucosa and gain entry in the bloodstream to become systemic (Cotran et al., 1999).

Bacteria have some especially insidious tricks up their sleeves to cause severe disease! First, let us define virulence and pathogenicity. *Pathogenicity* is the ability of any agent to produce disease in the host. *Virulence* is the measure of severity of the disease. Bacteria enhance their virulence (disease severity) in several ways. Some species have "virulence genes" that encode proteins that enhance the ability to adhere to, invade, and/or deliver toxins into the target cells or tissue. Virulence factors can also be encoded by plasmids and bacteriophages (viruses that infect bacteria). Both of these are mobile genetic elements that can spread horizontally between bacteria and pass different virulence factors. In this manner, a nonvirulent bacterial strain can become a virulent strain. Similarly, certain plasmids or transposons that encode resistance to antibiotics can transfer this ability to another strain and turn an antibiotic-susceptible bacterium into an antibiotic-resistant strain (Cotran et al., 1999).

Even more interesting are the tactics bacteria have evolved when they are in very large groups. The first is the phenomenon of quorum sensing. This is a signaling tactic wherein many individual bacteria coordinate and regulate gene expression such that as their density increases, they induce expression of virulence factors at high concentrations. This provides an advantage for the bacteria because the huge concentration of virulence factors overwhelms the host. Similar to quorum sensing, large congregations of bacteria can, as a group, "autoinduce" secretion of certain peptides that stimulate toxin production.

Another tactic bacteria have evolved to evade destruction by immune systems (and human medications) is to form a biofilm. A biofilm is a community of bacteria that live in a viscous layer of extracellular polysaccharides, lipids, and proteins that adhere to host tissues, devices, or surfaces in the environment. The composition of the biofilm enhances microbe adherence, protects them from host immune mechanisms, and increases their resistance to antibiotics used during treatment. Bacterial biofilms are notoriously difficult to eradicate and are often the reason for the recurrence of infections (this is one of the reasons why thorough cleaning of surfaces in managed care is critical!).

Step 3: Replication and Release from the Host

A pathogen's life cycle relies on the release of its offspring from the host's body to infect new hosts. This can be accomplished by skin and/or feather shedding, coughing, sneezing, urinating, and defecating, during sexual contact, or by insect vectors. Some microbes excrete spores and cysts into the environment. These forms can survive in the environment for a long time. Other excreted microbial offspring are more fragile and require direct contact/passage to their next host (e.g., person to person or animal to animal). Once shed from the host into the environment, the microbe can be acquired/taken in by other animals/humans. Some new hosts will get the full-blown disease, but others may be asymptomatic carriers (the microbe has infected them, but they show no clinical symptoms). A microbe released from an animal that passes to and can infect and cause disease in humans is known as a *zoonotic* pathogen. If a microbe passes from humans to animals, it is known as a *reverse zoonotic* pathogen. Disease from pathogens can be more complex than this, but let us leave it here for now and summarize this part.

The outcome of pathogen entry and infection is determined by the ability of the microbe to infect, colonize, and damage host tissues balanced against the ability of the host defense mechanisms to eradicate the pathogen and/or prevent its successful entry. Host barriers include innate and adaptive immune defenses. Innate defenses are the physical barriers, phagocytes, other generalized immune cells, and plasma proteins. Adaptive immune defenses are specific to the pathogen. The response of the adaptive immune response increases in magnitude, speed, and effectiveness with successive exposures to the same pathogen/microbe. This is why vaccination is very effective in mitigating infection and/or the severity of clinical symptoms.

There is an evolutionary battle between the pathogen and its hosts. From the pathogen's perspective, it wants to invade, replicate, and spread its offspring so that more hosts can be infected. You can see a balance between the severity of the disease and its host. If an infection comes on so strong that it kills its first host, the pathogen will not be able to spread its offspring to new hosts. The evolutionary balance is that the pathogen still infects the host, but because of mutations, the strain that survives usually results in less severe or no disease (e.g., persists in a latent/nonactive state) in a host. Less severe disease symptoms in the host allow the pathogen to replicate and release its offspring to infect new hosts (because the host has not died). In the case of latent infections, the pathogen may be reactivated if the host becomes immunocompromised, stressed, or ill. As we will see in more detail later, emerging and reemerging infectious diseases are increasing with climate change and affect all species.

Literature Cited

Borrel, G., Brugere, J. F., Gribaldo, A., et al. (2020). The host-associated archaeome. *Nature Reviews Microbiology* 18:622–636. https://doi.org/10.1038/s41579-020-0407-y.

Buschang, K. E., Bennett, J., Lagrue, C., et al. (2025). Global analysis of *Toxoplasma gondii* prevalence in wild avian hosts: Effects of phylogeny, ecology, and detection methods. *International Journal of Parasitology* 55(13):721–729. https://doi.org/10.1016/j.ijpara.2025.06.007.

Cotran, R. S., Kumar, V., and Collins, T. (1999). *Robbin's Pathologic Basis of Disease*, 6th Ed., pp. 3–42. Philadelphia, PA: W.B. Saunders Company.

Darwich, L., Cabezón, O., Echeverria, I., et al. (2012). Presence of *Toxoplasma gondii* and *Neospora caninum* DNA in the brain of wild birds. *Veterinary Parasitology* 183(3–4):377–381. https://doi.org/10.1016/j.vetpar.2011.07.024.

Doneley, B. and Xie, S. (2025). *Avian Medicine and Surgery in Practice*, 3rd Ed. CRC Press.

Elwell, C., Mirrashidi, K., and Engel, J. (2016). Chlamydia cell biology and pathogenesis. *Nature Reviews Microbiology* 14:385–400. https://doi.org/10.1038/nrmicro.2016.30.

Section 2

Health Assessment and Management

5

Clinical Pathology and Diagnostics

Clinical pathology is a field of medicine that deals with the diagnosis of disease based on lab analyses of bodily fluids such as blood and urine. It also includes bacterial culture and sensitivity, cytology, molecular pathology, and immunologic assays (such as serologies). Evaluation of these samples provides diagnostic information on the health (or disease etiology) of the animal. The major areas of evaluation include hematology, blood chemistry, serology, microbial culture, hormone or other protein evaluation, and urinalysis. Baseline (reference) ranges for these parameters for various bird species are published in the literature. It is important to understand that there may be variations in the reference ranges depending on the laboratory used, method of analysis, population sampled, and number of animals used to establish those ranges. While there may be statistical differences, the ranges may not be biologically different.

Blood

Before we go on to discuss diagnostics using blood, it is important to understand some basic information about blood collection and blood tubes. Blood chemistry, serology, and most other analyses in mammals are performed using the *serum* portion of the blood. Serum is the liquid portion of clotted blood once the cells have been separated and settled out of the fluid (e.g., by centrifugation). The red blood cell (RBC) will settle on the bottom half of the tube because they are denser than the serum. *Plasma* is the clear fluid resulting from centrifugation of nonclotted blood and the sample most often used in birds. The difference between serum and plasma is the presence of various coagulation factors in plasma where they are absent in serum (because they were used to clot the blood). In general, for most species, using plasma to evaluate chemistries or serologies will give similar results. However, there are certain parameters that may be different. For our purposes, understanding that plasma and serum are different fluids and are obtained from different blood tubes is sufficient.

The different types of commonly used blood collection tubes are shown in Figure 5.1. Blood tubes that contain anticoagulants are purple (or lavender) and green top tubes. The purple top is basically the standard tube for hematology. The red, tiger, and yellow top tubes

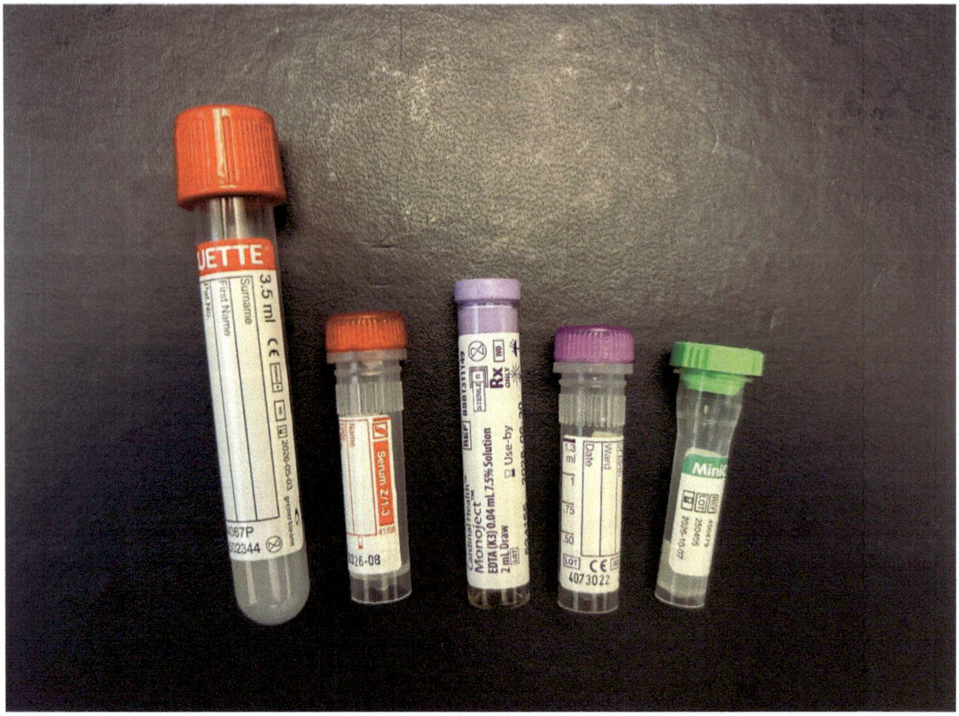

Figure 5.1 Blood tubes for the collection of large and small volumes. Red top tubes have no anticoagulant and are available in multiple sizes (3.5 and 1.3 mL volumes shown). Lavender top tubes have EDTA anticoagulant and are available in multiple sizes (2 mL and 500 μL volumes shown). Green top tubes contain lithium heparin anticoagulant and are available in multiple sizes (volume of 0.9 mL shown). *Source:* Photograph by author.

do not contain anticoagulant; therefore, the blood will begin clotting when added to the tube. The difference between the red, tiger, and yellow tube types is the presence of a gel in the tiger and yellow top tubes, which is absent in the red top tube. This gel is of intermediate density than the cells and liquid portion of the blood. As such, when the tube is centrifuged to separate those compartments, the gel settles in between them. This is important because if not fully separated, the RBC will continue metabolizing and utilizing glucose and some electrolytes in the whole blood, resulting in artificially lower values for these substances.

Improper or aggressive handling of blood tubes can affect blood parameters. Purple and green top tubes should be gently inverted back and forth a few times to ensure the anticoagulant contacts the entire blood volume in the tube. Anticoagulated whole blood should appear fluid and not clumpy. Clumps indicate clotting has occurred, and that sample would be unsuitable for hematologic analyses. Samples should be analyzed, centrifuged, or prepared for storage (if analyzed later) in a timely fashion. Delays can result in variable results (e.g., from continued consumption of analytes by RBC as mentioned above) and/or degradation of the sample. Samples should be refrigerated until analyzed within the day. Freezing of serum or plasma is often done when analysis is delayed. One freeze–thaw cycle usually minimally impacts blood parameters regardless of the length of time the sample was frozen. However, repeated freezing and thawing will affect sample values. Frozen whole blood is not useful for hematologic or biochemical analyses.

Finally, handling of the animal from whom the blood is drawn can affect the blood sample values. If the animal is stressed and resistant to restraint, their stress response will be evident in the blood. Increased corticosterone and/or other hormones will mask the baseline, unstressed condition of the animal. Stress is not usually an issue in animals trained to participate in medical procedures in zoos. However, in health assessments of free-ranging animals, there is no way to avoid this stress. Comparisons between managed care and free-ranging animal blood parameters should take this difference into consideration.

Hematology

Hematology is the study of cells in whole blood. Whole blood is circulating blood directly obtained from a blood vessel and is neither centrifuged nor allowed to clot. If left to sit in the blood tube, the blood will clot on its own (as it should or else when injured, blood loss would continue unimpeded). The cell types present in the blood are RBCs (also known as *erythrocytes*) and white blood cells (WBCs, also known as *leukocytes*). There are various proteins present in blood. Some are anticoagulants to help blood clot, while others are proteins of various functions, hormones, and antibodies. We will talk later about the importance of proteins in the blood.

To evaluate blood cells, the blood needs to be collected in a tube that contains an anticoagulant, such as heparin (in a green top tube) or ethylenediamine tetraacetic acid (EDTA in a lavender top tube; Figure 5.1). In birds, an EDTA tube is preferred. If the blood is allowed to clot, the anticoagulants will trap the blood cells in the clot, and the cell count will be inaccurate. Smaller blood collection tubes are often used especially for small birds/animals. Ideally, a blood smear should be made soon after blood collection. A blood smear (Figure 5.2) is made by smearing a drop of blood on a glass slide such that a single layer of cells is created from which to count the cells. The count can be made using a regular light microscope on high power (40× ocular) or under oil immersion (100× ocular with a drop of oil). The latter should be used by those less familiar with blood cell types, while experienced slide readers may use the 40× ocular. (I should say here that the eyepiece of microscopes typically has 10× magnification, so the magnifications are really 400× and 1000×, respectively.)

The blood smear permits counting (or estimating) RBC and WBC total count, count and type of individual WBC types, estimation of platelets, evaluation for the presence of abnormal RBC or WBC, and evaluation for the presence of blood parasites. There are far more RBCs than WBCs (the number of RBCs is in the millions as compared to WBCs, which are in the thousands). Figure 5.3 is a high-power view of various WBC types.

The size, color, and shape of RBC can be highly diagnostic (Figure 5.3). Mature avian RBCs are approximately 8–15 μm in length, elongated cells with oval nuclei. The cytoplasm has a homogeneous, reddish hue when stained with routine laboratory stains (such as Diff Quik®, Wright Giemsa). Cells that appear as slightly larger RBCs with a more basophilic tinge to the cytoplasm are likely immature RBCs, also known as *reticulocytes* (Figure 5.3). To obtain the most accurate count of reticulocytes in blood, a reticulocyte stain (e.g., new methylene blue) can be used on a separate smear. Normally, in birds 1–5% of RBCs are reticulocytes. RBCs with heterogeneous staining (polychromasia – various colors/shades)

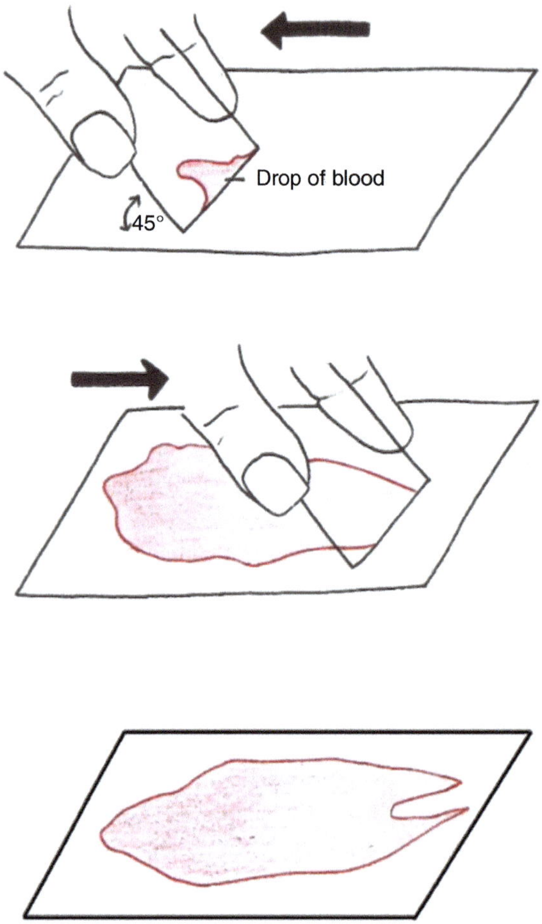

Figure 5.2 Diagram of how to make a blood smear. Place a small drop of blood on a clean slide. Using a slide, place the edge of the slide onto the blood spot at a 45° angle and move it backward 1–2 mm (top picture). Then push the slide forward (middle picture) spreading the blood. Note the reddish color fades as you slide (bottom picture). The relatively cleared area in the center of the smear reflects a monolayer of cells, which is the desired area for microscopic viewing.
Source: With permission of S. Mannone.

or anisocytosis (various sizes) indicate that the RBCs are not normal. These are signs of a disease process in the animal. There are normal species variations. RBC numbers increase with body mass and in diving birds. RBCs are also more elongate in shape if the species is a long-distance migrant or lives at high altitude (Scanes, 2022).

In addition to RBC counts, one can derive additional information. *Hemoglobin* concentration can be quantified using a hematology analyzer. The amount of hemoglobin dictates the oxygen-carrying capacity in the blood. RBCs low in hemoglobin typically appear paler on routine staining. *Hematocrit* (HCT, also known as packed cell volume) is the percentage of RBC in the blood. This parameter gives information regarding the relative amount of RBC. If the RBC count is low, the HCT will also be low. Normal species variation also occurs in HCT. In birds, HCT has been shown to be greater in adults than in juveniles, greater in migratory than in nonmigratory birds, higher before migration than after, and

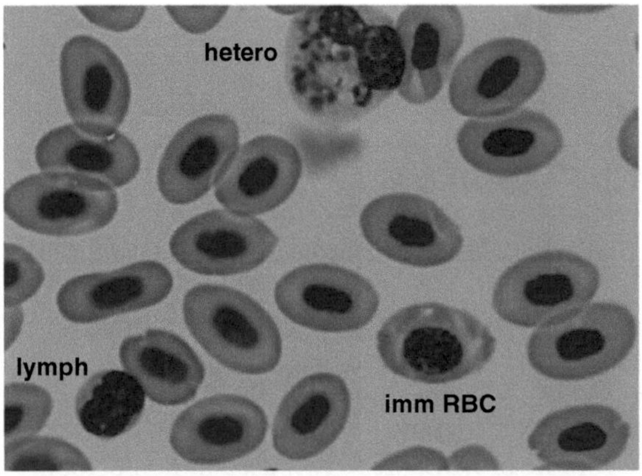

Figure 5.3 Blood smear from a bird. (A) High-power (1000×) view of a monolayer of mature RBC (oval cells with pale reddish-brown color cytoplasm) and WBC – hetero = heterophil; lymph = lymphocyte; imm RBC = immature RBC. Note the darker grayish cytoplasm of the immature RBC compared to the mature RBC. *Source:* Photomicrographs by J. Zaias.

increases with hypoxia (Scanes, 2022). HCT also varies with body size – larger birds have a lower HCT than smaller birds (Scanes, 2022).

The smaller size and/or paler coloration of the RBC indicate some level of decreased hemoglobin and/or iron concentration within the RBC, which is often seen coincident with decreased RBC, HCT, and is consistent with anemia. Anemia occurs when there is not enough RBC and/or hemoglobin within them, which results in decreased oxygen circulation in the peripheral blood. Clinically, the animal may be lethargic or not be able to maintain a sustained and/or high level of activity. Once recognized as anemia, the potential etiologies for anemia can be investigated (Box 5.1).

Box 5.1 Algorithmic approach to understanding anemia

Generally, there are two underlying conditions that can lead to anemia

Continuous blood loss — Failure to make and/or replenish new RBCs

The general etiologies (or causes) for each of these are different. When viewed in this light, the approach to identifying the ultimate etiology is straightforward.

- Continuous blood loss can be due to:
  - rapid blood loss in severe injury (before the body has regenerated the lost blood),
  - slower blood loss conditions such as bleeding ulcers or infectious hemorrhagic gastroenteritis in the gastrointestinal tract (GIT),
  - presence of RBC parasites,
  - failure to effectively clot (clotting agent deficiencies) such that smaller injuries can lead to massive blood loss.

(Continued)

Box 5.1 (Continued)

- Failure to make/replenish RBCs can be due to:
  - decreased or lack of hormonal stimulation such as in chronic renal failure (the kidneys stop making the hormone erythropoietin, which stimulates RBC production),
  - problems in the bone marrow that affect/deplete RBC precursor cells (including marrow cancer and toxins).

There are three calculated indices that can be used to characterize the RBC by size, HCT, and hemoglobin concentration. These are mean corpuscular volume, which is the ratio of HCT/RBC that gives information on the volume of RBC. Mean corpuscular hemoglobin is calculated as the ratio of hemoglobin/RBC. The mean corpuscular hemoglobin concentration is calculated as the ratio of hemoglobin/HCT and gives information on the hemoglobin concentration of the RBCs. These, along with reticulocyte count, can help characterize anemia.

Platelets (*thrombocytes*), players in blood clotting, can be observed on a blood smear (Figure 5.4). Platelets are small basophilic (blue-purple color) cells that look similar to lymphocytes but are smaller and have minimal to no obvious cytoplasm. These should be numerous on the smear. Platelet counts are calculated on hematology analyzers, but by analyzing a blood smear, an experienced technician can estimate if the platelets are low. Thrombocytes originate from thromboblasts in bone marrow or other organs (spleen or liver) that participate in erythropoiesis (RBC production) when needed.

RBC and thrombocytes are also active in the immune response! In addition to phagocytosis, both can produce inflammatory cytokines, nitrous oxide, and anti-microbial peptides, and RBC can participate in apoptosis (Cai and Wang, 2025; Scanes, 2022). Mammalian RBCs (which lack nuclei) also assist in immune function by recognizing and binding to pathogens and phagocytizing them. Avian (and mammalian) RBCs facilitate transcription, translation, and support expression of proteins important in the immune response (Cai and Wang, 2025; Kumar et al., 2025). Data suggest that metabolic activity in avian RBC mitochondria can be modulated to cope with environmental stressors (Cai and Wang, 2025).

Total WBC numbers can be easily counted or estimated. The number of each of the WBC types can be assessed by counting and noting the type of WBC out of 100 WBCs on a blood smear. This percentage multiplied by the total number of WBC can give the actual number of each type of WBC. There are five common types of WBC (heterophils, lymphocytes, eosinophils, monocytes, and basophils; Figure 5.4), and each responds to specific inflammatory or disease etiologies.

Lymphocytes are the most numerous WBC in circulation in birds (Figures 5.3 and 5.4b). They participate in the adaptive immune response. These are the B and T cells of the immune system. Special immunohistochemical staining is required to differentiate B and T cells from each other. For the purposes of a WBC count, distinguishing B from T cells on a blood smear is not needed. Mature lymphocytes are circular (7–15 μm in diameter), of similar size to RBCs but smaller than heterophils and have circular, dark nuclei with light blue cytoplasm. Often, there may be only a wisp of cytoplasm visible in the cell in some mature lymphocytes. Immature lymphocytes, called lymphoblasts, are larger than mature

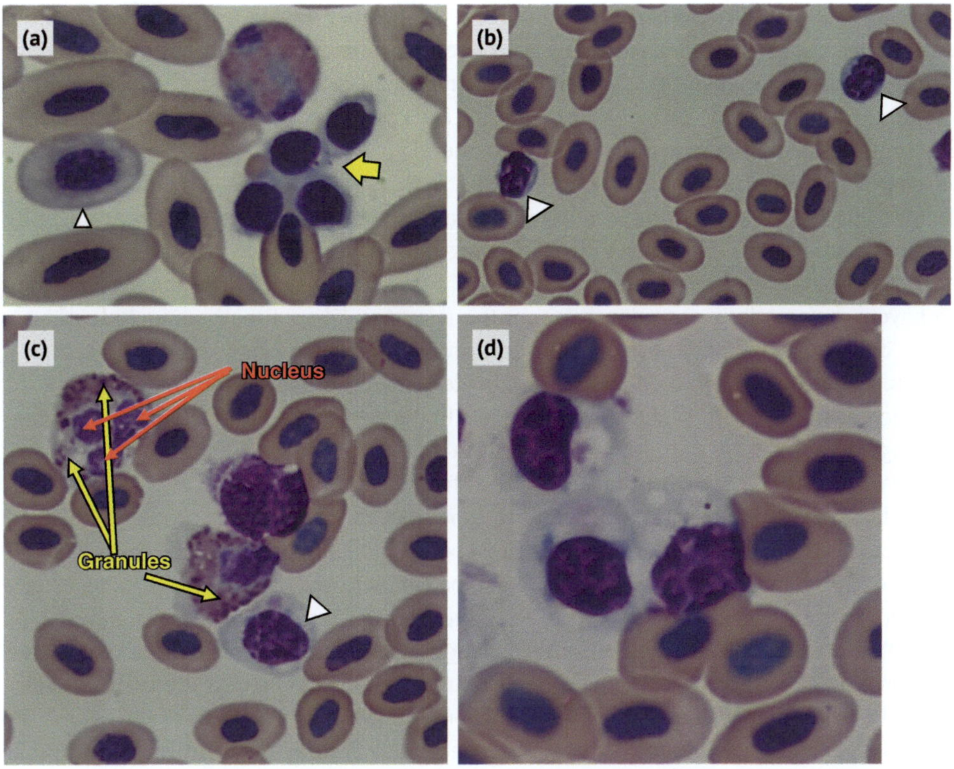

Figure 5.4 Blood smear from a bird. (a) A clump of avian platelets (yellow arrow). Slightly oval cells, but much smaller than RBC. Note the immature RBC to the left (white arrowhead). The large cell above the platelets is a heterophil with indistinct cytoplasmic granules. (b) White arrowheads point to two mature lymphocytes. Note the minimal blue cytoplasm visible. (c) Heterophils with cytoplasmic granules (yellow arrows). Red arrows highlight the multilobulated nucleus. White arrowhead indicates a large lymphocyte. Note the size relationship to the RBC (oval cells). Lymphocyte is of similar size. Heterophils are larger than RBCs. (d) Three large monocytes. Note the white "circles" in the large cytoplasm. These are vacuoles suggesting these cells are activated (1000×). *Source:* Photomicrographs by author.

lymphocytes and have a well-defined light blue cytoplasm. The presence of lymphoblasts in circulating blood is not a normal finding and warrants further investigation.

Heterophils are the second most numerous WBC in circulation in birds and are part of the innate immune response (Figure 5.4c). Heterophils are 9–15 μm in diameter and have reddish cytoplasm with a polymorphonuclear (various shaped nuclei) nucleus; that is, the nucleus can have many folds and shapes (multilobulated vs. a round nucleus). As the heterophils mature, the nucleus becomes thinner and folds on itself. Heterophils are the first responders. Increasing numbers of heterophils are seen with acute inflammation and bacterial infection. Their functions include phagocytosis (it is the main phagocytic cell), attracting lymphocytes, releasing anti-microbial peptides, killing by oxidative burst, and participating in acute inflammatory responses.

There are two other types of polymorphonuclear WBCs – eosinophils and basophils. The nuclei of these cells are similar in shape to those of heterophils. The difference lies in their cytoplasmic granules. Eosinophils contain orange, round granules that release histamine when stimulated. Eosinophils typically increase in number with allergies or when there are high loads of parasites in mammals, and likely in birds as well, although this has not been fully defined (Scanes, 2022). The orange granules make them distinctive. The other polymorphonuclear WBC is the basophil. These cells have dark blue vacuoles that release inflammatory mediators in acute and chronic allergic diseases.

Monocytes are the largest of the circulating WBCs reaching 15–22 μm in diameter (Figure 5.4d). They can be approximately twice as large as lymphocytes. They are usually round or irregular in shape with a kidney- or irregular-shaped nucleus and clear cytoplasm, sometimes with vacuoles. While monocytes are part of the innate immune system, they also have a major role in the adaptive immune response. Their functions include phagocytosis, chemotaxis, release of cytokines, and production of nitrous oxide (Scanes, 2022). When recruited to an inflamed tissue, monocytes will differentiate into macrophages or dendritic cells and aid in phagocytosis (internalizing debris or pathogens) and immune signaling. Monocytes are seen in increasing numbers with chronic inflammation.

Analysis of a blood smear is not technically difficult, but it does take practice! Having pictures of the blood cell types, knowing their sizes relative to the other cell types, and using a good microscope are a must. Cell counting must be done on a part of the slide that has a cell monolayer – that is, one layer of cells. This will be evident when scanning the slide, as you will no longer see cells atop one another. Also, the edges of the slide should not be used, as they often may be clumpy or have cells that are ruptured and in abnormal configurations due to the smear-making process. The main features used to identify the cells are their size relative to RBC and other WBC, the nucleus shape, and the color and features of the cytoplasm (Figure 5.3). Differential counting of the WBC needs to be done systematically to ensure that the same area is not counted more than once. This is usually done by following a specific path along the slide. For more details, see clinical pathology or hematology text references.

Chemistries

Blood chemistries involve the evaluation of proteins, enzymes, and electrolytes present in the serum or plasma. In birds, the use of lithium heparin tubes are the preferred collection tube for chemistry analyses. Various enzymes specific to different organs can be found in the bloodstream at low levels. If these values are elevated relative to baseline values, this denotes substantial cell necrosis in the tissue/organ, resulting in enzyme leakage out of the cell (remember the discussion of cell death in Chapter 1). Let us review the basic components (and their diagnostic relevance) of a typical blood chemistry analysis. It is critical to be aware of life history factors that affect some parameters, for example, growth, migration, and fasting. These, of course, are not always relevant for animals in managed care. However, for the assessment of wild or rehabilitation animals, these factors are critical to know.

Blood glucose levels in birds are at least twice as high as in mammals (200–400 g/dl; Van de Weyer and Tahas, 2024). If the value is low, blood handling and transport conditions should be evaluated to ensure the lower value is not due to RBC consumption of glucose (which would occur if centrifuge time was delayed).

After food consumption and digestion, glucose levels will increase in the blood. Glucose is used to produce ATP, which is required for cellular functions. When sufficient glucose is taken in, the excess glucose may be stored in the liver in the form of glycogen. In times of even more excess glucose, the glucose may be stored as fat. During times of fasting (such as can occur during migration), the body accesses glucose from these stores (e.g., glycogenolysis). When glycogen is depleted, body lipids will be mobilized and broken down (lipolysis) to produce free fatty acids that can be used to generate glucose by other pathways. In the extreme case of starvation, after lipids are broken down, the body will resort to breaking down muscle to generate glucose for energy. Life history physiology is critical in understanding the interaction between glucose (carbohydrates), lipid storage, and metabolism, and interpreting these various parameters in the blood.

Uric acid levels are one tool to evaluate kidney function. However, depending on the diet of the bird, the uric acid level can vary. For example, in carnivores, uric acid is higher than in granivores. In addition, the hydration status of the animal needs to be assessed. If the bird is dehydrated, the uric acid would be artificially increased. Hydration can be assessed by evaluating total protein and glomerular filtration rate at the same time as uric acid evaluation. Alternatively, the animal can be rehydrated, and then uric acid can be assessed. In chronic renal disease, animals will become anemic, have increased electrolyte levels, reduced glomerular filtration rates, and abnormal findings on urinalysis.

To evaluate pancreatic infection or disease, levels of amylase and lipase are measured. Both amylase and lipase are enzymes produced by the pancreas for the digestion of carbohydrates and lipids (fats), respectively. If these are elevated in the blood, this suggests cell death with leakage from the pancreas due to infection and/or necrosis.

The main electrolytes evaluated in blood are calcium, sodium, chloride, potassium, and phosphate. Electrolyte levels in the blood are regulated by the kidneys in otherwise healthy animals. Certain diseases (enteropathies or diseases of the intestinal tract) and symptoms (e.g., diarrhea) will result in loss of, or changes in, electrolytes. In extreme cases, imbalances in electrolytes can have negative effects on organ function. The kidney is responsible for balancing and adjusting which and how much electrolyte is reabsorbed into the bloodstream or eliminated in urine.

As there are many functions of the liver, there are various blood chemistry parameters (and combinations therein) that will indicate liver disease. These include, but may not be limited to, alkaline phosphatase, alanine aminotransferase, creatine phosphokinase, glutamate dehydrogenase, albumin, and certain proteins. Some of these are more specific to liver function than others, and some may be related to dysfunction in multiple organs. Liver function may be best assayed by levels of what it produces (albumin and many other proteins). Albumin is easily assayed in chemistries. In severe, chronic liver disease, animals will have decreased albumin production resulting in decreased serum albumin (hypoalbuminemia). With chronic kidney disease, the albumin is lost in the urine. We will discuss albumin and proteins more in a later section.

Since there are species-specific, individual, sex-specific, and life-history specific differences in all of these parameters, a constellation of changes is usually more predictive of disease than a single abnormal variable. This chapter is not intended to define how to diagnose specific diseases from abnormal blood values. Rather, it is intended to help the user understand the underlying precepts – why blood diagnostics are valuable, how these abnormalities can be detected, and why they are important.

Serology

Serology is the evaluation of antibodies in the peripheral blood. The presence of antibodies targeting specific pathogens/agents indicates that the animal was exposed to and mounted an immune response against that agent. In birds, these tests are usually done using a plasma sample. The basic technique involves exposing the plasma to a multiwell plate or slide, which is coated with the agent in question. If the animal contains circulating antibodies against the plated antigen, the antibodies will bind to it. The bound antigen–antibody complexes can be visualized using a color tag (e.g., ELISA tests, like those used on pregnancy or COVID home tests) or by counting radiation from a radioisotope tag. The relative measure of antibody concentration is denoted as a *titer*. A positive titer is one that is greater than baseline. The higher the titer, the stronger the immune response. A single serology can only indicate that the animal was exposed to the pathogen in question (unless the titer was very high). To understand if the exposure is current or in the past, a second serology titer should be analyzed 2–3 weeks after the first. If the second titer increases, this denotes an active infection because the body has increased the antibody response. If the second titer is lower than the first, this denotes a recent infection that is resolving. The titer is waning as the infection is controlled. If the second titer is the same as the first, this suggests exposure was not very recent but at some undetermined time in the past. This analysis holds true when assessing IgY antibodies (or immunoglobulins). IgY antibodies (analogous to IgG in mammals) are the most common circulating antibodies in peripheral blood. There is a progression of antibody generation when a new pathogen is encountered. IgM is the first type of antibody formed by the body upon first exposure to a new pathogen. If IgM is measured directly, a single positive titer will indicate active infection. IgY is the "stable," long-lasting type of antibody, which is most commonly assessed.

Proteins

Proteins in the blood function to maintain colloidal osmotic pressure of the blood, bind and transport compounds like hormones, and are involved in inflammatory responses. The main protein in the blood is albumin. Albumin comprises about 60% of the blood proteins and is produced by the liver. Acute phase proteins (APPs), also produced by the liver, comprise up to 20% of the proteins in blood. They are involved in the inflammatory response. Elevations in these proteins indicate an acute inflammatory response. The other major group of blood proteins are gamma globulins, which are immunoglobulins or antibodies. They comprise approximately 20% of blood proteins.

Total protein and albumin levels can be assessed as part of a blood chemistry panel. However, understanding the level of gamma globulins and APPs in addition to albumin can provide valuable diagnostic information. An increased APP fraction indicates acute inflammation. A very high gamma fraction would be due to a large increase in antibodies (IgY). A normal total protein level does not necessarily imply that the component protein types are normal in value. The albumin could be decreased, and the gamma globulins could be very elevated, yet the total protein value could appear normal. To assess the protein components, protein electrophoresis is used. This technique separates proteins by size using an electrical charge. The protein fractions are then quantified as a percentage of total protein. Changes in the protein fractions can lead the clinician toward an etiology for the inflammation observed. In addition, electrophoresis can be used to track the resolution of an inflammatory event by monitoring the changing protein fractions as they return to baseline.

APPs are proteins released during acute infection, inflammation, neoplasia, trauma, and stress. They are well conserved across species and are secreted within 48 hours of insult. APP are accepted parameters to diagnose and follow prognosis of infection and inflammation in companion animals and birds (Lee et al., 2024; da Fonseca et al., 2023; Desoubeaux et al., 2022; Cray, 2021; Delk et al., 2015; Cray et al., 2007, 2013). The three most frequently assayed APPs are C-reactive protein, serum amyloid A, and haptoglobin. These proteins can be assayed on a clinical chemistry analyzer or using serum protein electrophoresis.

Blood proteins are the primary regulators of osmotic balance in circulation. Essentially, a normal level of proteins in the blood is required to "hold" (or "keep") the fluid portion of the blood inside the vessels. Electrolytes also regulate osmotic balance in birds. In diseases that result in hypoalbuminemia (low albumin in the blood), fluid can leave the vessels and enter the body cavity. When fluid enters the coelomic cavity, it is called *ascites*. In liver failure, albumin production decreases. In chronic kidney failure, albumin is lost in the urine. In both situations, ascites can result.

While there are hematology and chemistry analyzers that can be used to analyze blood samples, there are simple and quick ways to get critical information on health. We discussed the ease of making blood smears to estimate RBC and WBC, assess the morphology of the cells, evaluate the WBC types, and search for the presence of blood parasites. The only equipment needed for this is a microscope and slides.

There is an easy way to measure the total protein and HCT. A capillary tube filled with a small volume (max 100 μL) of blood can be centrifuged. The resulting separation of RBCs to the bottom of the tube can be measured as compared to the total volume of blood (in the capillary tube) to yield a percentage of RBC (the HCT; Figure 5.5). To measure the total protein, after centrifuging, the tube can be broken just above the level of the RBCs. The plasma in the upper part of the tube is put on a refractometer (Figure 5.6), and the total protein is read off a scale in the refractometer. These quick and easy tests can give an early indication of disease.

Hormones and neuromodulators can also be measured in blood. Usually, analysis of these involves different techniques than those discussed above. Since these tests are not as common as chemistries or serologies, many managed care facility labs may not perform them in-house, and often these samples will be sent to outside labs. Sampling and interpretation of hormones and neuromodulators can provide a lot of good information, but they require an understanding of how and when they are secreted for accurate interpretation. Some hormones are continually (or constitutively) secreted, and some are secreted in pulses. Some are secreted in the morning (diurnal) and others in the evening (nocturnal). Understanding these patterns is critical to ensure the sampling times accurately reflect the average level and not the peak (highest level) or nadir (lowest level) of secretion. Samples to be collected over multiple days should be collected at the same time each day to avoid interpretation errors.

Most, if not all, managed care facilities have diagnostic labs with equipment and supplies to run standard hematology and biochemistry, urinalyses, and basic cytology. Depending on the size of the facility, the veterinarian and/or veterinary technician manage the

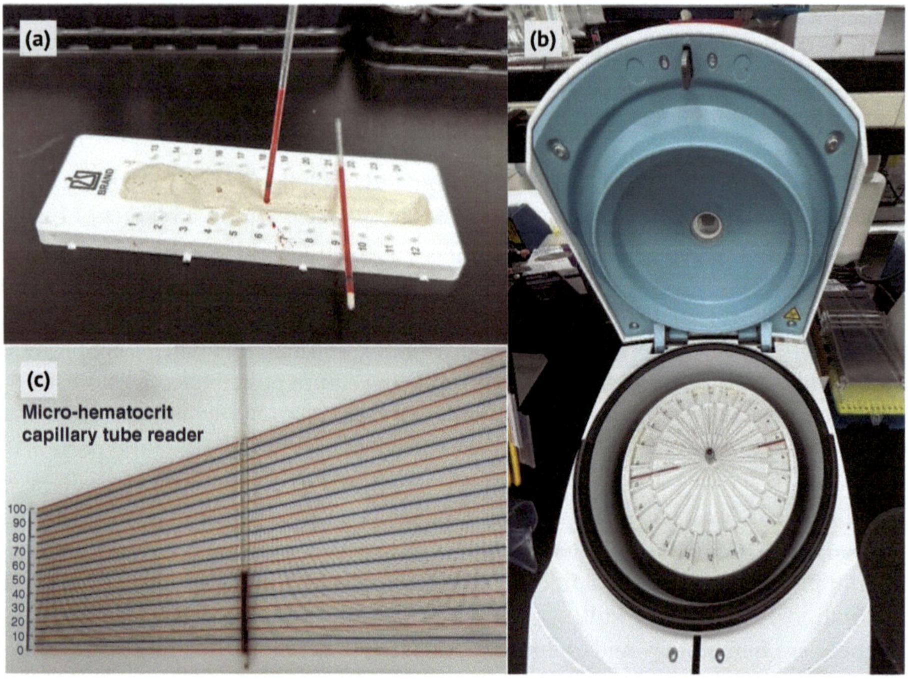

Figure 5.5 Capillary tube method to determine the HCT. (a) Two capillary tubes filled with fresh, noncoagulated blood. One end is placed in clay to prevent spillage out of the bottom. Yellow arrowhead indicates clay at the bottom of the tube. (b) The capillary tube is placed in a microcapillary centrifuge. (c) After centrifugation, the capillary tube is placed on a micro-HCT reader card to ascertain the HCT. Note the demarcation (black arrow) between the packed RBCs and clear serum. *Source:* Photographs by J. Zaias.

diagnostic testing. Alternatively, diagnostics can be sent out to local clinical pathology labs and/or specialists. Some facilities have "point of care" analyzers. These are small, mobile chemistry analyzers that can give a rapid (1 min) readout of select parameters from a small volume of blood. Generally, these instruments are expensive and may not be able to read out all parameters; however, they are very useful in critical care situations and for small birds. Because there may be some differences between analyzer types (for example, between the point of care analyzers and the larger countertop chemistry analyzers), comparing data from the same equipment will give a more accurate picture of any changes.

Hormone and neuromodulator levels can be affected by stress, various sampling procedures, and handling techniques. In mammals, assessing estrogen, testosterone, progesterone, luteinizing hormone, and follicle-stimulating hormone levels are used to interpret reproductive status; however, hormone assessment doesn't work in birds to determine reproductive status. Stress can be assessed by cortisol, epinephrine, and adrenocorticotropin hormone levels. Metabolic hormones include corticosterone, thyroid hormones (T3, T4), thyroid-stimulating hormone, and aldosterone. The normal baseline values of many of these hormones for many species of parrots and other species are known. Consult standard avian medicine tests for these data. However, there is still a lot yet unknown in this area.

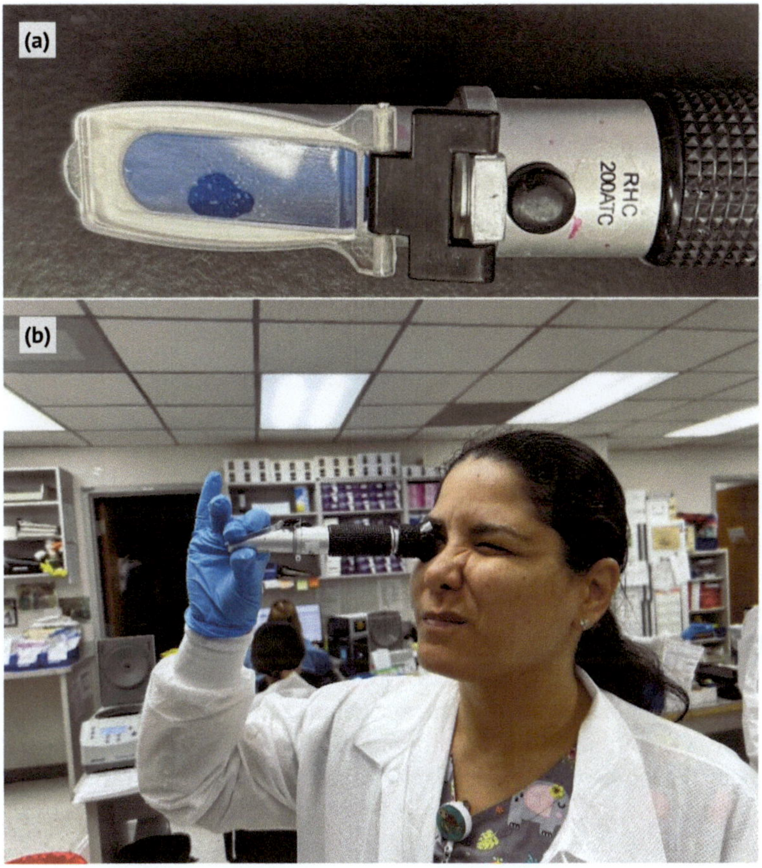

Figure 5.6 After the HCT is measured off the centrifuged capillary tube, the tube should be broken in half just above the demarcation between the RBC and serum. A drop of serum should be placed on a refractometer (a). Then the total protein can be read by looking through the refractometer (b). *Source:* Photographs by J. Zaias.

Urinalysis

Urinalysis is the analysis of urine. A urine sample can be obtained by collection of the white portion of the excrement or by passing a catheter up the cloaca and urodeum. The concentrating ability of the kidneys can be measured by evaluating the specific gravity (or concentrating ability) of the urine. The normally functioning kidney will produce urine with a normal range of specific gravity. In kidney failure, the urine would be very diluted (specific gravity lower than normal) because the injured kidney would be unable to reabsorb water, and the water would be excreted in urine. You probably have noticed a darker yellow color in your urine after exercise or when you are dehydrated. In this situation, your body responds by retaining/reabsorbing water. After you drink some water, your urine will return (be diluted back) to a pale-yellow color.

The pH of urine can be measured. The amount of protein, glucose, and the number of cells can also be measured. Normally, these should not be present in the urine. Increased protein in urine (proteinuria) suggests kidney damage (the tubules are not reabsorbing the protein). High urine glucose (glucosuria) suggests excessive glucose circulating in the blood (such as in diabetes in humans) or failure of the tubules to reabsorb. The presence of WBC in urine suggests inflammation, and the presence of RBC suggests bleeding. Sometimes crystals or small stones can be microscopically observed in the urine. The composition of these is important to determine etiology and define treatment. Finally, rare tubular casts (cylindrical protein structures) may be seen. These represent kidney tubular pathology. Any of these abnormal findings would be followed by other tests for kidney function and/or renal imaging (e.g., ultrasound).

Fecal Samples

Analysis of feces is a standard practice to detect the presence of GI parasites. In some species that preen themselves or others, external parasites may also be detected in feces. The collection of fecal samples is usually minimally invasive. The difficulty of fecal collection in aquatic species is to be able to identify from which individual it originated and to collect it rapidly before it dissolves or gets too diluted in the water. The fecal sample is placed in a specific solution (or liquefied), and a small sample is spread on a slide. The slide is evaluated for cells and parasites (eggs, larvae, or, more rarely, adults). Parasite eggs can be identified to species level and/or general type of parasite. With an understanding of the type and life cycle of the parasite detected, medication and treatment frequency/schedule can be initiated.

Understanding the life cycle of the parasite is important because some of the commonly used antiparasitic medications only work on the larval or adult forms. If a parasite infection is detected by identifying eggs, then there must be adults generating the eggs. The first dose of treatment would effectively kill the adults and any larval stages. However, the eggs remaining in the animal would be unaffected and grow into larvae and/or adults. Therefore, a second treatment is needed to kill the new larvae or adults before they lay eggs. Thus, the timing of development from egg to larvae to adult is critical to identify the next treatment time.

Other information can be harnessed from feces, such as hormones. The hormone itself may not be present, but metabolites of the hormone will be. All chemicals get metabolized in the liver. The result of metabolism is usually modification(s) of the parent compound into its metabolites. These can be excreted from the body through the urine and/or feces. The concentration or amount of the metabolite in a fecal sample will be related to the initial amount of the parent hormone and the GIT transit time. The metabolites, ratios of metabolites relative to the parent compound, and the rate of metabolism need to be known. The GI transit time is the time it takes from something to be ingested until excreted in feces. This time will vary with species and between carnivores (faster transit) and herbivores (slower transit). Therefore, the transit time gives the window of time that the metabolite has accumulated in the feces. For example, if the transit time is six hours, then any value measured in the feces represents the accumulation within the past six hours. In addition, another important consideration here is that the metabolite will be at a lower concentration than the parent compound. So, appropriate equipment/technology (e.g., high-performance liquid chromatography, HPLC) must be used to be able to measure the lower levels.

Feces can be analyzed for the presence of blood. If obvious, red blood is seen on or in the feces, this suggests that the source of the blood is relatively near the cloaca/vent. Fecal tests that look for "occult" blood (dark, black color) look for blood products after RBC breakdown. The presence of occult blood suggests the origination of the blood was farther away (higher up) in the GIT. One example of a possible etiology for a positive finding of occult blood in the feces would be a bleeding gastric ulcer.

Cytology

Cytology is the examination of cells. At its basic level, cytologic examination involves visualizing cells on a slide under the microscope. This evaluation involves identifying cell type, number, and any morphologic abnormalities. Cytopathologic techniques also include molecular-based analyses such as immunocytochemical staining, PCR, and single-cell analyses.

Cell samples may be obtained from any surface or cavity in the body. Typical cytological collections for routine health assessment may include fecal, nares/sinuses, feathers, and skin. Typical analysis of these samples includes evaluation of cell types, cell numbers, and the presence of bacteria, fungi, and parasites. If numerous (more than baseline) WBC cells are present, inflammation is present. If numerous (more than baseline) parasites are present, then there are higher-than-normal loads of parasites. Often fragments of plants or other debris may be seen. Baseline cytologic characteristics should be developed for each facility to be familiar with common background debris in your enclosures.

Cells from the lower colon, rectum, and/or cloaca may also be seen in feces. The cells may be normal or abnormal. Occasionally, cellular changes may indicate possible abnormalities and/or neoplasia. The cells can also be isolated and undergo molecular tests (such as polymerase chain reaction [PCR]). (This is the basis for human colon cancer testing using feces.) Finally, the feces can be analyzed for the type of food particles or digesta present in the fecal product. This can sometimes indicate deficiencies in certain types of digestive enzymes (e.g., pancreatic insufficiency disease).

Other Sampling Opportunities/Matrices

Collecting samples from an animal should always be done considering the health and safety of the animal and person(s) sampling. Ideally, collection using the least invasive technique should precede the use of more invasive techniques. Sampling animals in zoos/managed care is relatively stress-free because animals are trained to participate in medical procedures (Mattison, 2012). However, in free-ranging animals, the effects of stress from capture and handling would always be present.

Microbiome analysis is the evaluation and quantification of bacterial (and other microorganisms) species and numbers. While a full description of microbiome analysis is beyond the scope of this text, basically, analysis involves the use of PCR to identify the major bacterial genera, species, and relative numbers of each. Each part of the body (internal and external) has a "normal" resident population of microorganisms ("microbiome") as discussed in Chapter 4. Human biomedical research has shown that the GI and/or fecal microbiome content can be related to different diseases and pathologies. The same is also apparent in birds, as more and more studies study microbiomes (Trevelline et al., 2018). In eggs, the microbiome is deposited by the female during egg production. Thereafter, the microbiome will change with diet and interactions with other birds in the nest (Corl et al., 2024).

Saliva is not currently a popular matrix to sample birds; however, it is increasing in popularity. Saliva corticosterone levels were shown to be correlated with plasma corticosterone levels in wild and captive birds (Carbillet et al., 2024; Aota et al., 2023). In trained animals in managed care, this is a quick and relatively noninvasive procedure. Hormones and bacteriostatic agents (parent compounds or metabolites) can be assessed in saliva. The sample will require centrifugation. Because saliva volume is lower than blood, their concentrations would be low and require more sophisticated analyzers such as HPLC, which are not typically found in facility laboratories. The advantage of saliva analysis is the ease of acquisition in managed care animals. The disadvantages of analyzing saliva include the need for HPLC for analysis, dilution in the oral cavity, and the need to validate the relationship between levels in saliva and blood (the standard).

Feathers are a useful, minimally invasive matrix to sample. Feathers can be inspected for the presence of ectoparasites (e.g., feather mites and lice) and feather structure abnormalities. The feather pulp can be expressed, cytology prepared, and viewed under a microscope for the presence of quill mites. If any blood is present in the pulp, it can serve as an adjunct sample to check for blood parasites (González-Olvera et al., 2023). Feathers are made with keratin, which retains lipophilic compounds. Therefore, feathers can be assayed for hormones, contaminants, and heavy metals. The levels found therein would reflect accumulation since that feather erupted.

Muscle is a useful matrix for evaluation as it represents what is currently in the body. Muscle is very vascularized; therefore, what is in the blood can also be detected in the muscle. However, muscles are more invasive to collect and pain medication is mandatory. Muscle tissue is easily collected during a necropsy.

Thermal body temperature monitoring is becoming an increasingly common diagnostic tool for health and stress diagnostics. Infrared temperature monitoring using thermal cameras is useful to diagnose inflammation from any cause (e.g., infection and trauma), hormones/estrous cycles, surface heat, and stress (Jerem and Romero, 2023; Cilulko et al., 2013). The advantages of this technique are that it can be done totally noninvasively, without any handling, and from a distance (not too far) away. Disadvantages include weather interference, if you cannot get close enough to get a good reading, and behavior of animals interfering with the optimal area to image. The use of thermal imaging on drones can be used potentially to document the number of animals in a particular location (e.g., forest) by seeing their heat signals.

A final word on diagnostics of body samples: newer technologies, such as the use of drones for remote sampling, have and will continue to broaden the information we can obtain from especially more remote species. Even in managed care situations, we can improve and grow our diagnostic breadth by partnering with scientists who have equipment such as HPLC so that we can analyze agents and/or metabolites in very low concentrations that we currently cannot do in-house. There is so much more to learn.

Literature Cited

Aota, I., Yatsuda, C., and Izawa, E. I. (2023). Salivary corticosterone measurement in large-billed crows by enzyme-linked immunosorbent assay. *Journal Veterinary Medical Science* 85(1):71–75. https://doi.org/10.1292/jvms.22-0383.

Cai, F. and Wang, Y. (2025). Immune functions of avian erythrocytes: A comprehensive review from basic biology to pathogen-induced responses. *Frontiers in Immunology* 16:1675279. https://doi.org/10.3389/fimmu.2025.1675279.

Carbillet, J., Saks, L., and Sepp, T. (2024). Salivary corticosterone reflects plasmatic levels in a wild seabird. *General Comparative Endocrinology* 345:114390. https://doi.org/10.1016/j.ygcen.2023.114390.

Cilulko, J., Janiszewhi, P., Bogdaszewski, M., et al. (2013). Infrared thermal imaging in studies of wild animals. *European Journal Wildlife Research* 59:17–23. https://doi.org/10.1007/s10344-012-0688-01.

Corl, A., Charter, M., Roxman, G., et al. (2024). Social, environmental, and developmental factors affect the microbiota of barn owls (*Tyto alba*) in a cross-fostering experiment. *Animal Microbiome* 6:77. https://doi.org/10.1186/s42523-024-00365-w.

Cray, C. (2021). Protein electrophoresis of non-traditional species: A review. *Veterinary Clinical Pathology* 50(4):478–494. https://doi.org/10.1111/vcp.13067.

Cray, C., Arheart, K. L., Hunt, M., et al. (2013). Acute phase protein quantitation in serum samples from healthy Atlantic bottlenose dolphins (*Tursiops truncatus*). *Journal of Veterinary Diagnostic Investigation* 25:107–111. https://doi.org/10.1177/1040638712467986.

Cray, C., Rodriguez, M., and Zaias, J. (2007). Protein electrophoresis of psittacine plasma. *Veterinary Clinical Pathology* 36(1):64–72. https://doi.org/10.1111/j.1939-165x.2007.tb00184.x.

da Fonseca, L. A., Montiani-Ferreira, F., Soto, J., et al. (2023). Comparison of agarose gel and capillary zone electrophoresis methods with preliminary reference interval generation using capillary zone electrophoresis in bald eagles (*Haliaeetus leucocephalus*). *Veterinary Clinical Pathology* 52(3):452–460. https://doi.org/10.1111/vcp.13210.

Delk, K. W., Wack, R. F., Burgdorf-Moisuk, A., et al. (2015). Acute phase protein and electrophoresis protein fraction values for captive American Flamingos (*Phoenicopterus ruber*). *Journal Zoo Wildlife Medicine* 46(4):929–933. https://doi.org/10.1638/2014-0191.1.

Desoubeaux, G., Cray, C., and Chesnay, A. (2022), Challenges to establish the diagnosis of aspergillosis in non-laboratory animals: looking for alternatives in veterinary medicine and demonstration of feasibility through two concrete examples in penguins and dolphins. *Frontiers Cellular Infection Microbiology* 12:757200. https://doi.org/10.3389/fcimb.2022.757200.

González-Olvera, M., Hernandez-Colina, A., Chantrey, J., et al. (2023). A non-invasive feather-based methodology for the detection of blood parasites (*Haemosporida*). *Scientific Reports* 13(1):16712. https://doi.org/10.1038/s41598-023-43932-y.

Jerem, P. and Romero, L. M. (2023). It's cool to be stressed: Body surface temperatures tract sympathetic nervous system activation during acute stress. *Journal Experimental Biology* 226(20):jeb246552. https://doi.org/10.1242/jeb.246552.

Kumar, S. D., Ghosh, J., Ghosh, S., et al. (2025). Emerging concepts in the molecular cell biology and functions of mammalian erythrocytes. *Journal of Biological Chemistry*, 301(4):108331. https://doi.org/10.1016/j.jbc.2025.108331.

Lee, L. K. F., Hipfner, J. M., Frankfurter, G., et al. (2024). Baseline health parameters of rhinoceros auklets (*Cerorhinca monocerata*) using serum protein electrophoresis, acute phase proteins, and biochemistry. *Frontiers Veterinary Science* 11:1379980. https://doi.org/10.3389/fvets.2024.1379980.

Mattison, S. (2012). Training birds and small mammals for medical behaviors. *Veterinary Clinics North America Exotic Animal Practice* 15(3):487–499. https://doi.org/10.1016/j.cvex.2012.06.012.

Scanes, C. G. (2022). Blood. In: *Avian Physiology*, 7th Ed., C. G. Scanes and D. Dridi (eds.). pp. 293–326. Academic Press.

Trevelline, B. K., MacLeod, K. J., Knutie, S. A., et al. (2018). *In ovo* microbial communities: A potential mechanism for the initial acquisition of gut microbiota among oviparous birds and lizards. *Biology Letters* 14(7):20180225. https://doi.org/10.1098/rsbl.2018.0225.

Van de Weyer, Y. and Tahas, S. A. (2024). Avian diabetes mellitus: A review. *Journal of Avian Medicine and Surgery* 38(1):21–33. https://doi.org/10.1647/AVIANMS-D-22-00057.

6

Medical Care and Health Assessment of Birds

In this chapter, we will explore the basics of health care of birds in managed care/zoos, rehabilitation, as pets, and in free-ranging populations. (We will not discuss poultry farm animals here.) The basic underlying concepts are similar, but the details differ. One important distinction is that medicine, health care, and rehabilitation in managed populations are centered on the individual. However, in free-ranging populations, the health assessment is usually focused on the population level. The main components of medical management include environmental evaluation (referred to as husbandry in managed care or captivity), animal observation, physical examination, sample collection, assessment of these data, and ultimately a plan of care.

Animals in Managed Care

Life in zoos or other captive situations is well controlled for the most part. Animals are treated when ill, followed closely until the illness is resolved, provided with nutritive food, and given stimulation for enrichment. These features are the basis of preventative medical care. The other major component affecting health is husbandry, or the environment in which the animals live. Consider what it would be like for you to live in a dirty home. If you or your pets live in an unsanitary environment, your likelihood of getting sick would be higher than if you/they lived in a more sanitary environment. Living outside in the environment is uncontrolled in general. Therefore, in managed care, we try to manage the aspects of their environment that we can to optimize health and well-being. In the United States, as of June 21, 2023, the USDA regulates the medical care and husbandry of birds in managed care for birds used in research, for exhibition, and for pet sales. It defines minimum standards for husbandry and medical care that must be followed (Animal Welfare Act (AWA), subpart G). This document can be downloaded for free from the USDA website.

The AWA requires minimum standards for transportation, handling, feeding, facilities, and medical care of warm-blooded vertebrates. Facilities housing birds should be in good repair, have sanitizable surfaces, and perimeter fencing or containment to prevent escape or entry of unwanted animals or humans. If pools of water are present, they should be of sufficient circumference and depth to allow the species to approximate their normal swimming behavior. The water must have the appropriate temperature and salinity, continually monitored for changes, and documented. If the pool is indoors, the ambient air must be well-ventilated and of appropriate temperature, including an appropriate energy source and power backup. The sanitation of the land, water, food preparation area, and adjacent walkways should be frequently checked for unwanted microorganisms and thoroughly cleaned on a regular basis. As social species, birds should be housed with other conspecifics ideally. Food should be stored and prepared in specific ways to minimize contamination and inadvertent bacterial growth (especially during thawing). Veterinary care should be provided by veterinarians with experience in caring for the species in the facility. Recordkeeping should be meticulous, frequent, and complete.

Any solid or land surface should be constructed from a sturdy, nonporous (no holes) material so that cleaning and sanitizing are most effective. Cleaning frequency, agents used, and testing for sanitization effectiveness must be done and recorded (per USDA). For species housed indoors, the circulation of air within the enclosure must also be controlled, monitored, and minimum air exchange rates (rate of air entry and then exit from the enclosure – or air changes/hour) must be maintained to ensure adequate ventilation of clean, fresh air. Lighting in indoor enclosures is also important. If there is no illumination from outside, the internal lighting must reflect (as closely as possible) the light intensity, color spectrum, and photoperiod of the animal's natural environment. All these parameters must have monitoring devices (including systems to alarm when parameters are out of range) and regular documentation per USDA.

In food preparation, food storage, and areas immediately adjacent, similar requirements exist for sturdy, nonporous flooring and walls, and frequent sanitation. Food freezers must be documented to be at appropriately cold temperatures and have a system for alarming should the freezer fail. This is to protect the animal from improperly thawed frozen food, which may contain harmful bacteria or bacterial overgrowth that can make the animals ill. The thawing procedures mandated by the USDA are specific and designed to minimize contamination during the thawing of frozen seafood. On a regular basis, frozen fish or other frozen food should be sent for analysis of nutritional content (fat, carbohydrates, and protein) and tested for toxins or agents that can cause illness. All table/counter surfaces must be stainless steel (or similar) to prevent rust and for ease of sanitation. Food is sorted based on caloric intake for each animal as determined by their age and health status (e.g., growing young, laying females, incubating females, or ill birds). Cleaning and sanitizing the kitchen often takes as much time as preparing and feeding the animals. Again, cleaning and sanitizing the food area must occur after each feeding and be documented.

Other environmental factors need to be considered depending on the species and location. Structures or awnings to provide shade from the sun are commonly used. Attention to adjacent city lights and noise is important. Walkways and observation areas for visitors and staff are important. They should be positioned in ways to optimize function but minimize impact and intrusion on the animals. Last, but not least, exterior fencing or enclosure walls should preclude the entrance of unwanted intruders, both animal and human.

With the environment as clean and safe as it can be, there is a much lower chance of injury or disease. With preventative medicine and diagnostics, the chance of disease is reduced and, if present, can be addressed at an early stage. So, let us move on to preventative health care.

Preventative Health Care

A key component of continuing medical care is the individual's medical and social history. Ideally, the age and previous history of the animal are known. If not, careful observation is important to become familiar with the animal. We have a good handle on their current health status because of the detailed attention the animals get from zookeepers, veterinary technicians, and/or veterinarians. Health care includes the overall wellness of the bird in its environment. Overall wellness of birds includes information or indicators (positive or negative) of their environmental "quality," nutritional and medical status (e.g., from bloodwork), physical health, behaviors, and cognitive/mental enrichment and/or stimulation. Medical and nutritional status can be obtained/tracked in the veterinary medical record which per AWA should include blood work and amount of food consumed.

All health assessments or examinations begin with observations – observations of the animal's behavior, condition, activities, movements, etc. By and large, most of these observations originate from the zookeepers/caretakers who interact with them often multiple times a day. Zookeepers are often the first persons to identify an "issue" with an animal. Reports that animals are "not acting right" and not interacting with other animals as they usually would are typical subtle hints that something is not quite right with the animal – either physically or "emotionally." Through reinforcement training, zookeepers and veterinary technicians have the opportunity to put their hands onto the animals – look in their beaks, at their eyes, at their feathers, and body for marks or lesions without stress. Zookeepers should watch the animals eat to see if they have trouble eating and how readily they accept and/or manipulate the food. Preventative medicine in managed care benefits from the ability to train the animals, train them to be handled (if possible), allow sample collection, access to a scale, etc. Making these activities part of their natural behavioral repertoire permits more accurate data collection because the animal is not stressed during the sample collection. This also provides an easy way to get a close-up look all over the body. Generally, there are no other animals as well observed and cared for as animals in managed care except our own pets!

To deduce the overall wellness, evaluating or quantifying various parameters repeatedly can demonstrate patterns of change over time. Together with this information, the bloodwork data can clarify and/or confirm if an illness is present or not. Notations of animal wellness can be done formally using a worksheet (spreadsheet, etc.) or informally via individual notations in the medical record. It is most instructive to use a worksheet-type system to maintain consistency, especially if veterinarians change over time. Table 6.1 is an example of a health worksheet that may be used. It can be tailored to specific species or types of birds, but the same one should be used repeatedly in the same individual or species. The wellness worksheet involves criteria/measures that can be assessed from an in-hand or "visual-only" evaluation (obviously not too far, but away from the bird so it acts normally). At selected intervals of time, the individual can be scored as indicated on the worksheet and compared over time. The lower the score, the more "normal" the health and the better the welfare. If the score increases over the year, then there is something going on that is affecting health or wellness, and vice versa. Behavior of the animal is another critical part of wellness. Behavioral assessment can be added to this welfare sheet or can be done using a separate sheet that can be applied regularly. Ethograms are assessments of the amount of

Table 6.1 Details of semiquantitative scoring for avian condition assessment in managed care or in captured birds. This matrix can be modified/tailored for specific species or for use in the wild populations. Suggested parameters for use in wild populations are denoted by "W." Examples of what constitutes a score of 1 (best) to 4 (worst) are described.

Health index feature	1	2	3	4
Body condition[a]	Normal; BC score 3	Thin or fat; BC score 2 or 4	Very thin or very fat; BC score 1 or 5	
Eyes	Normal – bright, clear	Mildly sunken, squinting, mild-mod cloudiness	Moderate to markedly sunken, lot squinting, cloudy cornea, ocular discharge, and around eye	
Nares	Normal, no discharge	Clear nasal discharge	Yellow or greenish color discharge,	Previous + unequal size nares
Beak	Equal length top and bottom	Mild (<25% area) broken or cracked edges	Marked (>25%) Broken or cracked edges, unequal length bilaterally	Previous + scaliness
Appetite/food consumption	Normal	Eats no more than 85% of food offered (leaves ≤ 15% food uneaten)	Eats no more than 75% of food offered (leaves ≥25% food uneaten)	Not eating at all
Feathers[b]	Normal order, shininess	≤25% or less of feathers untidy, dull, broken	Greater than 25% until, dull, broken	
Skin lesions	No lesions	Abrasions present	Ulcerations present[c]	
Skin inflammation[d]	None	<20% of surface area inflamed and/or mildly increased temperature	>20% of surface area inflamed or very increased body temperature	
Itchiness	None	<20% observation time spent scratching	>20% time spent scratching	
Ambulation and balance	Normal and balanced	Mildly abnormal and imbalanced	Very abnormal and imbalanced, uses wings to balance	Previous + circling
Respiratory effort	Normal	Mildly increased effort	Marked increased effort with abdominal component	Previous plus tail bobbing
Coughing	None	Coughing < 25% observation time	Coughing > 25% observation time	

Health index feature	1	2	3	4
Posture	Normal	Slumped, single wing droop	Both wings drooped or down	

a. Body condition can be evaluated by body condition score (see Figure 6.3).
b. Feather condition can be evaluated by direct visualization or photography; molt stage or cycle should be clarified/noted.
c. Ulcerations contribute to loss of body fluids. Depending on the bird's size, these may be a major health concern.
d. Skin inflammation can be evaluated by thermography or direct visualization and measurement.

time spent in different behaviors. There are various styles for which to conduct these, but the same style/sheet should be used for an individual or species, especially if they are new to the facility. Various examples of this type of assessment have been published (Main et al., 2012; Mels et al., 2023; Justice et al., 2017).

Visualization of the bird from a distance is the first part of an examination. The general appearance, posture, condition of feathers, fecal/urine droppings, vocalizations, behaviors, and watching the bird walk or fly (or training them to do so on command) are useful. Locomotor evaluation is useful medically because it permits visualization of motor skills, neurologic state, and physiologic responses to activity (e.g., time to recover from activity and respiratory effort). The position of the wings at rest should be symmetric between the left and right wing. If one wing hangs lower or is not neatly folded against the body, this indicates a wing droop and suggests some injury to that appendage (Figure 6.1). If evaluating an aquatic or partially aquatic species, observing them in the water can indicate if they are listing (leaning) to one side or the other or sitting too high or too low in the water. Observing aquatic species movement on land is also important. Walking on land without the aid of buoyancy can reveal weight-bearing deficits or lameness that may not have been apparent while swimming. Observe the eyes, nares, and head for discharge, matted feathers, asymmetries, etc. If the bird walks in an uncoordinated manner, neurologic issues should be considered.

If possible, the regular enclosure/cage should be examined to see excrement (urine and feces). As you can imagine, excrement characteristics can reveal a lot about the bird's health. Table 6.2 lists the most common features of normal and abnormal excrement and possible etiologies. In this same vein (no pun intended; but "vane" is the body of the feather... ok), characteristics of normal or abnormal feather features and their potential etiologies are listed in Table 6.3.

Understanding how to handle birds is important. The ribs and chest area cannot be compressed! If so, the bird will not be able to breathe. The strongest and most dangerous parts of the bird must be controlled or restrained to prevent injury. The beak may be a weapon. Long, thin, pointy beaks can poke handlers in the face/eyes; therefore, they need to be held closed (Figure 6.2). Large parrots or raptors have extremely strong beaks with pointy tips (albeit turned downward). The feet and claws are also weapons as raptors use them to catch and kill prey. The correct protective equipment is needed. Thick leather gloves are used for raptors to restrain the legs, and wrapping a towel around the bird carefully will control the entire bird. Care must be taken to tuck the wings in normal anatomical position before

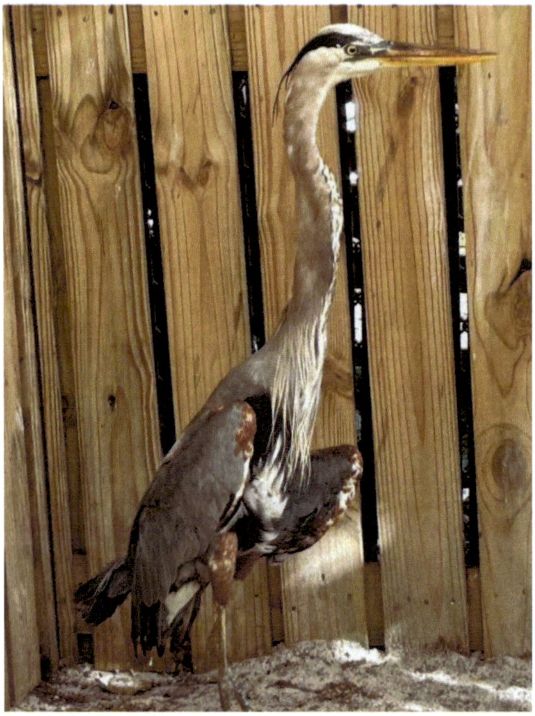

Photo by author

Figure 6.1 Wing droop in a Great Blue Heron. Note the left wing is positioned lower than the right wing.

Table 6.2 Fecal/urine characteristics and likely etiologies in birds.

Feces	Urine	Likely diagnosis/etiology
Formed, homogenous, brown-green color	White, slightly moist	Normal
Unformed	White, slightly moist	Diarrhea
Presence of undigested food	White, slightly moist	GIT problem
Blackish-dark color	White, slightly moist	Melena
Formed, homogenous, brown-green color	Green	Liver disease
Formed, homogenous, brown-green color	Thick, pasty	Dehydration
Normal with fresh blood	Normal with fresh blood	Cloacal problem

Source: Adapted from Doneley and Xie (2025).

wrapping or picking up the bird. Birds with long necks (or legs) may require an additional person to help unless the bird is anesthetized.

Hands-on inspection all over the body is important, as some abnormalities cannot be seen but can be felt. Training birds for handling and medical procedures is critical and the

Table 6.3 Assessment of feathers and skin.

Observed condition	Potential etiologies
Untidy plumage	Bird is unable to preen; or general feather Dystrophy disease
Not shiny color or wrong color	May be lack of powder down; possibly a pigment deposition issue
Feather damage	
Chewed or broken feathers	Overgrooming; self-mutilation; or malnutrition
Retained sheath; pulp twisted feather	Feather shaft abnormality; viral disease; feather dystrophy
Stress line(s) evident	"“break” in feather vane; if present on many feathers, problem may have been in the recent past

Source: Adapted from Doneley and Xie (2025).

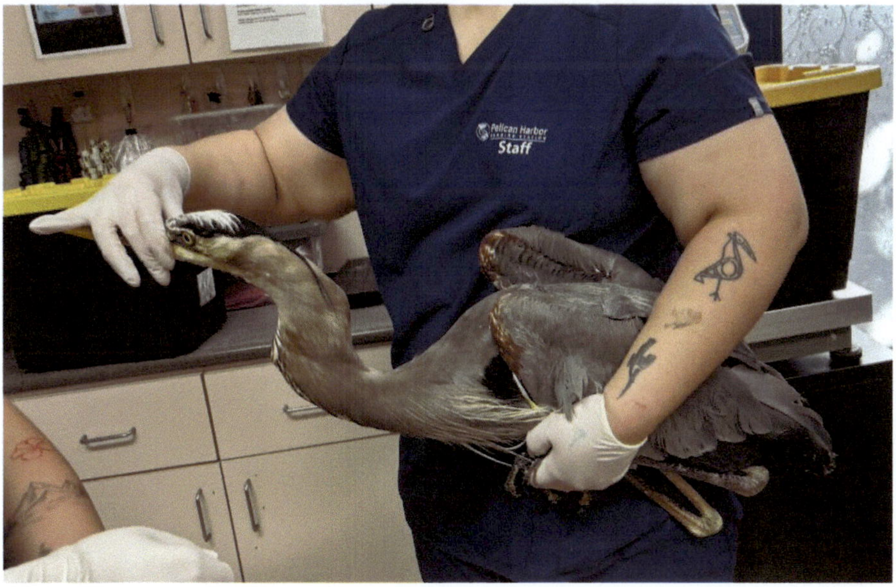

Photo by author

Figure 6.2 Restraining birds, especially large birds or those with long, pointy beaks, requires holding the beak with the other arm wrapped around the body. Note the wings are in a normally folded position tucked alongside the body.

key to good preventative care in captivity (Daugette et al., 2012; Mattison, 2012). In-hand physical examinations are performed at regular intervals as defined by the facility veterinarian using the USDA regulations as minimum standards. Physical examinations may include body weight and condition, examination of the body, extension of the wings, auscultation of the heart and lungs, body temperature, close examination of feathers, non-feathered areas, bottom of the feet, palpation of the coelom, and examination of the vent.

Sample collection may include blood, nasal exhalation or nares swab, fecal sample, and any other sample that may be deemed necessary (see Chapter 5). Periodically, other diagnostic modalities may be performed. Ultrasonography, endoscopy, radiography, or CT scans may be done on an as-needed basis. Anything that is done to the animal must be recorded in an individual's medical record that remains with the animal always (per USDA).

Body weight and condition can be evaluated in a couple of ways. The easiest way to monitor body weight is to train the animal to get onto and off a scale. Training to adopt a steady body position facilitates accurate body weight. If obtaining body weight is not possible, assessing body condition is important. Body condition can be characterized by the relative fatness of the body, applying a semiquantitative score to the keel area (chest) (1 = emaciated, 3 = normal, 5 = obese). Figure 6.3 illustrates body condition images of the keel of a bird. Recall that the keel is the site of attachment of the pectoral muscles. Evidence of bony protrusion of the keel indicates slight thinning or minor weight loss, and in cases of severe weight loss, the keel protrusion will be pronounced. If no protrusion is seen and the bones can be palpated under the skin, this is considered a normal body condition. If the bone cannot be seen or palpated at all, then this represents a fat or obese animal. If food is adjusted

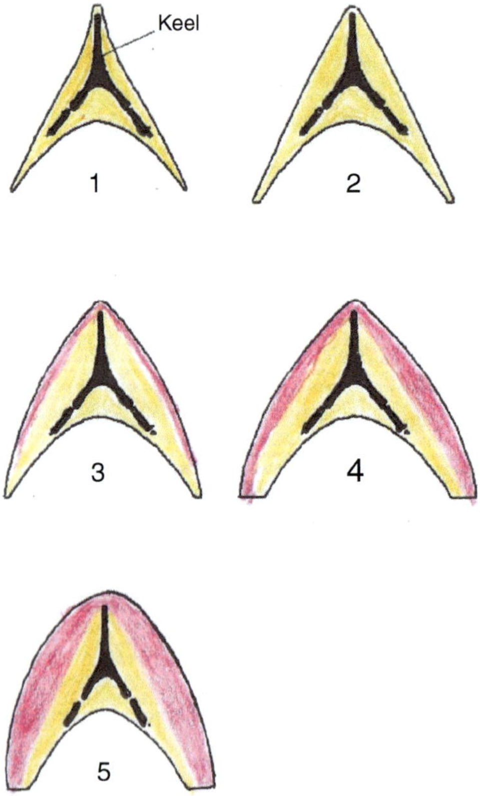

Figure 6.3 Assessment of body condition by examination of the keel musculature. 1 = very thin. Keel is felt and seen prominently. The pectoral muscles are concave laterally on the keel. 2 = pectoral muscles less concave but still thin. 3 = normal conformation. 4 = muscles start to obscure keel on palpation, appear more convex. 5 = obese conformation. The pectoral muscle is bulging, making it difficult to palpate the keel.

over time, the body condition will reflect that change assuming all else is normal. Regular body weight or condition assessment is usually done at least twice a year. It may be indicated more frequently in growing animals, geriatric animals, ill and recovering animals, or in nesting females. This frequency should be determined by the facility veterinarian.

If skin lesions or abnormalities are noted, they should be described: length, width, color, raised or flat, shape, and location. Using these features, they can be monitored over time for changes in these features. If skin sampling is needed, flat lesions can be scraped (using a scalpel blade) to provide the cells to be examined under a microscope or for culture. If the lesion is raised and liquid, it may be aspirated (insertion of a needle and withdrawal of the liquid inside) for cytology and/or culture. If a lesion is raised and firm, a biopsy may be warranted. These are all determinations made by the facility veterinarian. However, zookeepers and other staff can observe, describe, and document these lesions over time, which can provide useful diagnostic information. There is a tendency for people to mistakenly "interpret" a lesion instead of simply describing it. Interpretational comments include the use of the words "abscess" or "tumor" when describing a mass or raised lesion. This can be misleading. The interpretative comments should be used only when diagnostics are done to ascertain what the lesion truly is. One can never be wrong simply describing, but one can be frequently wrong if interpreting before sampling.

If there is feather loss or poor feather quality, the molt schedule of this individual or species should be checked. Feather loss will occur during molting, and this is normal. If the feathers are dull in color, broken, untidy, etc., outside of molting, this suggests that something is wrong. In addition, feather samples can be collected and examined microscopically for the presence of mites or lice. If significant dermatologic issues are suspected, a skin biopsy may be warranted.

Auscultation of lungs, air sacs, heart sounds, and rates provides critical information. Auscultation (listening with a stethoscope) requires practice. Heart sounds should be consistent across beats. The flow of air on inspiration and expiration can be smooth (normal) or "rough" (abnormal). Respiratory effort is a term describing the amount of effort exerted by the animal at each breath. This is assessed by observing the animal. Normally, a slight body movement in the thoracic region may be visualized with each breath. If the entire abdominal area moves, the chest rises significantly, and the tail bobs with each breath, this indicates marked respiratory effort, which is not normal and is severe. Previous activities of the animal must be known because after exercise or strenuous activity, the respiratory effort would normally be increased. So, context is important.

Sites of blood collection are the same among birds; however, depending on the bird's size, use of some sites may be more preferable or easier to safely access than other sites. The R Jugular vein, basilic vein (which is ventral to the ulnar artery on the underside of the wing), and the medial tibiotarsal vein (in larger birds) are common sites (Figure 6.4). The most important aspect of blood collection is training. Training the animal to stay still in a particular position and permitting a needle to be inserted smoothly. Bird veins are very thin and can rupture easily. Use of a heparinized syringe to prevent clotting during collection may be required in certain birds. The relaxed state of the animal during routine blood draws allows for accurate physiological data. If stressed, the animal's blood will reflect a stress physiology, which is not their usual physiological state, and it may mask illness. For hematology sampling, an EDTA tube is preferred. For chemistries, a lithium heparin tube is preferred.

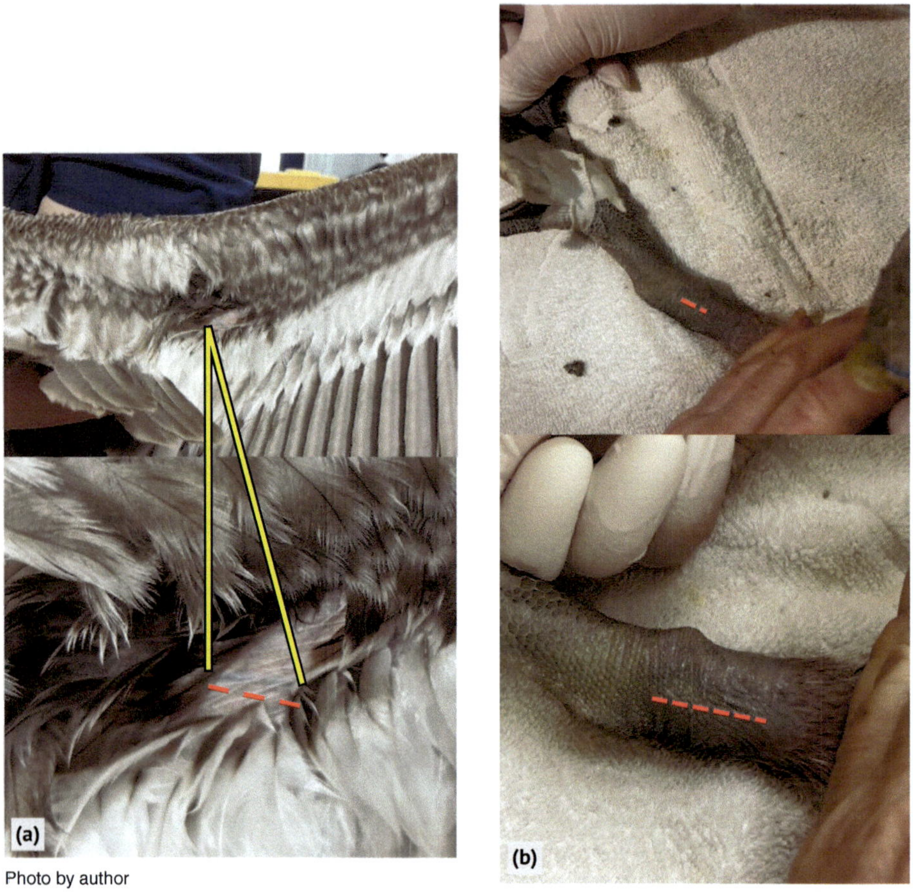

Photo by author

Figure 6.4 Sites of blood collection. (a) Ventral surface of the extended wing of a pelican. Yellow lines indicate enlargement of the area of the ulnar vein, which lies in the "wrist" area (in between where the primary and secondary feathers are). After wetting it with water or alcohol, the vein is visible running horizontally. A dashed red line underlies the vein. (b) The medial metatarsal vein runs along the medial surface of the metatarsal joint. A dashed red line underlies the vein.

Analysis of nasal contents/fluid or via exhalation/sneeze represents the state of the upper and possibly lower respiratory system. A very thin (pre-moisturized with sterile saline) swab can be gently inserted into the nares of a trained or restrained animal, or if the animal is sneezing, a slide or swab can be placed near the nares to catch the fluid sneezed out. Alternatively, the choana can be swabbed. The bird's mouth should be held open to provide good visibility of the anterior end of the choana for the collection (Figure 6.5). Cytologic analysis of the sample will define the cellular population and can show if there is an abnormal influx of inflammatory cells and/or the presence of bacterial overload or fungi. Culture of the sample is frequently done to ascertain the specific *species* (or *Genus*) of the bacteria present. These days, RNA-based identification (microbiome analysis) of genus and species (or family) of the bacterial microbiome can be analyzed. The relative value of using microbiome analysis versus routine bacterial culture will vary based on the reason for collection. Recall that there are normal resident bacteria in the nares and upper

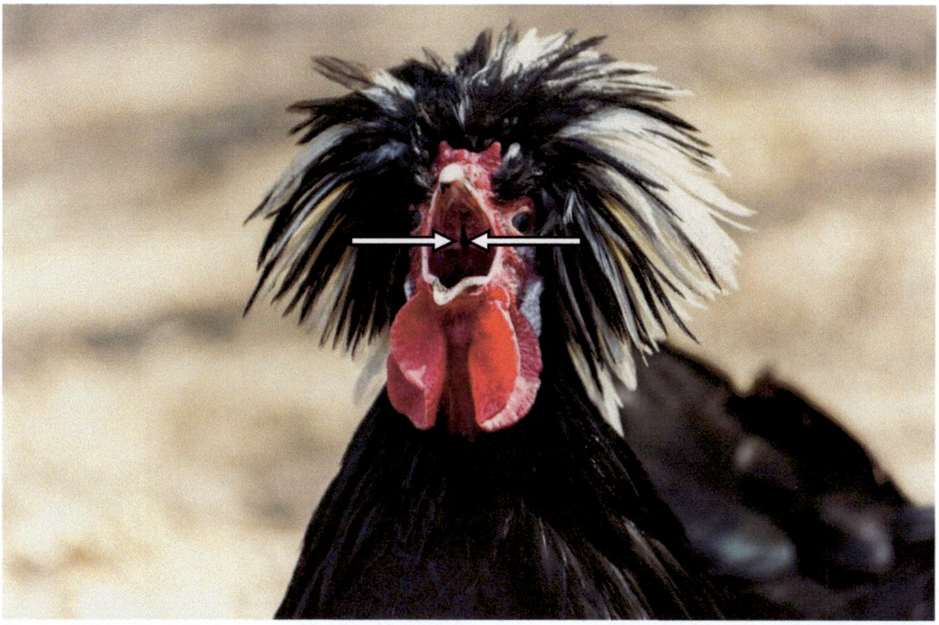

Shediva/Adobe Stock Photos

Figure 6.5 Polish chicken with its mouth wide open. Note the choana (arrow) located at the far end of the palate.

airways. Understanding how to distinguish those bacteria that are not normal resident flora is important. To devise a course of treatment, however, the process of bacterial identification, bacterial culture, and assessment of bacterial sensitivity to certain antibiotics is needed.

A sample of crop or gastric contents may be obtained via crop or gastric lavage (Figure 6.6). This involves inserting a plastic tube through the mouth down into the crop or stomach. Animals in managed care may be trained to allow this procedure, which can also be used to administer fluids (in low volumes), blenderized food, and/or medications if needed. The sample can be cultured and/or placed on a slide to view under the microscope.

It may be necessary to collect a fecal sample. The excrement as a whole, or the fecal part if you can decipher it, can be collected and sampled for cytology, presence of parasites, and/or culture. A cloacal swab may also be collected. This would be facilitated by training the animals or holding them still.

The least invasive methods of sample collection for diagnostics are usually preferred by humans and animals and can often be performed by nonveterinary personnel. Blood collection from trained animals is relatively less invasive because of the animal's conditioning; however, not all personnel may be permitted to collect blood samples. However, all could potentially collect a fecal sample and have it analyzed. These less invasive methods are also usually the most expedient – the results can be obtained faster.

The coelomic cavity should be palpated for masses, fluid (ascites), or signs of pain. The legs should be felt, and the bottom of the feet should be examined. Bumblefoot or other foot problems may be found (Figure 6.7); some species are more prone to this problem than others. Other samples, as mentioned in other chapters, can be collected that may provide

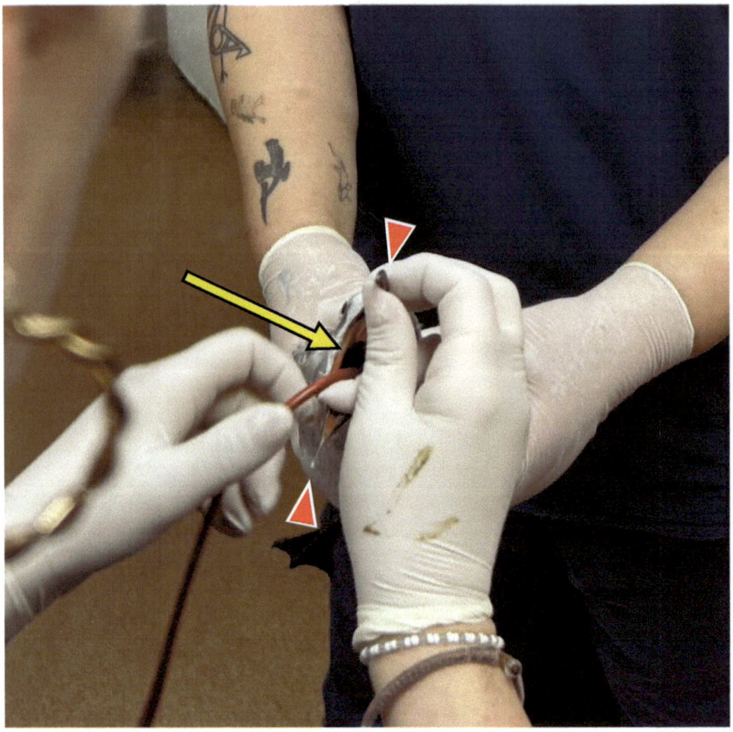

Photo by author

Figure 6.6 Common treatment modalities – Gavage. Tube feeding, also called gastric gavage, in a gull. The red rubber tube is inserted into the beak (yellow arrow), which is held open. Red arrowheads indicate upper and lower beak tips. The red tube would be attached to a syringe filled with a liquefied diet.

diagnostic support or provide less invasive ways to monitor and assess prognosis over time (how well the animal is responding to treatment and likely outcome).

Once the physical examination is completed and samples collected, the veterinarian and care staff evaluate the diagnostic findings and create an action plan for treatment or further workup if necessary. All the data are documented in the medical record, including any additional testing or plans for future diagnostics. This is all repeated annually or more frequently. In geriatric animals, preventative medicine and diagnostics are the general rule. Examinations and blood work are performed frequently to be able to detect and treat any abnormal findings as early as possible. The timetable for repeat examinations may also be sped up if animals have an illness or previous conditions of concern. The medical plan should be specific to each animal.

As in other companion animals, vaccinations are a part of the regular preventative health plan for pet birds, birds in managed care/zoo settings, and, of course, in poultry production. Pet bird vaccinations will include vaccines for diseases that are zoonotic, plus those of common bird diseases. In zoos, avian vaccines will likely also include those that target diseases to which they may be exposed living outside (e.g., West Nile virus). In poultry production, there are anywhere from 10 to 20 vaccinations that may be given, and they may start vaccinating at the egg stage (Table 6.4) (MSD Veterinary Manual, 2024; Scanes and Christiansen, 2020)! Vaccines can be administered under the skin, in the muscle, via nasal

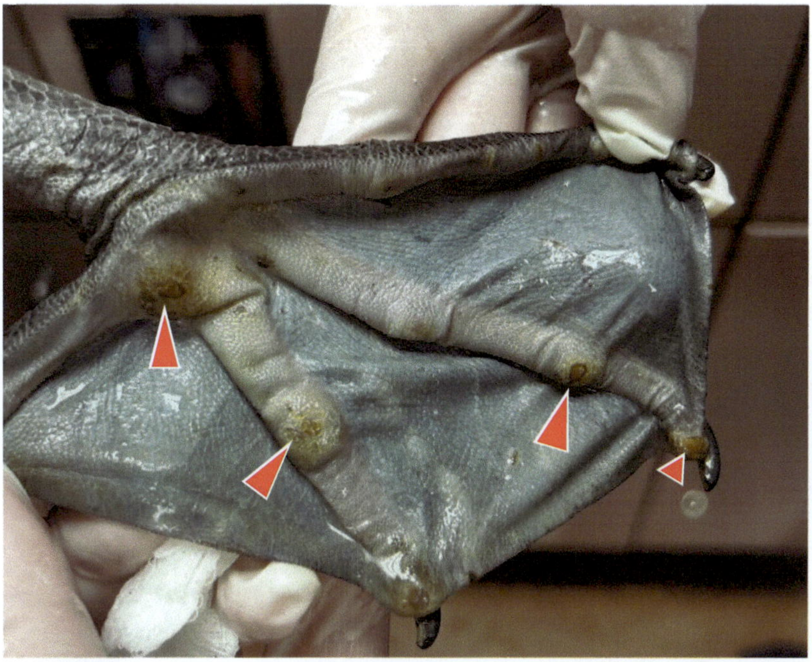

Photo by author

Figure 6.7 Examination of the bottom of the feet. This is the underside of a foot from a Brown Pelican. Note the mildly raised yellowish and brown bumps at the metatarsal (foot bone) joints (red arrowheads). These are early lesions of "bumblefoot." This is a condition where the underside of the feet becomes inflamed and infected, often resulting in very large and painful lesions.

Table 6.4 Vaccination schedules. Laying hens have a more intensive vaccination protocol because they live up to 1.5–2 years. Broilers raised for meat are harvested at 6–7 weeks of age.

Disease/agent	Age	Layers	Broilers	Zoo	Pets
Marek disease	Days 17–19 of incubation	Y			
	1 day		Y		
Polyomavirus[a]	3–4 weeks				Y
Newcastle virus, Infectious bronchitis virus	2–4 weeks	Y	Y		
	5 weeks	Y			
	8–10 weeks	Y			
	12–14 weeks	Y			
	16–18 weeks	Y			
Encephalomyelitis,					
Fowl pox, Mycoplasma	10–12 weeks	Y			
	18 weeks	Y			

(*Continued*)

Table 6.4 (Continued)

Disease/agent	Age	Layers	Broilers	Zoo	Pets
West Nile virus				Y	
Avian influenza[a,b]				Y	

Source: Adapted from MSD Veterinary Manual (2024).

a. Annual booster vaccination.

b. Influenza virus vaccination is variably approved for use in the United States and recommended for use in Europe.

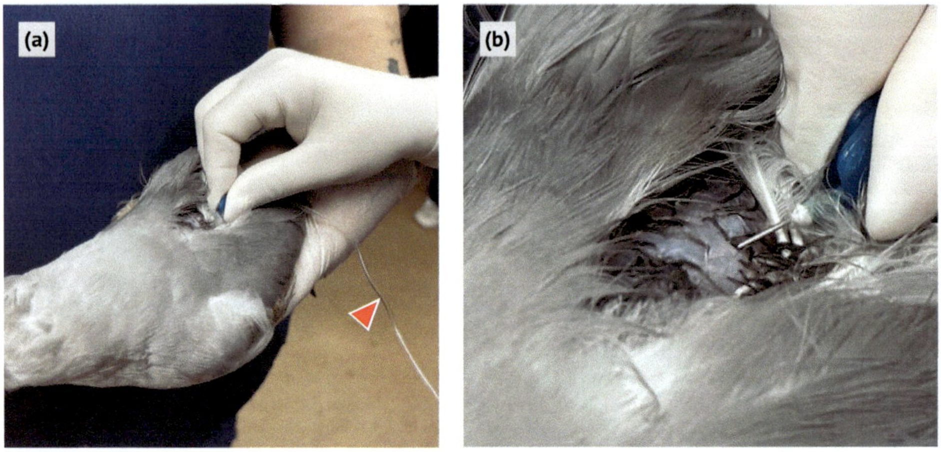

Photos by author

Figure 6.8 Common treatment modalities – subcutaneous fluid administration. (a) Interscapular subcutaneous fluid administration (on the back, in between the shoulders). Note the clear tube on the right side (red arrowhead); this would lead to a syringe with the fluid (sterile NaCl) to administer. (b) Close up of the needle under the skin. A slight elevation/expansion of fluid from under the skin is visible.

spray/inhalation, or directly injected into the egg. Depending on the species and age of the animal, the frequency and type of vaccine may change. Vaccinations against some diseases are under development now, but more work needs to be done in this arena. Potential vaccination of wild populations is discussed in Chapter 12.

Basic Treatment Modalities

Medications, fluids, vitamins, and other supportive therapies can be administered by oral dosing, injection in the muscle (IM), subcutaneous (SC or SQ; under the skin; Figure 6.8), intravenous (IV) (which is the most direct route for effect), transdermal (across the skin), or inhaled across the respiratory tract. The locations for IV instillation are similar to the sites of blood collection. IV injections may not always be possible, however. An alternative route is instillation into the tibiotarsus bone shaft *(intraosseous)*, usually using a catheter. Detailed instructions/recommendations for this procedure can be found in avian medicine texts (e.g., Doneley and Xie, 2025).

Injection into the muscle (preferred site is the pectoral muscle) ensures rapid uptake into the bloodstream because the muscle is very vascularized. If the bird is small, splitting the dosage between two sites would be less painful for the bird. Subcutaneous injections take a bit longer to absorb into the bloodstream, but are easy to do. The inguinal areas (ventral aspects of the pelvic region) or the interscapular region are preferred sites. This technique is not effective if the animal is dehydrated. You will see the liquid bolus, but it will be slow to absorb (decreased in size).

The oral route (PO or "per os") is one of the most common and easiest routes to administer medications and/or fluids. Commonly, medications may be inserted or mixed into the food and swallowed while feeding if the food items are large enough. Crushing pills and dissolving them in water can be given PO using a syringe. Crop gavage is the technique where the liquid, liquefied food, and/or medications are delivered through a tube placed down into the crop. Animals in managed care may be trained to receive (accept passage) an orogastric tube down to the stomach. In addition to medical use, giving fluids by this method can be used in emergency situations.

Transdermal absorption is a route available for some medications. The avian skin is thin so absorption would be quick; however, the skin may become irritated, inflamed, or worse if the medication is irritating. Finally, nebulization is an easy technique that can be used to treat respiratory diseases. Mixing the medication in sterile saline and nebulizing it (similar to how it is done in human humidifiers/nebulizers) allows the bird to calmly (without handling) take the medications. If able, the bird may be placed on a perch into a fish tank or plastic chamber that is closed with only a port open for the nebulization to enter the chamber. This passive route is safe for birds and humans, and the animals get the benefit of the humidification into their respiratory tracts as well.

Rehabilitation Medicine

Health care in a rehabilitation context is like managed care; however, you start with a possible disease or trauma and an *unknown* medical history. Because of this unknown medical history, the animals should be treated as if they are "infectious," that is, as if they have a disease that is easily transmissible to other animals (and possibly humans). If animals are rehabilitated in or near a managed care facility, the rehabilitated animals must be far enough away from facility/zoo animals of the same species and family; the outflow water of their pool (if aquatic species) must be discharged in a way that it will not mix with water servicing facility animals nor dumped directly into adjacent bays or oceans (if applicable). All equipment and supplies used in rehabilitation should be separated and not shared with facility supplies and equipment. People who care for the rehabilitation of animals should ideally be different people than those working in the main bird facility. If they cannot be different people, then staff should work in the facility (known health status) animals first, then tend to the rehabilitation (unknown health status) animals, and then go home and shower before returning. The flow of traffic is always "known to unknown" or "clean to dirty."

All equipment, including staff clothing and footwear, in rehabilitation areas should be thoroughly sanitized and cleaned daily. The rehabilitation space should be kept completely clean every day. This is because if infectious agents are splashed on staff or equipment, then allowed to dry out, they can potentially aerosolize with strong winds and/or rain or be carried on clothing or equipment.

Medical care is basically similar. Observations, body condition, physical exam, blood work, etc., all need to be done. However, now we are dealing with wild animals who are *not* trained to cooperate and are often in critical condition. These animals require people to hold them. If an animal is in critical condition and very weak, it may put up less of a fight when handled; such animals will be the ones who require the most medical care. If weighing the animal is not possible, the use of body condition indices is useful for condition assessment. The weight can be estimated to calculate drug dosages.

In rehabilitation care, regardless of the species, most animals will initially be experiencing several conditions, including, but not limited to, shock, emaciation, dehydration, hypoglycemia (low blood sugar), trauma, infections, and parasites. The primary goals are to stabilize the animal and provide hydration/fluids, glucose, and probably pain medications. The most direct route to administer fluids is through the veins. However, in dehydrated birds, IV administration can be challenging due to the difficulty of accessing vessels. Usually, water with electrolytes or plain water can be provided subcutaneously or as oral fluid therapy (Figure 6.8). Sugar in the form of dextrose can be added to provide some energy. Once dehydration is more stable, then liquefied food mixed with water can be administered through a syringe or direct feeding. Very emaciated animals may need to be tube fed (gastric gavage) to provide nutrient-dense food in small volumes. Animal handling to pass a tube into the stomach includes not only holding the animal but also having someone hold its beak open (if a large animal) so that the tube can be passed down into the esophagus. The bottom line is that all this handling and sampling is very stressful for the animals as well as the humans. Sometimes, there needs to be a trade-off between handling to obtain a sample versus leaving the animal alone (not handling it) because of the induced stress.

When samples are collected from animals in rehabilitation, in addition to the regular blood work, the blood should also be tested for antibodies to some known pathogens (appropriate for that species) and potential zoonotic pathogens. Zoonotic pathogens are those that can be transmitted from animals to humans. At first blood draw, serology (or PCR) for detection of antibodies (or the agent itself) to these pathogens is crucial so that the veterinarian can adequately protect staff in case there is confirmation of zoonotic agents or any other agents of concern. Personnel protection should be worn from the moment the rehabilitation process begins until it is verified (by repeat testing) that the bird is negative for potential zoonotic agents. Personnel protection equipment (or PPE) includes, at a minimum, face masks to cover the mouth and nose, wearing gloves, and eye protection (goggles or glasses). Scratches or sores on arms and legs – any open wound on skin (including cuticle lesions of nail biters) – provide pathways for pathogens to enter and therefore should be covered.

Prophylactic treatment of the animals should start as soon as possible after stabilization. Antiparasitic medications may be given to decrease parasite loads. High parasite loads often accompany dehydrated and emaciated animals. If lesions, or other causes of infection, are observed, antibiotics are started. These need to be broad-spectrum antibiotics that can kill gram-positive and gram-negative bacteria. This may require more than one antibiotic. When samples are analyzed, the treatment regimen can be revised to match the sensitivity of the bacterial species cultured. This often takes several days, so the prophylactic treatment must be strong to get the animal treated through the first 4–7 days. As antibiotics kill the pathogenic bacteria, they also kill and wipe out the normal commensal bacteria of the intestine and elsewhere. This sets up conditions that are perfect for opportunistic fungal infections to grab hold. Thus, monitoring for these infections and providing antifungals or probiotics may be needed. Medication schedules may vary depending on the size of the individual, if the animal can be sedated or not, and/or medication dosing schedules.

If any obvious external lesions are present on the animal, treatment can begin after a day or so. Close examination of the skin (plucking feathers may be needed) under the feathers is needed. Skin lesions, especially full-thickness wounds (e.g., full skin sloughing) and ulcerations, if present, should be managed as rapidly as possible since large open lesions permit fluid and protein loss, compound dehydration, and increase the risk of secondary infection. Once the animal is more stable and rehydrated, more intensive debridement (removal of dead tissue) or even minor surgical repair of deeper lesions can be done if needed.

Once the illness and disease etiology are positively identified, additional treatments and medications can be added or changed. Blood values of electrolytes and protein levels dictate fluid therapy. All this time, vitamins, probiotics, prebiotics, and natural feed additives may help increase digestibility and weight gain.

Depending on the age and species, the animal may be a candidate for release back into the environment. In this case, as soon as the animal is strong enough to maintain itself and fly, more and more hands-off time is needed so that the animal does not acclimate to humans. Food can be placed in an area/position that is easy for the bird to access and ideally as similar to their natural foraging approach as possible. Eventually, if an insectivore is getting close to being ready for release, live insects should be added into the feeding regime so that the animal reacclimatizes to pursuing and capturing live prey.

Treatment continues until the eradication of the disease. Before release, it would be prudent for the animal to be off antibiotics for some time to lower the potential of contributing to antibiotic resistance in local bacteria. This time period is called the withdrawal time. Often, this time period is a few weeks, but it may differ for each drug and species and is based on how long it takes to clear the drug from the body. Because poultry producers abide by withdrawal guidelines, they have data on withdrawal times that rehabilitators can apply to other species of birds before release. If a tag/monitor will be placed on the bird to track it post-release, this should be done right before release.

In rehabilitation medicine, there are a lot of unknowns at first, but many unknowns remain even if the animals are set to be released. What if the animal has become somewhat acclimated to humans even though attempts were made to minimize human contact? What if there are other infectious agents that could be spread from this released bird to other wild birds? Will this animal survive? Will it get hurt or get preyed upon by large predators? Can it still hunt/collect food? Often, we will not know for certain. There are not a lot of data published on the success of avian rehabilitation and post-release success. These data are critically needed as we are likely facing more and more birds that will require rehabilitative care given anthropogenic and climate changes (Pyke and Szabo, 2018). Banded California pelicans (*Pelecanus occidentalis californicus*) released after rehabilitation between 2009 and 2019 were found to have a 70% likelihood of survival if they were up to one year of age, while older pelicans had 80% likelihood of survival (Duerr et al., 2023). Increased survey efforts from 2015 to 2019 indicated that average longevity post release was 5.7 years, and some birds were resighted at ages of 13 years and older. This is great! From a population and environmental health perspective, though, it would be great to also know what pathogens they were exposed to at arrival to rehabilitation, prior to release, what pathogens were normal for that area, etc. These kinds of data would help us understand any unintended disease impacts on the wild population and conspecifics.

Data on the success of rehabilitation (irrespective of release) and characterization of numbers and species that arrive at rehabilitation centers are slow to emerge as well. Data from a local rehabilitation center between 2017 and 2024 in Miami has an overall 36% release rate of animals after birds arrive at the center alive (Costa, Zaias unpublished data). The release rates differed for different species and varied across years with brown pelicans having a 55% release rate while double crested cormorants had the lowest release rate (16%) and seagulls' rates were intermediate (36%; Costa, Zaias unpublished data). There are various factors that contribute to rehabilitation success and post-release survivorship, including location, food guild and foraging mode, species, and habitat. Much more data are needed to make educated decisions regarding rehabilitation plans (Cope et al., 2022).

Rehabilitation of any animal is very rewarding! Not only does one get to help save an ill animal, but rehabilitation also provides unique opportunities for people to handle or engage with different species. It also can be a fruitful portal for knowledge gain in the field and for the species treated. While "in hand," we can apply successful medical treatments and see improvements and healing in the short term. But once the animal is released into the wild, we have no idea whether that short-term gain will translate into longer-term survival. That is why tagging is so important. We can monitor animals for a period of time post-release. Some tags can even provide basic physiologic parameters (heart rate, respiratory rate, temperature, etc.), in addition to location. Some can provide more detailed information on where animals are moving and/or feeding. These tags/monitors may be costly, but the information gained is critical.

In situations where the animal cannot be released, before rehabilitation ensues, a plan for which facility/zoo will ultimately house the bird is ideal. In these cases, the same health care plan begins. After initial medical problems are resolved and there is no evidence of unfavorable pathogen exposure, then continuing treatment plans leading up to transfer to final destination (if needed) are decided. In this scenario, however, personnel or volunteers working with the rehabilitating animal can continue to maintain appropriate and safe contact and interaction with the animal. Acclimation to people is now not a problem! Frozen or nonliving food can continue to be fed, and medication can be continued as needed. Withdrawal time is no longer an issue.

General Signs of Illness and Common Conditions

Birds are notorious for not showing pain or illness! This is a protective instinct called "masking phenomena" (Doneley and Xie, 2025). This is typical of all prey species. If they show signs of weakness, they will get preyed upon. Therefore, more subtle signs must be noticed to identify a disease as early as possible. By the time a bird shows signs of disease, such as inappetence (off feed), changing behaviors, lethargy, and/or altered posture, fluffed up feathers, eyes closed, and evidence of pain, their disease process is far, far along. Lameness or limping clearly indicate potential bone break or trauma, which can be defined by radiographs.

Daily food intake is a useful indicator of illness and should be recorded. If food consumption is not usually directly observed in its entirety by staff, then the weight of the initial amount and then remaining food can be measured to determine how much the bird is eating (assuming they are alone in an enclosure). This would be noted in the animals' records, and close observation over the next several days would provide evidence of continued inappetence (or reduced intake) or not. If it persists, then diagnostic workup on the animal is warranted.

Common conditions (not including poultry farms) can vary between species and housing conditions (one to a few birds vs. large flocks). Traumatic injuries are more likely to occur in flocks. Depending on management practices, common disease etiologies can include malnutrition, vitamin deficiencies (or excesses in some cases), trauma, viruses, bacteria, parasites, and, in longer lived birds, neoplasia. Common clinical signs of these diseases include abnormal feathers, loss of feathers, pruritic (itchiness), and/or feather dystrophies, beak overgrowth or misalignment, foci of inflammation, raised lesions, crusty or scaly lesions, inanition, and lack of movement (will not fly nor walk). These signs may reflect local or systemic disease.

For skin or feather issues, feathers should be checked for mites, lice, or other parasites. The molting history should be discussed to see if there is evidence of molting irregularities or lack of molting. If molting irregularities are suspected, nutrition and hormone levels should be evaluated. Treatments of lesions would be based on their severity. The basic tenets are similar – debride the lesion (remove the dead tissue), clean, apply wound care, and provide antibiotics to control secondary bacterial infection.

Clinical signs of an eye condition usually include blepharospasm (blinking), eyelids closed, corneal edema (swelling), and potentially overt ulceration and/or abscessation. Trauma to the eye may result in cloudy appearing eyes, with areas of opacity, possibly with redness and overt vascularization, epiphora (excessive tearing), crusty periocular debris, and periocular matted feathers. The latter two signs indicate likely secondary infection, likely from bacteria. General treatment would include antibiotic ophthalmic drops, possibly a topical ophthalmic analgesic (blepharospasm and closed eyes suggest a painful eye). Systemic antibiotics may be required, especially if there is ulceration, if blepharospasm is severe, and if it is difficult to open the eyelids to treat topically. Cataracts of the lens may be observed. A veterinary ophthalmologist may be needed in certain situations.

Respiratory tract diseases may present with audible breath sounds, discharge from the nares, possibly matted feathers around the beak, and/or unequal and/or swollen nares. Diagnostics include evaluation of the respiratory rate, respiratory effort, blood work, culture of discharge, sinus lavage, bronchoscopy, radiographs, and/or CT (if possible). General treatment could include steroids to reduce inflammation, antibiotics, and/or agents that maintain open airways. These could be administered orally, by injection (depending on the species), or by aerosolization/nebulization.

Remaining Systems and Geriatric Care

In captivity, diseases in the other major organ systems are more rare. Regular diagnostic checkups and monitoring can demonstrate any changes in these systems that require additional workup. As our populations in zoos and other managed care facilities are aging, more attention is being paid to geriatric care, in part drawing from data in human medicine.

Defining "old age" in birds depends on the species' lifespan, so it will vary. The basic premise is routine diagnostics and examinations (including radiography and/or ultrasound), but on a more frequent basis as they age. Behavioral and cognitive testing as indicators of potential neurologic disease may be prudent to do regularly. These testing modalities should permit early detection of any impending serious conditions more prevalent in aged animals (e.g., neoplasia). Surgical management of disease (e.g., tumor treatment) is expected to improve as anesthetic procedures/agents improve in avian medicine.

Free-ranging Avian Capture, Release, and Health Assessments

Mark and recapture projects are great opportunities to assess the health and resilience of bird populations over time, especially when they live in areas heavily impacted by anthropogenic or climate effects. To perform these studies, permitting may be required. In addition to basic anatomic, demographic, and population information, the birds can be sampled to assess health. The birds would undergo the same basic approach to medical care – physical examination, measuring or weighing, condition assessment, and diagnostics (from blood collection, collection of other samples, sample collection for contaminant levels, and genetics, etc.). The difference in this scenario is that the data collection must be quick and efficient to minimize handling time and thus animal stress. This process may involve a large team of people to carry out a smooth and successful capture and release. Each animal may be individually tagged and/or fitted with a device to track their location, etc. Repeat annual projects can then track animal health year after year. These types of studies are the basics of conservation physiology.

Although the data are collected on individual animals, the outcome information is presented as population-level data. Demographics of the population captured include the number of males and females, relative ages, and sizes. Prevalence information (e.g., number of diseased animals vs. healthy animals) can be ascertained. The prevalence of disease types and whether they vary by sex or age group can also provide more detail on health. The number of offspring hatched and surviving in the current season provides an estimate of reproductive output for that population in that location. These capture sessions collect data on only a sample of the population. Previously collected information on animal movements in areas where captures may take place can provide information on whether these areas are utilized similarly by all ages and sexes, or if some sexes or age groups prefer this area. Assuming random and equal representation of animals, the data collected can reflect true population characteristics.

Resampling year after year can provide information on population size, changing demographics, and animal movements. Prey/food sampling is a useful adjunct to these types of studies so that population trends can be analyzed relative to resource availability. Year after year, long-term data can show trends in survival rates over time and aging survivorship. It can verify relatedness by observing nesting attempts and fledglings by animals that were formerly caught. Additionally, data about the environment, contaminants, and habitat quality can be evaluated over time, especially if compared to other capture-release studies from "cleaner" or "more polluted" areas. Box 6.1 discusses other issues related to capture and release studies.

Box 6.1 Capture and release projects on birds – thoughts

The capture, collection of data, tagging, and release studies are gold mines for data collection! They are extremely stressful for animals and humans – from the actual capture in the net to the handling and pressure to process them quickly. The benefits to the population (and species) for conservation, management, and learning about the animals are clear. But what benefit are these studies to the individual animals that are sampled? Can (or should) the individual animal captured be medically treated by the veterinarian(s) on the study if there is some obvious lesion that can be addressed? Can (or should) the animals be vaccinated for particular diseases if an appropriate vaccine exists? Can (or should) an animal in very poor condition be euthanized right then if a serious or fatal condition is observed during the workup? Can (or should) we conduct these types of projects on species of concern or endangered species (there is always a risk to the individual animal)?

If the answer to these questions is "no," then we should ask ourselves, are the population data obtained from these live capture and release projects worth the stress it places on the individual animals that are caught? What about the stress on the adjacent animals that escape capture? Is there any longer-term consequence to the capture, such as avoidance of that area for some time after the capture? If the capture site was a prime foraging area, what effect could that have on the population as a whole? Repeat capture of animals suggests that any negative effects over time are not prohibitive. However, other questions remain. I assert that there is no single "correct" answer. Just a lot to think about.

Health assessment projects on free-ranging animals can provide a wealth of information on natural diseases and physiology that may never be experienced by animals in managed care. However, not all species can be easily captured, especially those that frequent dense forests or distant locations. Thanks to newer innovations, aerial photogrammetry is a method for obtaining various types of data from animals noninvasively. The photographic/video data are analyzed using computers, and the resulting data can be validated for several species.

There is a potential benefit to individuals in managed care from wild animal data. For example, data from elderly free-ranging individuals can provide "relative" baseline values for this age group, which can be used as comparative data for elderly birds in managed care (and vice versa). Perhaps an elevation in a certain parameter is "normal" or common in free-ranging geriatric animals. If this were unknown, then this elevation may be viewed as abnormal in the captive animal, where it is more "normal" or common in its free-ranging counterpart. I said "relative" baseline values in quotations earlier because comparing blood data between animals in managed care versus free-ranging populations is hindered by stress changes (which can be observed in blood data) resulting from capture-related stress. Even with this caveat, these "baseline values" are likely useful to be aware of.

Finally, the benefits of in-depth studies on free-ranging populations of especially high-trophic-level bird species can also contribute to human health. Many species of long-lived birds are apex predators (e.g., albatross and raptors) and are considered to be sentinels of the marine and terrestrial environments they share with human populations (Liguori et al., 2026; Pacyna-Kuchta and Roman, 2026). Changes in the health of these sentinel species due to changes in the environment allow us to better understand and manage any potentially negative impacts on animal and human health. Collaborations and data sharing between different disciplines can help us manage or mitigate health and environmental impacts on threatened bird species (Chen et al., 2024; D'Elia, 2010). While this occurs in various places, more of these types of data are needed urgently.

Literature Cited

Chen, F., Jiang, F., Ma, J., et al. (2024). Intersecting planetary health: exploring the impacts of environmental stressors on wildlife and human health. *Ecotoxicology and Environmental Safety* 283:116848. https://doi.org/10.1016/j.ecoenv.2024.116848.

Cope, H. R., McArthur, C., Dickman, C. R., et al. (2022). A systematic review of factors affecting wildlife survival during rehabilitation and release. *PLoS One* 17(3):e0265514. https://doi.org/10.1371/journal.pone.0265514.

Daugette, K. F., Hoppes, S., Tizard, I., et al. (2012). Positive reinforcement training facilitates the voluntary participation of laboratory macaws with veterinary procedures. *Journal of Avian Medicine and Surgery* 26(4):248–254. https://doi.org/10.1647/2011-056.

D'Elia, J. (2010). Evolution of avian conservation breeding with insights for addressing the current extinction crisis. *Journal of Fish and Wildlife Management* 1(2):189–210. https://doi.org/10.3996/062010-JFWM-017.

Doneley, B. and Xie, S. (2025). *Avian Medicine and Surgery in Practice*, 3rd Ed. CRC Press.

Duerr, R. S., Jaques, D. H., Selby, B. G., et al. (2023). Medical history and post-release survival of rehabilitated California Brown Pelicans *Pelecanus occidentalis californicus*, 2009–2019. *Marine Ornithology* 51:157–168.

Justice, W. S. M., O'Brien, M. F., Szyszka, O., et al. (2017). Adaptation of the animal welfare assessment grid (AWAG) for monitoring animal welfare in zoological collections. *Veterinary Record* 181(6):143. https://doi.org/10.1136/vr.104309.

Liguori, G., Castagna, F., Bava, R., et al. (2026). Raptors as sentinels: Unveiling the environmental and health risks of pfas contamination. *Toxicologic Mechanisms and Methods* 1–24. https://doi.org/10.1080/15376516.2026.2643909.

Main, D., Mullan, S., Atkinson, C., et al. (2012). Welfare outcome assessment in laying hen farm assurance schemes. *Animal Welfare* 21:389–396.

Mattison, S. (2012). Training birds and small mammals for medical behaviors. *Veterinary Clinics of North America: Exotic Animal Practice* 15(3):487–499. https://doi.org/10.1016/j.cvex.2012.06.012.

Mels, C., Niebuhr, K., Futschik, A., et al. (2023). Development and evaluation of an animal health and welfare monitoring system for veterinary supervision of pullet farms. *Preventive Veterinary Medicine* 217:105929. https://doi.org/10.1016/j.prevetmed.2023.105929.

MSD Veterinary Manual (2024). *Merck Manual*. Rahway, NJ: Merck & Co.

Pacyna-Kuchta, A. and Roman, L. (2026). Seabirds as sentinels for per- and polyfluoroalkyl substances exposure - A global analysis after year 2010. *Environmental Pollution* 389:127368. https://doi.org/10.1016/j.envpol.2025.127368.

Pyke, G. H. and Szabo, J. K. (2018). Conservation and the 4 Rs, which are rescue, rehabilitation, release, and research. *Conservation Biology* 32(1):50–59. https://doi.org/10.1111/cobi.12937.

Scanes, C. G. and Christensen K. D. (2020). *Poultry Science*, 5th Ed. Waveland Press, Inc.

7

Reproductive Health and Management

Reproduction and life history are critical pieces of information for health and species conservation. The various species of birds encompass a wide array of reproductive and developmental differences; therefore, since some are K-selected species (long-lived, extended parental care), conservation efforts must take into consideration the longer generation times, longer interclutch intervals, migratory behavior, and mating locations. Long-term studies on free-ranging/wild populations have yielded reproductive details for many species and families of birds. Detailed data have also been acquired from species kept in managed care such as zoos, aquaria, or wild animal parks. Understanding the reproductive details and differences between species is important for monitoring reproductive rates in free-ranging populations as well as for population management in managed care.

Avian reproduction is basically similar across species. Reproductive cycling in all species begins with the stimulus of increasing *photoperiod*; that is, increasing amount of light in the day. Light is sensed by the pineal gland in the brain, which then triggers a signal to the hypothalamus. Releasing hormones are sent from the hypothalamus to the pituitary gland at the base of the brain, which then secretes stimulating hormones to act on target organs (e.g., ovary or testes) to produce and secrete hormones into the bloodstream. This system works on a negative feedback loop such that when the end hormone is at sufficient levels, the hypothalamus is signaled to stop the releasing hormone, which stops the secretory cycle.

The female reproductive cycle involves follicular development, ovulation, egg laying, and then anestrus (the period between egg-laying bouts). Gonadotropin-releasing hormone (GnRH) is released in a pulsatile fashion by the hypothalamus and binds to the pituitary gland. In response to this, follicle-stimulating hormone (FSH) is secreted and stimulates the ovarian follicles. At this juncture, vitellogenesis begins under the stimulation of rising estrogen, LH, and androgens (Hrabia, 2022). *Vitellogenesis* is the synthesis and deposition of yolk precursor proteins into the preovulatory follicle (starting with the largest follicle). At this point, the oocyte in the follicle undergoes the first half of meiosis and appears as a small white circle called the "germinal disc" and sits on top of the yolk (Figure 7.1; Hrabia, 2022).

The *infundibulum* of the oviduct draws in the oocyte, and it is here that the second meiotic division of the ova occurs, followed by fertilization (Figure 7.2). The zygote then moves down the oviduct to the *magnum* region. Here, layers of albumin are added around the zygote over 2–3 hours' time. Then, the developing egg moves down to the *isthmus* of the

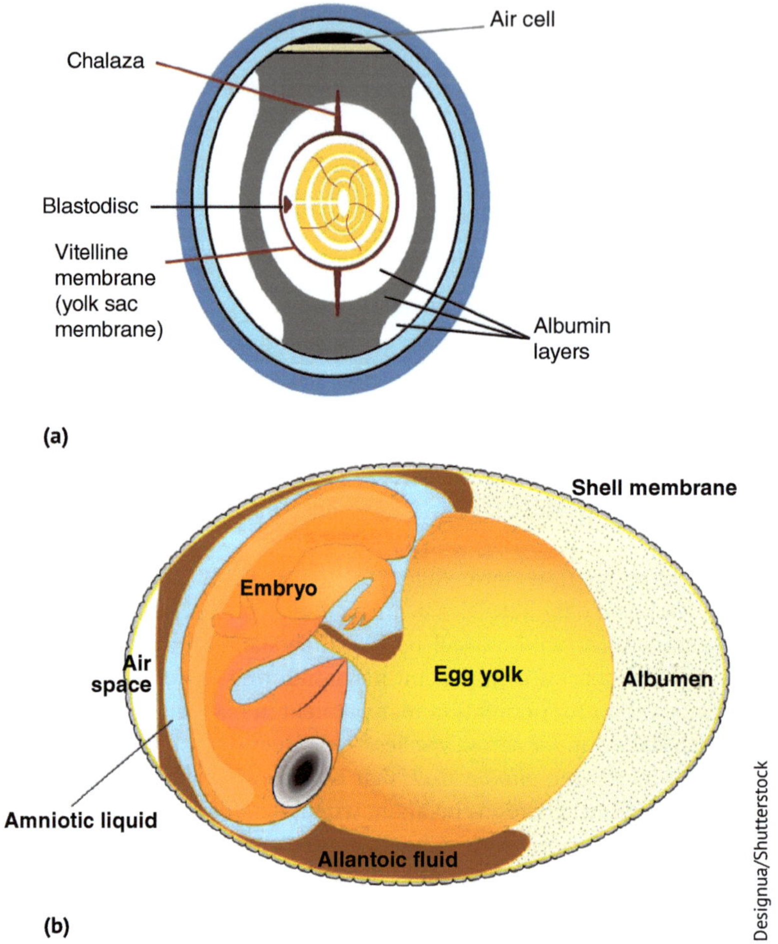

Figure 7.1 Bird egg in detail. (a) Embryo soon after laying. (b) Embryo in the second half of incubation.

oviduct. Here, the keratin shell membrane is added; this takes 1–5 hours. The *shell gland* (*uterus*) is next in line, and it is here that the calcareous shell and aqueous albumin are added. From here, the egg moves down into the vagina and then the cloaca for excretion. The entire cycle takes approximately 24 hours. Most species lay an egg every day to complete the clutch; others lay every second day until the clutch is complete (Hrabia, 2022; Faaborg, 2020).

In males, testosterone is necessary for the production of sperm in the testes and for mating behavior. In seasonally breeding species in response to increasing daylight, testosterone will begin increasing before the breeding season to stimulate hyperplasia and development of the seminiferous tubules, which ensures the male produces enough mature sperm. After the mating season, sperm levels will decrease, and the seminiferous tubules will regress. In females, the oviduct and uterus will also regress in the nonbreeding season (Faaborg, 2020).

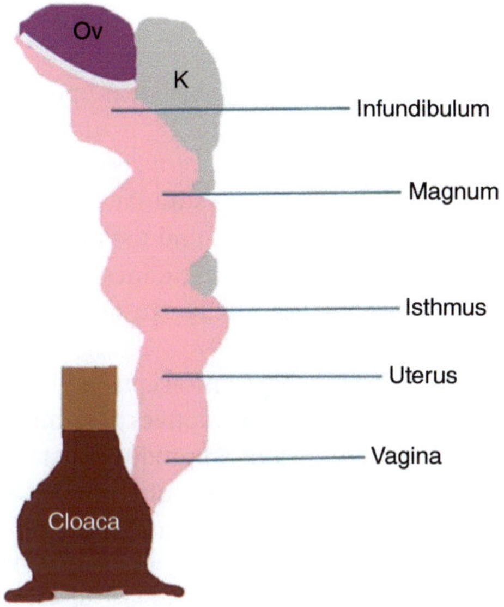

Figure 7.2 Diagram of the female reproductive tract.

Monitoring and Management of Reproduction

Reproduction in managed care can occur by natural mating between existing individuals in a given facility, transfer of males (or females) to a different facility for natural mating, or transfer of semen to inseminate a female in another facility. If the facility does not have unrelated mature eligible males and females, then sperm from unrelated males is an easy solution and enhances genetic diversity. Obviously, transporting frozen sperm is much easier than moving a live animal! Understanding the genetics and details of managing breeding colonies is critical, especially for threatened or endangered species.

The science of sperm cryopreservation in birds has advanced significantly over the past few decades but still has challenges (decreased sperm quality post thaw). Avian sperm morphology is not like mammalian sperm morphology. Avian sperm are quite variable in shape! In general, they are long, thread-like structures, many without a round or oval head like in mammals. Some appear spiraled or twisted, and the tails can be of variable length (Carballo et al., 2019). Data indicate that sperm morphologic variation is related to sperm competition and breeding strategy of the species (Carballo et al., 2019). What makes avian sperm so challenging for cryopreservation is that they have a high concentration of polyunsaturated fatty acids in the sperm membrane. Freezing then thawing for use in insemination causes oxidative damage to the fatty acids in the sperm and kills the sperm, leaving the resulting number of usable sperm extremely low (Perez-Rivero, 2025). While in the production world, managing poultry sperm has been well researched and developed, the same processes and techniques do not necessarily work well with other species' sperm! More research is needed on artificial insemination using frozen sperm in other avian species.

Prevention of Reproduction

If reproduction in managed care settings is not desired, then there are several options. Separation of males and females (either continual separation or only during mating season) will prevent mating and egg laying. Depending on the facility and bird species, this may or may not be easily accomplished. Female birds use various cues to stimulate egg laying. These include environmental factors like photoperiod, rainfall, etc. and the presence of a true or perceived mate. Hormones are poor indicators of egg-laying readiness; rather, in birds, behaviors are better indicators of impending egg-laying activity. (In mammals, female estrus can be tracked using hormones.)

The other method to prevent mating and egg laying is by using contraceptives (birth control). The main type of contraception is hormonal. Hormonal contraceptives are similar in concept to those used in humans – using hormones to induce a nonreproductive state. This form of contraception relies on accurate knowledge of reproductive and hormonal physiology. In birds, the main strategy is to give the females GnRH agonists such as leuprolide acetate and deslorelin acetate (Borsdorf and Petritz, 2025). These increase the GnRH signal in the body, providing a negative feedback signal to the gonads to decrease activity, which decreases folliculogenesis. However, even with hormone therapy, the environmental factors must also be managed for success. Hormonally induced decreased or delayed egg laying is reversible (Borsdorf and Petritz, 2025). While used mostly in female birds, this approach can also be used in males to suppress testosterone.

There are surgical options to inhibit reproduction, though these are irreversible. In theory, removal of the ovaries (*oophorectomy* or *ovariectomy*) would stop reproduction. However, the renal arteries are intermingled with follicles, which makes ovariectomy not feasible in birds. Removal of the oviducts and uterus (*salpingohysterectomy*) is more feasible in birds (Borsdorf and Petritz, 2025). This surgery can be used to irreversibly inhibit egg laying or to manage a disease or tumor in these organs.

Egg Development

Of all the incredible features of birds, the coolest one is the egg! (Well, flight is pretty cool too!). Earlier, we briefly reviewed the stages of egg development prior to egg laying. Let us dive a bit more into the egg, its development, and lay (no pun intended) the basics for how the environment can impact eggs and their developing embryos.

Under the stimulus of GnRH and LH, vitellogenesis begins. Recall that vitellogenesis is the synthesis and deposition of yolk precursor proteins into the preovulatory follicle. The yolk proteins include lipoproteins, very low-density lipoproteins (VLDLs), and vitellogenin, which are all produced in the liver. The yolk is deposited as yellow concentric layers around a protein core. This will be the main nutrient source for the growing embryo. The yolk will comprise 20–65% (depending on life history, see later) of the egg mass. At this point, the oocyte appears as a small white circle called the "germinal disc" (Figure 7.1). The germinal disc comprises just 1% of the egg's total volume but contains all the DNA and 99% of the organelles (Hrabia, 2022).

Next, the germinal disc becomes surrounded by layers of ovarian tissue. Upon integration of the yolk proteins, the entire follicle will enlarge, and the oocyte will undergo the first half of meiosis. Luteinizing hormone (LH) begins to increase, and at its peak, the follicle ruptures releasing the oocyte (= *ovulation*). The top part of the oviduct, the *infundibulum*, contains cilia which draw the oocyte into it. Mating occurs around this time (although females can store sperm in an alcove of the cloaca for a while), and this is when the second half of meiosis occurs. Then the oocyte and sperm fuse to form a *zygote*. At this stage, the sex of the embryo is determined by the female gamete contribution. Females have ZW and males have ZZ chromosomes. (Note, the pattern is opposite to that in mammals. Male birds have the pair of same chromosomes, whereas in mammals, females do.)

The zygote proceeds down the oviduct to a thickened area called the *magnum* (Figure 7.2). Here, albumin layers are deposited. Albumin (the "egg whites") layers surround the yolk and consist of protein and water. There are three distinct layers of albumin. The innermost layer closest to the yolk is thick and viscous and anchors the yolk to the egg. The middle layer is thicker and even more viscous. The outer layer is thin and watery. The function of the albumin is to provide an aqueous environment for the developing embryo, prevent desiccation, provide some anti-bacterial molecules (such as lysozomes and ovotransferrin), and serve as an additional nutrient source (Hrabia, 2022; Svobodová et al., 2019).

After a couple of hours, the zygote with its new layers moves to the *isthmus*, where the keratin shell membranes are added. The inner keratin membrane is apposed to the albumin and serves to contain the aqueous portion of albumin. The outer, thicker membrane will anchor the egg to the outer shell. At the blunt end of the egg, the layers separate to form the air space from which the embryo will breathe. During embryonic growth, as the yolk is absorbed, the air space will enlarge accommodating the increase in respiration as the embryo enlarges (Mueller et al., 2022).

From here, the egg moves into the uterus, which in birds is called the *shell gland*. Here is where the calcareous shell is added, so it is an appropriate name. The shell is a protein organic framework in which inorganic minerals (98% calcium) bind. They align in a particular arrangement, which creates small pores at the shell surface. These pores allow gas exchange (oxygen in, carbon dioxide out) but are small enough to prevent water loss. Outside the shell is a thin cuticle. It is this cuticle layer that one sees, and it may be of different colors and textures depending on the species. The cuticle is water repellent. From here it moves down to the vagina and then to the cloaca for release. Mucous lubrication helps the egg move through the tract (Hrabia, 2022; Faaborg, 2020).

Vessels develop on the surface of the yolk sac, which are responsible for transporting nutrients from the yolk to the embryo during development (Figure 7.1). Right before hatching, the embryo draws the yolk sac into its body to continue using it as a food source. Some chicks can live several days post hatching on this yolk sac remnant. The developing embryo also develops a sac to collect its waste. The hindgut membrane creates an outpouching, the *allantois*, which will collect and store waste from the embryo. Early on during incubation, the allantois serves as an additional respiratory organ; later, its only function will be waste retention. While in the egg, the embryo derives nutrients from the yolk, albumin, and also from the eggshell (Hrabia, 2022; Orłowski et al., 2019).

Incubation and Hatching

For proper development, the egg needs to exchange carbon dioxide for fresh oxygen, have a sufficient heat source to maintain the appropriate temperature, and the egg must be turned regularly altering the embryo's position. Optimal temperature for incubation is 37–38 °C. Egg temperatures of 43 °C or greater are lethal. Prolactin and estrogen levels are increased in females during incubation. If males contribute to incubation and/or additional parental care, prolactin is increased in them as well. The act of incubation will stimulate increased prolactin secretion (Hrabia, 2022). In females, the increased prolactin will inhibit GnRH and prevent egg laying.

So how do birds incubate eggs? Yes, they "sit" on eggs! But what is really happening is that they are contacting the egg with their *brood patch*. The brood patch is an area of the upper abdomen and lower chest skin which, under stimulation by prolactin and estrogen, loses its feathers, becomes edematous (enlarges and thickens due to fluid accumulation under the skin), and develops an increased number and size of blood vessels. These skin changes enable close and intimate contact with the eggs. The vessels transmit heat to keep the eggs at optimal developmental temperature (Hrabia, 2022). If the environmental temperature is cold, the incubation time will increase. If the environment is hot, parents may not keep skin-to-egg contact, but rather sit above the eggs to shade them. In addition, the parents can take up the heat from the eggs and dissipate it. There are various other strategies to keep eggs warm and/or cool them down including nest type and location.

Hatching success is highly dependent on the proper position of the embryo in the egg. One to two days before hatching, the chick will puncture the keratin membrane to get full access to the air space to get enough oxygen for breathing. Then, when it is time to leave the egg, the "egg tooth" on the beak will hit the eggshell to cause it to crack and open. This process is called pipping. By this point, the eggshell is very brittle as it has given nutrients to the developing embryo.

Nestling Care

Care of nestling birds after hatching varies with their developmental mode. *Altricial* species have nestlings with immature/undeveloped organs (except for the GIT), are unable to move about, feed themselves, or thermoregulate on their own. Examples of species with altricial young are many that build a nest (e.g., mockingbirds and parrots). *Precocial* species have young that hatch from the egg with fully mature organs, and they are soon able to walk, feed themselves, and thermoregulate. Examples of species with precocial young are chickens and other poultry. These are two ends of the spectrum, and there are variations in between (Faaborg, 2020). In general, altricial nestlings grow faster than precocial nestlings, although precocial species have a lot more yolk in their eggs (approximately 65% vs. 20%, precocial and altricial, respectively; Faaborg, 2020). Management of growth in broiler chicks is described in Table 7.1. It is obvious though that the amount of parental care needed for altricial nestlings is greater than for precocial nestlings. The parent(s) need to feed the nestlings, clean the nest (remove fecal matter), and defend the nest from predators. Depending on the species, parental care may last quite a long time and include other

Table 7.1 Growth of chickens raised for meat consumption. Note the decreased time until the chicks reach market weight over the years. Feed : gain ratio is the amount of feed needed to increase/gain body weight. The lower the ratio, the more efficient (and economic) the system is. This is due, in part, to genetic selection for increased growth rate and breast muscle weight (relative to body weight).

Year	Days to market	Weight (kg)	Feed : gain ratio
1935	98	1.3	4.4
1975	56	1.7	2.1
1995	47	2.1	1.95
2018	47	2.9	1.82

Source: Adapted from Scanes and Christensen (2020).

duties such as keeping them warm in freezing temperatures (e.g., in some penguins). Birds have a fledgling stage during which the nestlings leave the nest, complete flight feather growth, and learn to fly. The length of the fledgling period and transition to independence varies, as does the level of parental care at this time. This period of transition to independence is stressful as the fledgling learns to live on its own. In-depth discussion of parental care and breeding systems is beyond the scope of this text but is fascinating.

Female Health During Egg Laying Cycles

Egg development and laying are energetically expensive physiologic processes for females. Thankfully, in managed care, females are fed sufficient calories to manage the increased caloric burden required by these processes. However, during egg development and laying, the body's immune and hormonal systems do significantly change to accommodate nutrient mobilization for egg development. Awareness of these changes permits more accurate health assessment of, and preparation for, optimal female health and welfare.

Maternal investment in eggs is significant. The weight of a single egg represents up to 15–20% of female body weight (Faaborg, 2020). In smaller species, the egg weight as a percentage of female body weight is relatively greater than for larger species. This may not be energetically challenging for a large bird but is definitely so for a medium- to small-sized bird. Acquisition and storage of fats and proteins to deposit into the developing egg is critical to hatching success. Thus, as in mammals, the cost to the female may manifest in a trade-off between components destined for the developing eggs versus energy toward her own health/immune competence. This redistribution/trade-off of energy is extreme in laying (commercial) chickens. Table 7.2 demonstrates how egg production has evolved over time in the poultry industry. Quite remarkable!

Most of the detailed information on female health during egg laying comes from poultry, but the basics are applicable to other bird species. Experimental antigen challenges to females actively laying eggs versus non-egg laying females show that plasma from egg-laying females had a decrease in the T cell (cell mediated) arm of the immune system and an enhancement in the humoral and innate part of the immune system

(Schmucker et al., 2021). Further, within the oviduct, there is an increase in the concentration of proinflammatory cytokines and increased T cell recruitment (Nii et al., 2011). These findings indicate that the female's own immune system is changed to benefit the developing eggs. Experimental supplementation of calcium and vitamin D3 to egg-laying females resulted in increased estrogen, total protein, and globulin concentration in the females' plasma (Attia et al., 2020). The eggshell quality of these females was enhanced as was her laying performance. Data also confirm that a female can seed the egg with a sample of her microbiome before the eggshell gets calcified (Trevelline et al., 2018). What does all this mean? This information allows us to understand what relative levels of plasma/serum variables (e.g., calcium) and immunologic parameters are normal for a laying female. If levels of calcium are low, then we would want to monitor the female closely for egg binding or soft eggshells unless we supplement her with calcium and vitamin D3. If we do not know or understand the normal changes in the clinical physiology of females, then we may misinterpret those data or fail to act to supplement her if she is in poor condition.

The oviduct and uterus contain mucosal barriers that defend against and mitigate infections in the developing egg. These barriers are physical, chemical, biological, and immunological in function (Nii, 2022). Cells are tightly adhered to each other, preventing pores or points of pathogen entry across the mucosa. The oviduct mucus is viscous and contains antibacterial agents and antibodies. There is a normal microbiome that prevents foreign bacteria from crossing the oviduct mucosa (Nii, 2022). The mucosa also has immune cells that look out for and can instigate an inflammatory response if needed. (Gastrointestinal tract mucosa also has these components.) When estrogen increases in anticipation of egg production, these barriers are activated and develop to protect the impending eggs (Hrabia, 2022).

To create an egg in 24 hours, the female must have all the components the egg needs already in her body in a form ready to deposit into the egg and to make the eggshell. This involves mobilizing and moving nutrients, fats, calcium, etc. in her body. It is estimated that a female bird preparing to produce eggs typically has twice as much glucose, lipids, and other nutrients circulating in her plasma as in the nonbreeding season (Hrabia, 2022). Calcium is needed at such high levels that the blood cannot hold it all, and the female must mobilize more from her bones. The developing embryo derives calcium and other nutrients from the eggshell. Studies show decreasing nutrients in the eggshell and increasing nutrient levels transferred into the egg itself over incubation time in the western capercallie grouse (*Tetrao urogallus;* Orłowski et al., 2019). To prepare for this energy expenditure and metabolic increase, the female must build up sufficient fat stores (in the subcutaneous layer and liver) ahead of time. If the female is in good condition and able to adequately prepare for egg development, the eggs will receive the appropriate amounts of fats, proteins, etc. to feed the developing embryo until hatching. If the female is in poorer condition, then she may not be able to supply the eggs/embryo adequately to survive until hatching, only be able to supply fewer eggs sufficiently, thus reducing her brood size, or tap into her own body stores and muscle to supply nutrients to the eggs, but at her ultimate expense (e.g., she may not survive past this breeding attempt). Laying hens in poultry farms lay an egg almost every day of the year (Table 7.2)! How do they manage it?

The amount and quality of the nutrients and molecules allocated to the developing egg by female birds can have long-lasting effects on the phenotype and viability of her eggs. In general, and across various taxa, eggs that receive more nutrients and resources produce larger offspring that attain a larger adult size and have increased viability and

Table 7.2 Commercial laying hen annual egg production. Compare the numbers of egg production over the past 100 years. Breeding and genetic changes have decreased the time for estrus cycling to egg laying down from 24–26 hours to 12–16 hours after the dark cycle (using a 14 hour light to 10 hour dark light schedule).

	Egg/hen/year	Hen mortality (%)
1920	100	40
2015	265 (250–300)	<5

Source: Adapted from Scanes and Christensen (2020).

fecundity (Mousseau and Fox, 1998). Female birds may allocate resources differentially to their eggs within a clutch and across subsequent clutches depending on their condition, environmental conditions, and life history variables. Hammouda et al. (2012) found lower levels of antibodies in eggs belonging to female yellow-legged gulls (*Larus michahellis*) who were in suboptimal condition versus eggs from females in optimal condition. Laying order and sex of the embryo can also impact allocation to eggs. Experimental exposure to sheep red blood cells (SRBC) should induce antibody production against them. In female zebra finches (*Taeniopygia guttata*), the level of maternal anti-SRBC antibodies significantly decreased with laying order (greatest concentration in first laid eggs, lowest in last laid eggs) among eggs bearing sons; there was no relationship with laying order in female embryos (Martyka et al., 2010). In this example, females differentially allocate antibodies to male eggs. Differential allocation of anti-bacterial agents to eggs can also be due to the egg's perceived reproductive value (or mate attractiveness). When the father of the eggs was more attractive, the female blue tit (yes, that is a real bird name! *Cyanistes caeruleus*) deposited more lysozyme into her eggs than females mated to "less attractive" blue tits (D'Alba et al., 2010). Females have been shown to invest in allocating increased antibodies to their eggs when the nest's bacterial population is more variable, thus augmenting their chance of avoiding infection (van Veelen et al., 2022).

In addition to immunomodulatory agents, hormones/androgens deposited can also influence egg development. Groothuis et al. (2005) showed that environmental factors affect androgen and cortisol levels in females. She can then pass the androgens into her eggs to modify and enhance embryo phenotype depending on the environment and/or sex of the egg. The effects of androgens in developing embryos are varied but include postnatal changes such as antioxidant/anti-bacterial effects, muscular development, sexual selection, and mate choice (Parolini et al., 2018). Experimental augmentation of testosterone in the yolk of yellow-legged gull (*Larus michahellis*) eggs led to embryos with larger body size but smaller brain size (Parolini et al., 2018). This was a terminal experiment, so the postnatal effects of these changes were not evaluated. To throw in another variable, eggs contain enzymes to metabolize maternal steroids, and metabolism levels can vary with laying order, which would adjust the actual concentration within a given egg (Kumar et al., 2018). So, supplementation of eggs with hormones and other agents can be very complex.

In general, sequential egg laying provides the opportunity for the female to depurate (dump, get rid of) any toxins or contaminants in her body. In marine mammals, firstborn calves suffer a greater mortality from higher levels of contaminants than subsequent offspring (Wells et al., 2005). A similar situation appears to be true in some avian species.

For example, mercury levels in quail eggs laid first in a clutch had higher mercury levels than levels in the later eggs of the clutch (Beccardi et al., 2025). The horrible irony is that a female in good body condition can unknowingly harbor a lot of organic contaminants (or other pollutants) in her nicely built-up fat stores. These then pass into the developing eggs, which can potentially result in pathology and/or death of the egg/chick!

We also need to address the negative effects on population growth and reproductive success. Reproductive disease/pathology that results in decreased reproductive success in birds can occur due to contaminants, infectious agents, and/or random variation/genetic abnormalities. Reproductive failures, pathologies, and diseases typical of mammals are also seen in birds. These include decreased fertility and survivorship at any life stage, pyometra (bacterial infection in the uterus), anatomic abnormalities in any part of the reproductive tract, and reproductive tract cancers (Doneley and Xi, 2025). Most of the avian reproductive disease/pathology, including decreased reproductive success, that are seen in the wild today are likely related to environmental contaminants alone or in combination with infectious pathogens and climatic changes. These factors will be discussed in subsequent chapters.

Studying Reproduction in Wild Populations and Application to Conservation

The increase in the number of threatened and/or endangered species has led to many efforts (successful and unsuccessful) to raise birds in managed care/zoos or other facilities with the intent of releasing the young and repopulating the troubled population. One of the earliest attempts to raise birds in captivity and then release them back to the wild that I recall involved the California condor (*Gymnogyps californianus*). By 1991, the Fish and Wildlife Service captured the remaining individuals from a crashing California condor population near Los Angeles (Klinger, 1991). Their numbers had severely dwindled due to anthropogenic impacts. After several years, they were ready to release some subadults to a location near the original population. In 2025, almost 35 years later, the reintroductions have been successful, are continuing, and the population is rebounding. We will return to this topic in a later chapter.

How can we apply the detailed knowledge of reproduction we have gathered from animals in managed care (and/or rehabilitation) to free-ranging/wild populations? In populations of species that we are able to repeatedly catch, sample, and release, we can collect samples for hormone and blood analyses; census the area for nests, vegetation, etc.; and collect the usual life history information (size, growth, sex, etc.) to provide a snapshot of reproductive health and status of individuals and population status. We can analyze those data in relation to environmental data (such as water/soil quality, presence of toxins or contaminants, prey abundance) to help us understand what factors may be related to the changes. In populations where we have the privilege of sampling over long periods of time (e.g., longer than at least one breeding season), we can track life history data in relation to changes in the environment over that same time period. This can paint a picture of the population in relation to environmental and anthropogenic impacts, which are invaluable for management and conservation efforts. Reproductive and growth data obtained from captive animals provide reference points to interpret data collected from wild birds of the same (or similar) species. Data gleaned from animals in managed care can and do benefit their free-ranging counterparts in this way. Data from wild birds also help birds in managed care in a similar way.

Literature Cited

Attia, Y. A., Al-Harthi, M. A., and Abo El-Maaty, H. M. (2020). Calcium and cholecalciferol levels in late-phase laying hens: Effects on productive traits, egg quality, blood biochemistry, and immune responses. *Frontiers in Veterinary Science* 7:389. https://doi.org/10.3389/fvets.2020.00389.

Beccardi, M., Bertram, J., Bouwhuis, S., et al. (2025). Experimental evidence for maternal offloading of mercury pollution via reproduction. *Environmental Pollution* 385:127121.

Borsdorf, M. C. and Petritz, O. A. (2025). Medical management of reproduction in birds. *Journal of Veterinary Clinical Exotic Animals* 28:107–125. https://doi.org/10.1016/j.cvex.2024.07.006.

Carballo, L., Battistotti, A., Teltscher, K., et al. (2019). Sperm morphology and evidence for sperm competition among parrots. *Journal of Evolutionary Biology* 32(8):856–867. https://doi.org/10.1111/jeb.13487.

D'Alba, L., Shawkey, M. D., Korsten, P., et al. (2010). Differential deposition of antimicrobial proteins in blue tit (*Cyanistes caeruleus*) clutches by laying order and male attractiveness. *Behavioral Ecology and Sociobiology* 64(6):1037–1045. https://doi.org/10.1007/s00265-010-0919-y.

Doneley, B. and Xie, S. (2025). *Avian Medicine and Surgery in Practice*, 3rd Ed. CRC Press.

Faaborg, J. (2020). *Book of Birds – Introduction to Ornithology*. Texas A&M University Press.

Groothuis, T. G., Müller, W., von Engelhardt, N., et al. (2005). Maternal hormones as a tool to adjust offspring phenotype in avian species. *Neuroscience and Biobehavior Reviews* 29(2):329–352. https://doi.org/10.1016/j.neubiorev.2004.12.002.

Hammouda, A., Selmi, S., Pearce-Duvet, J., et al. (2012). Maternal antibody transmission in relation to mother fluctuating asymmetry in a long-lived colonial seabird: The yellow-legged gull *Larus michahellis*. *PLoS One* 7(5):e34966. https://doi.org/10.1371/journal.pone.0034966.

Hrabia, A. (2022). Reproduction in the female. In: *Avian Physiology*, 7th ed., C. G. Scanes and D. Dridi (eds.). pp. 941–986. Academic Press.

Klinger, D. (1991). California condor to return to the wild in 1991 as Fish and Wildlife service announces "The condor is back!" USFWS 91-44, News release.

Kumar, N., van Faassen, M., Kema, I., et al. (2018). Early embryonic modification of maternal hormones differs systematically among embryos of different laying order: A study in birds. *General Comparative Endocrinology* 269:53–59. https://doi.org/10.1016/j.ygcen.2018.08.014.

Martyka, R., Rutkowska, J., and Cichoń, M. (2010). Sex-specific effects of maternal immunization on yolk antibody transfer and offspring performance in zebra finches. *Biology Letters* 7(1):50–53. https://doi.org/10.1098/rsbl.2010.0549.

Mousseau, T. A. and Fox, C. W. (1998). The adaptive significance of maternal effects. *Trends in Ecology & Evolution* 13(10):403–407. https://doi.org/10.1016/S0169-5347(98)01472-4.

Mueller, C. A., Burggren, W. W., and Tazawa, H. (2022). Reproduction in the female. In: *Avian Physiology*, 7th ed., C. G. Scanes and D. Dridi (eds.). pp. 1015–1098. Academic Press.

Nii, T. (2022). Relationship between mucosal barrier function of the oviduct and intestine in the productivity of laying hens. *Journal of Poultry Science* 59(2):105–113. https://doi.org/10.2141/jpsa.0210090.

Nii, T., Sonoda, Y., Isobe, N., et al. (2011). Effects of lipopolysaccharide on the expression of proinflammatory cytokines and chemokines and the subsequent recruitment of immunocompetent cells in the oviduct of laying and molting hens. *Poultry Science* 90(10):2332–41. https://doi.org/10.3382/ps.2011-01596.

Orłowski, G., Merta, D., Pokorny, P., et al. (2019). Eggshell resorption, and embryonic mobilization and accumulation of calcium and metals in eggs of wild and captive Capercaillies *Tetrao urogallus*. *Environmental Pollution* 249:152–162. https://doi.org/10.1016/j.envpol.2019.03.010.

Parolini, M., Possenti, C. D., Romano, A., et al. (2018). Physiological increase of yolk testosterone level does not affect oxidative status and telomere length in gull hatchlings. *PLoS One* 13:e0206503. https://doi.org/10.1371/journal.pone.0206503.

Perez-Rivero, J. (2025). Challenges in bird cryopreservation. *Cryo Letters* 46(2):74–81.

Scanes, C. G. and Christensen K. D. (2020). *Poultry Science*, 5th Ed. Waveland Press, Inc.

Schmucker, S., Hofmann, T., Sommerfeld, V., et al. (2021). Immune parameters in two different laying hen strains during five production periods. *Poultry Science* 100(11):101408. https://doi.org/10.1016/j.psj.2021.101408.

Svobodová, J., Šmídová, L., and Javůrková, V. G. (2019). Different incubation patterns affect selective antimicrobial properties of the egg interior: Experimental evidence from eggs of precocial and altricial birds. *Journal of Experimental Biology* 222(Pt 6):jeb201442. https://doi.org/10.1242/jeb.201442.

Trevelline, B. K., MacLeod, K. J., Knutie, S. A., et al. (2018). *In ovo* microbial communities: A potential mechanism for the initial acquisition of gut microbiota among oviparous birds and lizards. *Biology Letters* 14(7):20180225. https://doi.org/10.1098/rsbl.2018.0225.

Van Veelen, H. P. J., Salles, J. F., Matson, K. D., et al. (2022). The microbial environment modulates non-genetic maternal effects on egg immunity. *Animal Microbiome* 4:44. https://doi.org/10.1186/s42523-022-00195-8.

Wells, R. S., Tornero, V., Borrell, A., et al. (2005). Integrating life history and reproductive success data to examine potential relationships with organochlorine compounds for bottlenose dolphins (*Tursiops truncatus*) in Sarasota Bay, Florida. *Science of the Total Environment* 349:106–119.

Section 3

Environmental Challenges to Avian Health/Disease

8

Physical Anthropogenic Stressors – Climate Change, Habitat Fragmentation, Air Pollution, Fires, and Fisheries Interactions

Introduction

Physical anthropogenic effects on birds include hunting, overfishing and other fishery interactions, urban noise and light pollution, land use and fragmentation, and air pollution/fires. (Contaminants, heavy metal accumulation, pesticide/fertilizer use, pharmaceuticals in the water are discussed in the next chapter.) These events/actions change bird habitats, can result in interactions with humans or urban structures (power lines, building windows, wind farms, etc.), cause stress, and can compromise welfare. Some species have adapted fairly well to urban life by adapting new or alternative nesting sites and food items, and because some species are not as fearful of, or deterred by, humans as others (e.g., gulls and pigeons). The assumption is that urbanization and habitat fragmentation or change are stressful and negatively interfere with bird health and populations. First, we will go through climate and temperature changes, urbanization and habitat effects, air pollution, and finish with fisheries interactions.

Climate and Temperature Change

Temperatures have increased by 1.1 °C (1.9 °F) in the past decade, with the majority of the increase occurring during the last 50 years (Samset et al., 2023). This means that the rate of temperature change increased more rapidly recently than in the first 50 years. In the past 10 years though, the rate of warming has increased by almost 28% globally (Table 8.1; Samset et al., 2023). In addition to this general increase in global temperature, we have also had an increased number and intensity of heat waves (Frölicher et al., 2018). Storms occur earlier and/or later than they used to and last longer. Different weather patterns, like El Niño, La Nina, and cyclones are changing the "usual" climate conditions and impacting a major upwelling region off the Pacific West Coast of the United States, which in turn affects the upper trophic level species (Clairbaux et al., 2021).

Intense heat can be dangerous, as we know. Public service announcements on television, web, social media, and radio warn us to stay inside when it is extremely hot outside. What do birds do? Birds have thermoregulatory behaviors which allow them to minimize heat uptake and disseminate excess heat out of their body (recall Chapter 3). That is fine

Table 8.1 The rate of temperature increase per decade over the past 50 years.

50 years	20 years	10 years
1973–2022	2003–2022	2013–2022
0.18 °C ± 0.01	0.21 °C ± 0.03	0.23 °C ± 0.08

Source: Adapted from Samset et al., 2023/CC BY 4.0.

for short term. Dehydration from prolonged heat (aka heat stress) is a legitimate concern (Williams et al., 2012). Management of water loss is more challenging for larger bodied birds (because they have less surface area) and is predicted to lead to increased mortality (McKechnie and Wolf, 2010). There are other effects of a changing climate and increasing temperatures. While many speak of temperature increase as a future event, it has already caused negative effects globally (Ripple et al., 2025). Here is a sample of what we know to date about increasing temperature effects on birds.

Arguably, the most well-known consequence of global warming is that colder areas will not remain as cold for as long. Polar ice caps are melting. The poles already have reduced ice formation and shorter persistence of ice coverage due to melting. This affects prey abundance and/or density, especially if fisheries activity is also present and marine mammals are also competing for food. Black guillemots (*Cepphus grylle mandtii*) in the Beaufort Sea, Arctic, have suffered high nestling starvation and death (Divoky et al., 2015). The sea ice has been retreating much faster than before and arctic cod, the guillemots' primary prey, has significantly decreased in abundance. Arctic Brunnich's guillemots (aka thick-billed murre; *Uria lomvia*) and common guillemots (aka common murres; *Uria aalge*) also have declined in population size due to ice loss and increased temperature (Bonnet-Lebrun et al., 2022). Data from a terrestrial species, the bananaquit (*Coereba flaveola*), show that increased storm activity in the pre-breeding season led to lower population growth than in drier years with fewer storms (Boal and Bibles, 2025).

The population of little auks (*Alle alle*) in Greenland decreased to approximately 100 pairs in 2007 due to increased sea surface temperature (SST) and decreased ice (Jakubas et al., 2024). The entire species, though, is listed as "least concern" by IUCN as it is apparently able to manage environmental and prey fluctuations by flexible foraging habitats (Gremillet et al., 2012). Cassin's auklet (*Ptychoramphus aleuticus*) in the northern Pacific Ocean has adopted a "double brooding" strategy wherein they attempt a second breeding attempt in resource-rich years (Johns et al., 2022). This extra nesting has ultimately increased recruitment of breeders to the larger population, which has helped buffer against mortality in the harder years. In Europe, it is predicted that Eurasian oystercatcher (*Haematopus ostralegus*) adult survival will be increased while nest fecundity will be decreased with rising temperatures (van de Pol et al., 2010). These opposing effects should act to maintain population levels.

The largest recorded heatwave to date began in the Fall of 2014 in the NE Pacific Ocean. Temperatures were elevated (higher than three standard deviations above the mean) for two years. Over 62,000 common murres (*U. aalge*) beached dead and/or moribund (Renner et al., 2024; Piatt et al., 2020). This mass mortality event likely totaled almost a million murres, assuming only a mere fraction of stranded birds were found. Fewer adults led to decreased reproductive success and population decline. The increased SST, it is thought, disrupted the lower food chain dynamics leading to decreased prey for the birds. Data on the various murre breeding colonies in that region before, during, and after that heatwave indicate that the population has not recovered to their previous numbers. Murre levels are stable, and that area in the eastern Bering Sea can apparently now only support a lower carrying capacity given the precipitous decline in prey fish (Renner et al., 2024). The Pacific cod (*Gadus macrocephalus*) stocks decreased 80% and humpback whale (*Megaptera novaengliae*) numbers also decreased 20% during this heatwave (Renner et al., 2024). Heatwaves are already increasing in frequency, are lasting longer, and are predicted to accelerate (Frölicher et al., 2018).

Increasing temperatures also have indirect fitness consequences for birds. Red knots (*Calidris canutus canutus*) breed in the Arctic but migrate to the tropics for the winter. These birds' offspring were smaller than previously, with shorter bills and smaller bodies (van Gils et al., 2016). When they got to the winter grounds in the tropics, their survival rates plummeted because their shorter bills could not extract the more nutritious bivalves and they had to consume seagrass instead. Common loon (*Gavia immer*) populations are also negatively affected by the climate in the nonbreeding season (Saunders et al., 2021). Models of increasing temperature show decreased growth rate and body size in black-legged kittiwakes (*Rissa tridactyla*) and the glaucous-winged gull (*Larus larus glaucescens*) but not in thick-billed murres (*Uria lomvia;* Sauve et al., 2023). Consequently, the kittiwake and gull will likely suffer reduced survival. Wild zebra finches (*Taeniopygia castanotis*) decreased their brood visits with increasing temperature (Wheeler et al., 2025).

Another prominent effect of increasing temperature is expansion of habitats and home ranges. It is predicted that almost half of the galliform species in China will have significant range shifts due to increasing temperatures (Li et al., 2010). The range of temperate species is and will continue to increase to the north at 1.48 km/year and to higher altitudes with continued warming (Haase et al., 2025; Zhu et al., 2022; Srinivasan and Wilcove, 2021; Rushing et al., 2020; Lehikoinen et al., 2013; La Sorte and Thompson, 2007). Tropical species' ranges may condense but are not predicted to move northward. Instead, they are projected to suffer population declines and/or declines in species richness (Voskamp et al., 2022; Frishkoff et al., 2016). Data from Australia's rainforests suggest that with climate change endemic and high elevation bird species will decrease by half, while the lower altitude species will increase and move northwards (Williams and de la Fuente, 2021). Models evaluating reproductive output indicate that 57% of avian species will have a decreased number of offspring and species' ranges will decrease by 50% by 2050 (Jetz et al., 2007; Halupka et al., 2023). These numbers are devastating.

Species that are adapted to more variable climates are predicted to have greater thermal tolerances than tropical species (Khaliq et al., 2014). Similarly, species adapted to fragmented landscapes/areas should be generalist foragers, and their populations should have less population turnover due to climate change (Jarzyna et al., 2015). Time will tell if these predictions are correct.

We already have data that some species have shifted their phenology (timing) to begin breeding earlier than previously because of warming. Pied flycatchers (*Fideccula hypoleuca*) have shifted the date of breeding 10 days earlier in the period between 1980 and 2002 (Both, 2010). Eurasian coots (*Fulica atra*) advanced the start of their breeding season and the date of the median laying time, while the total length of the breeding season did not change (Halupka et al., 2020). Common goldeneyes (*Bucephala clangula*) breeding in higher latitudes started breeding earlier and extended their season. Data from 1995 to 2022 indicate that these birds use the start of ice break as their cue to start breeding (Poysa, 2025). However, despite attempts to adapt, their reproductive success has decreased with warming temperatures. Migrating European pied flycatchers *(Ficedula hypoleuca)* have differential plasticity and responsiveness to climate change. Populations at the northern edge of their range have advanced the start of the breeding season twice as much as those birds at the southern edge (8 vs. 3.6 days, respectively,) and they have increased reproductive success while the southern and central populations have not (Vega et al., 2021).

Changes in prey abundance due to melting sea ice and ice floe shifts can impact species abundance. While we know arctic seabird foraging is tied to the ice in some way, the details are important to understand. Evaluation of chemical signatures in eggs of thick-billed murres (*Uria lomvia*) indicated a significant reliance on the ice for foraging and that in years with more ice, murre eggs were larger and had a greater energy density than in years with less ice (Cusset et al., 2019). Interestingly the same was not true for common fulmars (*Fulmaris glacialis*) in the same area, illustrating that there may be very different outcomes and breeding decisions for different species (Gutowsky et al., 2022). The high reliance on sea ice for food and reproduction puts this species at potential risk of population decline due to continuing warming. Little auks (*Alle alle*) in the Arctic rely on zooplankton for food. In years when the sea ice retreats and the summer is ice free, the little auks change their foraging strategy and go to large coastal glaciers that become hotspots for feeding. The zooplankton there get stunned by the cold shock of water influx from the glacial ice and are easier to capture (Grémillet et al., 2015). This plasticity in their foraging strategy has allowed them to maintain their chicks' growth rate at little cost to themselves.

Species that migrate long distances are faced with different challenges than resident species or short distance migrants because they are far away from their destinations and do not know the status of their prey at the distant site. Sedentary and short distance migrants have prolonged their breeding season more than have long distance migrants (Halupka and Halupka, 2017). The Florida scrub jay (*Aphelocoma coerulescens*) (a nonmigratory, sedentary species) has advanced the start of their breeding season in warmer winters in central Florida (Barve et al., 2025). However, despite a longer season and increased nesting attempts, their fledgling success rate has been low.

One issue with shifting the timing to start reproduction earlier is that their new arrival time may not overlap with the abundance of their preferred food ("mismatch timing"). In Europe and Russia where the Pied flycatcher breeds, the population in the oak habitat had significantly fewer caterpillars (their preferred food) to feed on in the hotter years relative to the other habitat types (Burger et al., 2012). Long-distance migrating insectivorous species in the Netherlands suffered a decrease in abundance due to a timing mismatch relative to their insect food source (Both et al., 2010). Data on migratory species of waterfowl from Asia showed desynchronized timing in 12% of species making it challenging for them to find sufficient food (Wei et al., 2024). Changes in migration routes also impact the birds' energetic/energy needs. Adelie penguins (*Pygoscelis adeliae*) in Antarctica use ice movement to direct migration routes and end up traveling farther when they fly along the fjords (Jongsomjit et al., 2024). Endangered Atlantic puffins (*Fratercula arctica*) from large colonies or poor local winter conditions end up migrating farther and visiting less productive foraging areas (Fayet et al., 2017). The extra flight distance and increased foraging effort had a negative effect on reproductive success. For this already endangered species, expending this extra energy will not be sustainable ultimately.

Timing mismatches in migration also affects brood parasitism. The common cuckoo (*Cuculus canorus*) migrates on a timescale more similar to long distance migrants than shorter distance migrants (Saino et al., 2009). The cuckoo's parasitism rate decreased (fewer number of nests parasitized) because it could only parasitize the nests of the longer distance migrants as the timing was unfavorable to use shorter distance migrants' nests. For the cuckoo, this is a negative consequence as it leaves fewer eggs for the other species to raise. But for the population of birds that have fewer nests with cuckoo eggs in them, this is positive.

Several studies have documented morphological changes in birds with globally increasing temperatures. The ecological theories Allen's rule and Bergmann's rule predict that species adapted to warmer climates will have longer appendages and smaller bodies, respectively, to maximize surface area for cooling. Between 2007 and 2017, nestling tree swallows (*Tachycineta bicolor*) had increased body mass and developed longer wing length, which were positively associated with fledging success (Houle et al., 2020). During this period, the temperature and rain were increasing, and there appears to have been selection for those morphological traits. Similarly, Ryding et al. (2024) evaluated morphologic traits of museum specimens in a variety of Australian species from the past century. They demonstrated increased beak surface area, tarsus length, and relative wing length with rising temperatures demonstrating a shared convergent response to climate change. In contrast, a study examining body measurements from a database of almost 98% of all avian species found elongation of appendages only congruent with Allen's rule as did a study of Australian shore birds (Fröhlich et al., 2023; McQueen et al., 2024).

Are these phenotypic changes random or associated with heritable genetic changes consistent with natural selection? We do not know for certain. But there are some data that show clear relationships with genetic changes. Four decades of data on the hermit thrush (*Catharus guttatus*) show that a reduction in beak size is paralleled by changes in a particular allele associated with this trait (Adams et al., 2025). Bosse et al. (2017) have found a gene that is related to increasing beak length, and which is positively associated with reproductive success in great tits (*Parus major*). This change in beak length appears to be related to the utilization of bird feeders! In addition, genomic studies are uncovering linkages of morphological traits (including bill morphology and wing length) with particular alleles (Campagna and Toews, 2022). These data will allow us to rigorously test heritability and answer some of these questions.

The future of bird populations and biodiversity in the tropics is also heavily influenced by humans – land use, agricultural development, urbanization, etc. (Khaliq et al., 2023). These factors make it harder to predict population levels and health. The major health effects of increasing global temperatures will likely be due to the expansion of habitats and ranges of not only birds, but all species, *including* infectious agents of disease and their vectors! We will return to that in Chapter 10.

Urbanization and Land/Habitat Change

Urban sprawl is the effect of people living in cities and spreading out to create (or impinge upon) suburbs. Further spread impinges on rural communities and open land. Urbanization involves buildings, often tall apartment or office buildings with limited green space/grass associated with it. It involves lights (lots of lights!) shining on long

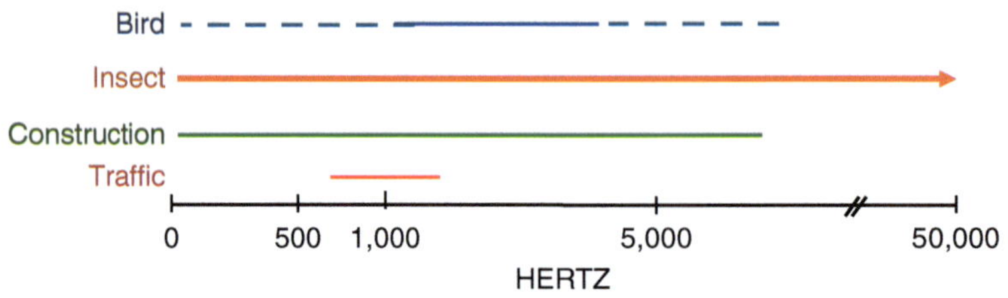

Figure 8.1 Frequency (hertz) of bird hearing relative to city noises and insect prey. Solid line for birds indicates the most common frequencies; dashed line represents less common frequencies.

into the night. It includes cars, trucks, fire engines, and other moving vehicles that are constantly making lots of traffic noise. Traffic and construction noise directly overlap with the hearing range of birds (Figure 8.1). (However, interestingly, burrowing owls, *Athene cunicularia*, in South Florida thrive around airport runways with deafening jet noise on a daily basis.) And along with noise, automobiles are very good at contributing to air pollution. Driving has become much more stressful for people (ok, for me), so it is reasonable to assume wild birds that live in urban areas also get stressed. And in fact, that is exactly what we are seeing.

Creating apartment buildings, office buildings, and roads involves the use of solid, impermeable materials. These materials absorb heat and contribute to local heating with heat literally radiating off the ground. In the mid to higher latitudes, this extra heat production may be nice. But in tropical and lower latitudes, more heat may be very stressful and cause heat stress and dehydration. In addition to heat production, buildings may act as barriers, and the cities can appear fragmented. Avian species that are more sedentary are more likely to respond to buildings as barriers to movement. Natural predators are usually absent within cities. But they are often replaced by new predators – domestic cats, corvids, and small mammals. Power lines and cables can also be places of injury to birds (Revorêdo et al., 2025).

What about interactions with people? Even increasing numbers of people in/near foraging habitats can be a problem. Consider gulls wanting to forage on a beach shoreline. This is nearly impossible for them to do if the beach is crowded with people. Depending on the location, the nearest other shoreline may be a long distance away. It pains me to even write this, but I have seen (in Miami) gulls scavenging food from a dumpster (Figure 8.2)! (This is apparently not uncommon. However, I am embarrassed for them!) AND not only are there peer-reviewed literature articles on gulls frequenting garbage landfills, but there is also one about a gull repeatedly riding in a garbage truck back and forth to a dump station (Cimino et al., 2025)!! (But I digress).

Very simply and succinctly, data indicate that land fragmentation, light at night, increased noise, and human proximity are all physiologically stressful and have negative reproductive/population consequences for most species. Human disruption of land even includes guano (seabird feces) harvesting which has resulted in disruption of food webs and breeding interference of seabirds (Box 8.1). On the other hand, we can potentially see early workings of natural selection on changing morphological traits in several avian species that have successfully integrated into cities. We can compare them with their rural population counterpart to assess the changes. This aspect is very cool!

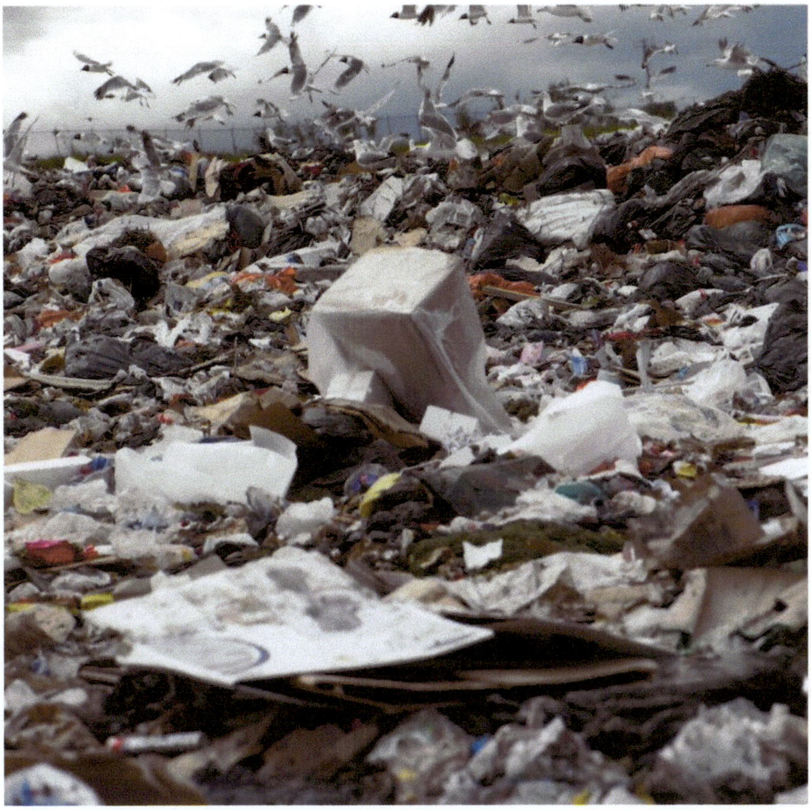

Figure 8.2 Seagulls at a garbage dump. Need I say more?

Box 8.1 Guano harvesting

Years ago, back to approximately 1000 AD, the Inca people were the first to recognize guano as an asset. Guano is fecal material (which appears white in color) from seabirds that roost and/or breed on mountain cliffs (and from bats in caves). The Inca discovered that guano was an excellent fertilizer for their food crops, and this contributed to stable communities at that time (Scarrow, 2021). So important was guano to their culture that they had a "law" forbidding people from harming or killing the birds that made the guano.

Speed forward to 20th-century humans. We, too, discovered the riches of guano; however, in our collection of it, we have destroyed roosting and breeding habitats of the very birds we depend on. Contrary to how the Inca people respected guano harvesting, modern humans relegate it to a menial task, low-paying job with poor working conditions and numerous safety issues. Dust from the harvesting contains microbes and spores which, if inhaled in large quantities, can make those workers ill. And we may be impacting local indigenous cultures in those areas.

Guano forms over years and years. It is rich in nitrogen and phosphorus nutrients. It has a definite ecological role in supporting microbial and insect communities (Justel-Diez et al., 2023). If overharvested, the local environment loses these nutrients,

(Continued)

Box 8.1 (Continued)

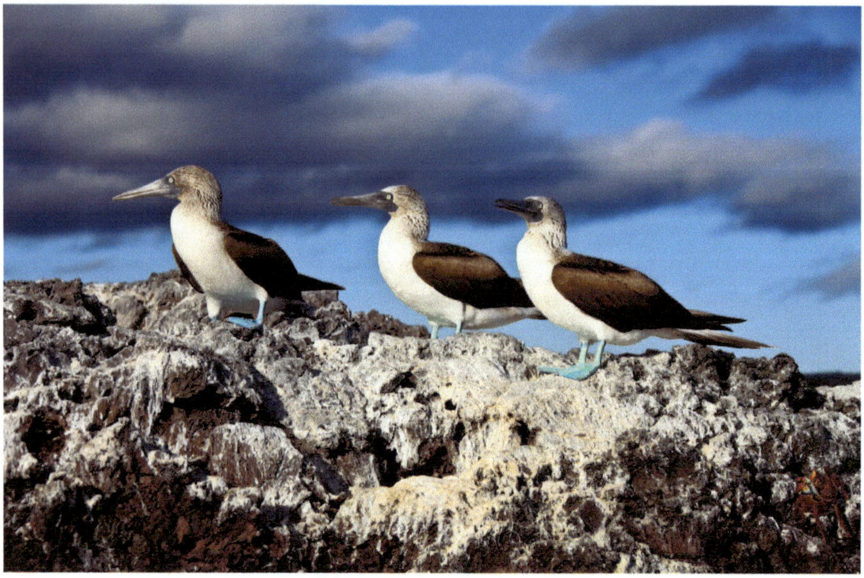

Blue-footed boobies standing on a cliff with guano.

affects food webs and productivity, and can contribute to land and soil degradation. So how can we more respectfully collect the guano? We can harvest guano in the nonbreeding seasons so as not to affect breeding success. We can also only partially harvest any single area and rotate areas so as not to deplete all the guano. Proper safety equipment and proper compensation will help the industry. And finally, perhaps we should include the local cultures in decision-making about guano harvesting? The ecological effect of guano in the oceans and on land is significant as a refuge for many birds and animals.

We do not yet know everything about the effects on urbanization on birds. Let's look at a sample of what we have learned so far about bird health and urbanization.

Light and Noise Pollution

Excess and continuous light (including light at night) and noise are referred to as light and noise pollution. Only in experimental exposures of birds can we begin to decipher the effect of light independent of noise and vice versa. In the urban environment, they are usually intertwined. Overall, urban environments seem to have negative effects on birds new to this environment. The urban environment has negatively affected survival in great tits (*Parus major*). Those raised in the urban habitat had shorter telomeres, evidence of oxidative damage in their cells, and reduced survival over the winter (Isaksson et al., 2024; Grunst et al., 2020; Injaian et al., 2019; Salmon et al., 2017). (Telomeres are the outer protective ends of the chromosomes. They normally shorten with aging, so shorter telomeres are interpreted as a shorter lifespan.) Tree swallow (*Tachycineta bicolor*) nestlings raised with continuous white noise had differential stress and immunologic responses. Lighter weight nestlings had lower plasma corticosterone and higher feather corticosterone than heavier nestlings (Obomsawin et al., 2021). In addition, their immunologic response when challenged was decreased relative to heavier nestlings. These data suggest that there may be some physiologic and/or immunologic stress/effect from noise in developing altricial young. Altricial nestlings cannot escape from background noise because they are confined to the nest until fledging time. A study of these species can provide lots of information on nestling developmental processes in response to urbanization.

Light into the night and on earlier in the morning can trigger release of reproductive releasing hormones and shift the timing of reproduction (Isaksson, 2018). Various studies have shown induction of metabolic enzymes in response to noise, specifically, military type noise did so more than road traffic or human activity noise (Amjad et al., 2024). Corticosterone levels were acutely elevated with increased noise in nestling tree swallows (*Tachycineta bicolor*) and in western bluebirds (*Sialia mexicanus*) both of whom had reduced nesting success (Injaian et al., 2019; Kleist et al., 2018). In addition to stress-induced increases in corticosterone, urbanization resulted in the increase of other stress markers. In six Brazilian bird species, increased noise resulted in an increased heterophil : lymphocyte ratio characteristic of a stress leukogram and increased haptoglobin in great tits (Ribeiro et al., 2022; Ziegler et al., 2021; Raap et al., 2017).

Land fragmentation and changes in tree cover affect densities of insects that prefer canopy cover (Viljur et al., 2022). This decreases the abundance of insectivorous and omnivorous bird species, thereby contributing to decreased species richness or diversity (Deng et al., 2025; Marquis et al., 2025; Senzaki et al., 2024; Morelli et al., 2023; Senzaki et al., 2020). A retrospective study on land use changes found that forest specialists and cavity nesters had reduced distributions while mixed forest and deciduous forest generalist species' distributions did not change (Regos et al., 2018). Larger and heterogenous parcels (larger "fragments") of forest land are correlated with species persistence and greater prevalence of native species (vs. exotic species; Arévalo et al., 2022; Fröhlich and Ciach, 2019; Michalski and Peres, 2017). Birds living in urban areas in Brazil had an increased heterophil : lymphocyte ratio stress response than did rural birds (Santos et al., 2025). In addition, this stress was negatively correlated with body condition, so the greater the stress response, the poorer the body condition.

Noise and light pollution were shown to cause decreased abundance of Eurasian coots (*Fulica atra*; Mathiaparanam et al., 2024). This effect was seen independently for light and noise and was magnified when evaluated together. Similarly, synergistic effects were seen in a study of 140 North American avian species (Wilson et al., 2021). Early developmental noise exposure to eggs during the last week of incubation in laboratory-reared zebra finches (*T. castanotis*) resulted in increased embryonic death, and the survivors had reduced reproductive success when they reached adulthood (Meillère et al., 2024). Great tits (*P. major*) laid smaller clutches and had poorer fledgling success in noisier than in quieter areas (Halfwerk et al., 2010). Budgerigar (*Melopsittacus undulatus*) breeders experimentally exposed to increased light at night had decreased egg production, and the eggs had low hatchability (Malek and Haim, 2019).

The most obvious problem of noise relates to interference of vocal communication (for intra and interspecific communication) and hearing (including for predator/prey detection). Studies have shown that birds can modulate the volume (amplitude), pitch, etc. of their song and calls in regard to environmental noise but results were variable and did not apply to all species (Cho et al., 2025; de Framond et al., 2025; Deoniziak and Osiejuk, 2021; Curry et al., 2018; Francis, 2015). Omnivorous birds were more sensitive to excess noise and selected foraging locations with less noise interference, likely to avoid prey detection issues (Francis, 2015). Tawny owls (*Strix aluco*) exposed experimentally to noise had difficulty locating prey with acoustic cues but compensated by using visual cues (Passarotto et al., 2025). In terms of predator detection, noise pollution can drown out alarm calls of an impending predator (Templeton et al., 2016; Matyjasiak et al., 2023; Jung et al., 2020). These effects will worsen with increasing temperature and humidity, as these factors aid sound in traveling farther.

Effects of noise on behavior have been observed. Western bluebird (*Sialia mexicana*) parents fed nestlings fewer times with short-term experimental exposure to noise (Ozkan et al., 2024). However, continual noise led to the opposite effect, suggesting responses to noise may differ if acute or chronic in nature. Activity patterns of great tits (*P. major*) in urban settings were modified relative to those of individuals in forest populations (Dominoni et al., 2020). Other studies have shown increased nest visits and vigilance behavior with increased noise (Duarte et al., 2023; Liu et al., 2022). Sleep patterns were also negatively affected in great tits (Ouyang et al., 2017). Noise and light pollution affected cognition, learning, and motor skills in experimentally exposed zebra finches (*Taeniopygia castanotis*) and western Australian magpies (*Gmynorhina tibicen dorsalis*; Osbrink et al., 2021; Blackburn et al., 2023).

So far, we have identified a lot of negative effects of city life on birds. But some species, such as pigeons, some sparrow species and European starlings, are good at adapting and have some positive experiences near people. Azure-winged magpies (*Cyanopia cyanus*) had less brood parasitism in urban areas compared to nests in rural areas (Liu et al., 2025). This was positively related to reproductive success and reduced energy expenditure, which suggests that urban areas may be refuges from parasitism behavior. Promising findings regarding plasticity and adaptation were noted in dark-eyed juncos (*Junco hyemalis*) in southern California. Bressler et al. (2020) note that nesting higher off the ground and on artificial surfaces led to increased fitness. They documented the same successful nesting features in both Los Angeles and San Diego populations and noted that successful pairs renested in similar locations on subsequent nesting attempts. These findings suggest plasticity and convergence of behavior across these two populations. Flexibility and plasticity are crucial for resiliency, which will be imperative for many birds.

Humans are great at helping birds by providing nesting boxes, bird feeders, and bird baths. And bird numbers shoot up! (There are few things are more exciting than seeing – and hearing- a huge flock of parrots flying around here in Miami!) When/if these species (some exotic, I know) can displace others, then alternative foraging habitats open up that they capitalize on. Without entering into the debate about "exotic" species' "rights," no matter what bird species are in our cities and feeding at our feeders, urbanization has created more foci of bird aggregations. Reduction of wetlands due to climate change, drying up wetlands, reclamation, and change to agriculture and farming land has also created areas of large avian aggregations. This is especially notable during migration when birds "stop over" at wetlands to eat, refuel, and/or rest. These areas create high-density situations, which can lead to intra- and interspecific competition for resources and are excellent conditions for density-dependent processes, such as pathogen spread, to thrive.

A single bird feeder cannot accommodate hundreds of birds at a time; however, repetitive visits by the same or different birds can lead to the same "aggregation" outcome as decreased wetlands. That outcome is an increased spread of infectious diseases. Infectious diseases, by definition, infect/go from one host to the other. The more dense or large the aggregation, the greater the potential disease spread/infection rate. Meta-analysis of terrestrial changes that resulted in avian aggregations revealed that 53% of scientific papers reported increased disease prevalence, while only 21% reported decreases in disease prevalence (Brearley et al., 2013). The data are accumulating.

I am not "blaming" birds, but data are very clear that migrating birds are the vehicles of infectious disease spread around the world (see disease Chapter 11). At areas of bird aggregation, feces, feather shedding, etc. can leave infectious particles on the ground for other individuals to unintentionally ingest or inhale. I am not advocating that we should stop using bird feeders. However, since many of the infectious agents in bird droppings can infect humans, we humans need to adjust how we manage (or clean) those feeding stations/bird feeder areas. In addition to disease particle transmission, many of the bacteria in feces may have "anti-microbial resistance" genes, which can horizontally pass to other local bacteria, furthering the spread of antibiotic resistance. Arguably, the biggest health threat to birds (and people) is these "new" aggregation areas. The infectious agent may be new to the area, and local birds may not have immunity to it. This can lead to mass mortality of local birds. People can be at risk also.

So, what can we do to mitigate bird (and human) disease in cities? Most humans live in urban areas. These issues will continue unless we advocate and make some changes. Some suggestions of what can be done are provided in Table 8.2.

Table 8.2 Actions to help mitigate bird issues with urbanization.

- A little "nature" outside the window is nice! We can clean the area below the feeder to avoid feces building up. Clean and disinfect the bird feeder on a regular basis. These actions will help decrease the potential for the spread of any agent.
- In high-density housing areas/apartment buildings, know your neighbors. If any of the closest ones are immunocompromised, then they would be the most at risk of getting sick. It isn't your responsibility, but it is considerate. And if you are immunosuppressed, wear a mask when cleaning those areas.
- Be active and good stewards of the environment. Donate to or assist in groups/activities that work with potential areas of bird aggregations, like wetlands. The larger those areas are, the lower the infectious rates will be because the density of individuals would be lower.
- Properly dispose of house waste and food items, especially into containers that seal well. Recycle whatever you can to reduce the load of waste. Excess food/food waste can be donated to local gardens for composting.
- Know where the nearest wildlife rehabilitation center is located.

Air Pollution/Fires

The canary in the coal mine – early in the 1900s, coal workers used to bring a canary in a small cage down into the coal mines in which they worked (Figure 8.3). This canary was their sentinel to detect for increased levels of odorless carbon monoxide and/or other toxic gases. If the canary showed any signs of illness (fell over, changed respiration, dropped dead), the coal miners would take this as a sign that it was not safe to remain down in the mine, and they would exit the mine at the surface. A bird – in this case, a canary (not sure why not a different species of bird) – was used because of birds' known sensitivity to airborne chemicals/toxins, their rapid metabolism, and rapid gas exchange in the respiratory system.

Air pollution, I would argue, is the worst of all the anthropogenic insults for birds. The birds can live and nest in a huge heterogeneous habitat, but they still must breathe the polluted air. Bird respiratory systems are very large and very sensitive to what is inhaled. Birds have a good respiratory immune response, but the area of pulmonary tissue and the increased efficiency of absorption of air particles can be a double-edged sword. If there is anything else other than oxygen in the air they breathe, that will cross into the bloodstream as well.

Enter human industrialization and development. Increasing air pollution from automobiles, construction, etc. Increasing numbers of wildfires and smoke. The ability of tiny pathogens to become airborne on a particle of dirt, sand, or a droplet of water. Do you see where we are heading?

Air pollution is a major public health concern for humans and animals and is predicted to continue increasing in the coming years. Between 2011 and 2020, the human mortality

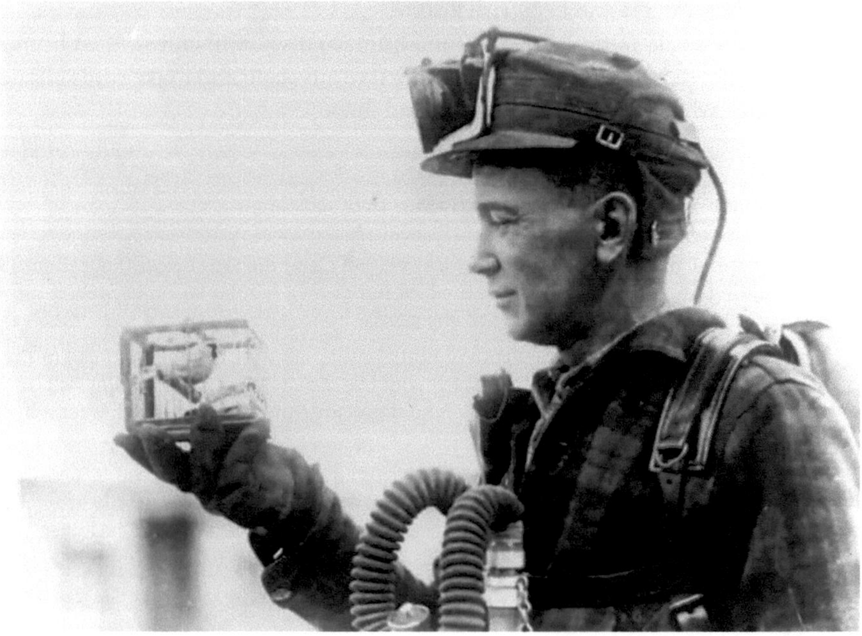

Figure 8.3 Mining foreman R. Thornburg shows a small cage with a canary used for testing carbon monoxide gas in 1928. *Source:* United States Bureau of Mines/George McCaa/Public domain.

rate increased by 73% per year due to smoke from fires (Qiu et al., 2025). The number of studies on the effects of air pollution on birds has risen significantly since 2000 (Sanderfoot and Holloway, 2017). Typical air pollution involves a mixture of gaseous substances, particulate matter (PM), and water vapor (Zhou et al., 2025). Natural sources that contribute to air pollution include fires, volcanic eruptions, winds, sandstorms, and sea spray from the oceans. Anthropogenic sources include combustible fossil fuels from cars, industry, agricultural practices, deforestation, and sewage treatment plants. There may be metals or other contaminants attached to droplets or PM. PM found in air pollution can range from 10 to 10^{-9} meters in diameter. Because of their size, the larger PM deposit in the nasal cavity or upper respiratory tract. However, the smaller diameter PM can penetrate farther down into the tract and potentially cause severe respiratory or other organ diseases.

Urban sprawl and human encroachment into new areas have and will increase the intensity of exposure to air pollution. Smaller PM in the air can stay aerosolized for weeks. Exposure to air pollution can cause mild health conditions in humans, such as allergies and rhinitis, or can result in more severe conditions such as pneumonia or potentially cancer by increasing DNA damage and altering telomere length (Sanderfoot Holloway, 2017). On the cellular and metabolic level, air pollution causes increased inflammation and oxidative stress, cell damage, immune suppression, and decreased pulmonary function among other changes (Radbel et al., 2024; Sanderfoot and Holloway, 2017). Allergens or infectious agents can attach to the particles inhaled and affect the health of the person/animal. Indoor air pollution derives in part from outdoor air pollution which enters the home, and from indoor appliances, compounds aerosolized from the operation of gas heaters, gas stoves, air conditioning, and activities such as tobacco smoking (Qiu et al., 2025). Tobacco smoking is likely the largest cause of indoor air pollution affecting birds. Not only does the smoke and its toxic constituents enter the respiratory system, but they can also adhere to the skin and negatively affect other body systems. These findings have been found in pet cats and dogs, but likely also extend to birds or other pets in a smoker's household (Smith et al., 2017; Knottenbelt et al., 2012).

In birds, the clinical manifestations of air pollution, cigarette smoke, and humidity extremes are similar to those in humans. These manifestations include inflammation of the nares (rhinitis), sinuses (sinusitis), trachea (tracheitis), and bronchial tree (bronchitis). In rhinitis and sinusitis, you will see discharge from the nares and may see the bird shaking its head, sneezing, or scratching and rubbing their faces (Doneley and Xie, 2025). The discharge may also be seen on the facial feathers below the nares, around the eyes, and the nares may be enlarged and swollen. In severe cases, the bird may have trouble breathing. Histopathologic examination of the respiratory tract in birds after chronic experimental exposure to vehicle emissions showed a reduction in the number and shortening of the tracheal cilia, increased mucus, and other alterations to the respiratory epithelium (Llacuna et al., 1993). Anthracosis (deposition of carbon particles) in the lungs from air pollution was found in 55% of zoo animals, 45% of companion animals, and 28% of wildlife species (Leya et al., 2023). The organ changes above would make it difficult to remove PM from the airway. In addition to the effects of PM, nitrous oxide and ozone in air pollution negatively affect cellular metabolism and defense mechanisms (Radbel et al., 2024).

Natural fires shape biodiversity in many forests and habitats. In fact, controlled fires (controlled or prescribed burns) are a tool to manage the health of an assemblage of vegetation by clearing decaying material and removing potential fuel that can feed a wildfire. With anthropogenic climate and land use changes, hotter and drier conditions are conducive to fires, which are predicted to be larger and more severe than natural fires. The changing abundance of forest species may be directly related to some aspects of fire, and avian abundances can severely decrease in large "megafires" (McGinn et al., 2025; García-Redondo et al., 2023). For example, greater sage grouse (*Centrocercus urophasianus*) experienced 40% adult mortality and 79% nest failure when fires in 2015–2016 burned the sagebrush vegetation that they depended on (Tyrrell et al., 2023). Severe fires, air pollution, and smoke contributed to mass mortality of migrating birds in the western United States (Yang et al., 2021).

Wildfire smoke is a complex mixture of PM, gases such as carbon monoxide and nitrogen oxide, and volatile and semi-volatile organic compounds, including acetaldehyde, chloroform, and formaldehyde. PM from wildfire smoke has a high content of elemental carbon, organic carbon, and heavy metals (Chen et al., 2021). From a literature review, data indicate that at least one variable associated with fitness and welfare in birds was negatively affected by smoke exposure (Barton et al., 2023). These variables include (but aren't limited to) DNA damage that can lead to cancer, reproduction, survival, altered pulmonary microflora, metabolic abnormalities, inflammation, and susceptibility to other lung diseases (Barton et al., 2023; Wang et al., 2023). Most of the pathology arises from PM. Experimental exposure of ducks to carbon nanoparticles resulted in liver pathology and initiation of apoptosis (Al-Badri et al., 2019). Furthermore, $PM_{2.5}$ (particulate matter 2.5 nm in size) has been associated with the acquisition of antimicrobial resistance genes, which can lead to increased secondary bacterial infections that are difficult to treat (Zhou et al., 2025). Twenty years of banding data found that there were two distinct behavior and health changes in birds exposed to fire smoke (Nihei et al., 2024). The "acute" effect from PM inhalation resulted in decreased activity of the birds (fewer were captured). In the "chronic" effect, activity rate returned to normal, but body condition decreased over multiple seasons. Finally, to add insult to injury, increased aridity and drought (which are projected to occur with climate warming) lead to increased PM in the air and also lead to more wildfires (Lee et al., 2025).

Small, lower severity fires can be useful to clear out the underbrush, and these may have little impact on the resident birds. Forest owls, especially small cavity nesting species, were not affected by small fires in California (McGinn et al., 2025). Wildfire can also destroy large stretches of land or forest. After the fire, new and invasive species can move in, displacing native species. This pattern can lead to a decrease in plant diversity and the homogenization of plants and animals. This then affects the community of invertebrates and seeds available for consumption (Tyrrell et al., 2023). Avian diversity can also change after fires and potentially be advantageous to certain species by decreasing the density of birds (decreased competition, greater food/bird) at that location overall (Rey et al., 2019). Alternatively, birds in smaller habitats, islands, and or in populations with genetic bottlenecks may suffer greater losses than in larger areas (Brown et al., 2013; Barbet-Massin and Jiguet, 2011). Species with strong site fidelity will also be more susceptible to population decrease if their habitat is burned and prey abundance and/or nesting habitat is decreased (O'Neil et al., 2020). Wildfires and smoke can alter bird movements and social networks (Johnson et al., 2023; Gosper et al., 2019).

Managing fires can have unexpected negative consequences. Polyfluoroalkyl substances (PFA) from the firefighting foam seeped into the sediment, killed invertebrate prey, and subsequently, the resident flamingo population there plummeted (Foekema, 2017). Flamingos returned the next year and fed in the toxic area again. The chronic effects of those PFAs on the flamingos are not known. In addition to adsorption of firefighting chemicals, the soil/sediment also suffers a decrease in nutrients, making it potentially substandard for foraging after fires (Sousa-Lima et al., 2025).

Some species of birds specialize in foraging in burnt forests. Black-backed woodpeckers (*Picoides arcticus*) specialize in burnt ponderosa pine forests (Hutto, 2008). Frank et al. (2025) found that fire-origin stands supported 8.8 more species than clear-cut stands immediately following disturbance (2–5 years), including a greater number of cavity-nesting species. Distinct bird communities in recently burned forests suggest that these areas may be especially valuable for promoting biodiversity.

In summary, wildfires are projected to increase in frequency and severity due to global warming and associated anthropomorphic changes. There are various factors that relate to whether the population of birds will increase or decrease, including habitat type, species biology, vegetation, etc., except of course if the fire was very severe. More data are needed to understand and predict how specific populations will respond and to understand the long-term effects of smoke inhalation and the contaminants in fire-fighting chemicals/agents.

Fisheries Interactions

Commercial and artisanal fisheries exist worldwide to supply seafood for global and local consumption, respectively. Annually worldwide, approximately 200 million tons of fish and seafood are fished and/or produced! This includes commercial "fish farming" – aquaculture – which may be located in oceans, bays, or on land. Commercial fisheries exist for various fish, invertebrate, and algal species. Due to overfishing of the oceans and new technological advances, aquaculture production now produces about half of the commercial seafood as do fisheries. The long-term sustainability of fisheries is complicated by climate change and anthropogenic changes (Cheung et al., 2025).

Fisheries equipment (nets and boats) often causes direct and indirect damage to piscivorous birds. There are various types of nets that are deployed to catch seafood, each with its own complement of negative consequences for birds (Figure 8.4). Large-scale fishery operations use purse seine nets and trawls mostly. Trawls, which are pulled along the sea floor, are the most common method used in industrial fishing. They account for approximately 25% of the total catch. Trawls at mid-water level catch an additional 10% of the total. Purse seine nets are the second most common and account for about 20% of the catch. However, nets cause more severe injury to the birds. Gillnets, long line, and pole and line fishing are the fishing types used more often in the smaller and artisanal fisheries. As is evident in the figure of the various fishing gear, all involve the use of fishing lines and/or nets. Fishing hooks and weights (sinkers) are used in pole and line and longline fishing. Different types of fish are caught by various techniques.

Birds take advantage of the fishing boats (and aquaculture pens) to get an easy meal (Figure 8.5). That is the positive part of the bird's interaction with fisheries! An easy meal often comes from the undesired seafood parts that are discarded from fishing boats during processing. However, there are various direct and indirect dangers (negative effects) to birds associated with fisheries operations. The main direct danger to birds is drowning from getting caught in nets and lines. Indirect negative impacts to birds include reduced

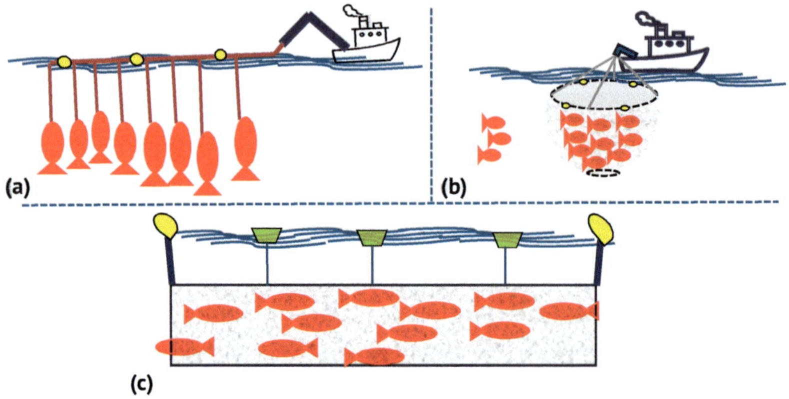

Figure 8.4 Fishing net types. (a) Longline fishing. Use for pelagic (mid-water) or demersal (bottom) fishing. (b) Purse seine net. Used for dense schools of a single fish species. (c). Gill net. A wall of net that hangs in the water. Not specific to species of fish. Size of mesh determines which fish are caught.

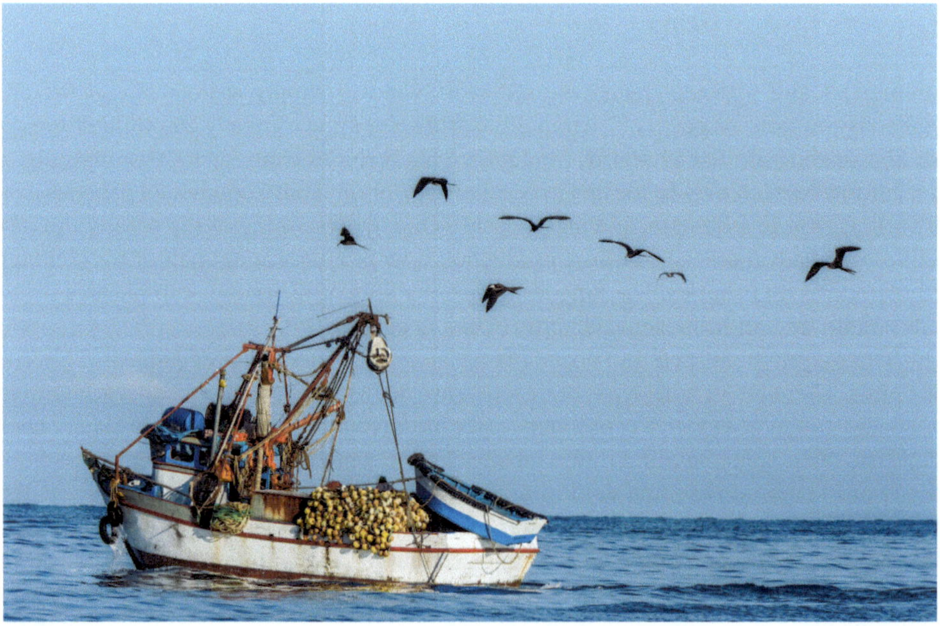

OSTILL/Getty Images

Figure 8.5 Fishing boat attracting birds.

prey abundance from overfishing and chronic effects from nonlethal injuries and stress from getting tangled in nets. Fishing lines, hooks, and sinkers from recreational fishers can also negatively affect birds. They can get entangled, injured, and/or swallow hooks and sinkers, potentially leading to lead poisoning (see below). Fishing gear is responsible for 83% of plastic entanglements in birds since 2014 (Ryan, 2018). Seabird entanglements have increased 16–25% since 2014. Let's look at the health effects of fisheries interactions in more detail.

Evidence of by-catch mortality is sometimes found at necropsy. Necropsy of gulls (*Larus* spp.) along the Norwegian coast revealed fluid in the lungs, edema, and multiorgan congestion. The birds were in moderate to good body condition. This is consistent with drowning (Christensen-Dalgaard et al., 2022; Ewbank et al., 2020). Other times, mortality is witnessed and/or inferred from the relationship between the birds' location and the boats' locations. More and more studies are finding significant overlap and co-occurrence between fishing boats and seabirds. Male and female Magellanic penguins (*Spheniscus magellanicus*) in Patagonia have differential foraging areas part of the year; however, there is considerable overlap of penguin foraging areas (no difference between the sexes) and fishery areas (Dodino et al., 2021). Southern giant petrels (*Macronectes giganteus*) forage in areas that overlap with fishery activity when feeding young (Blanco et al., 2022). Antarctic petrels (*Thalassoica antarctica*) and several species of Pygoscelid penguins are often found foraging in krill fishing areas adjacent to fishing boats (Hinke et al., 2017; Descamps et al., 2016).

Several studies have employed GPS-type tags on birds to monitor where birds forage and their relation to fishing boats. Individuals from three species of shearwaters (*Calonectris diomeda, C. borealis, C. edwardsii*) were tagged with instruments that could record adjacent boats' radar signals (Navarro-Herrero et al., 2024). Data from this study showed a high degree of association of birds with fishing vessels on fishing grounds but also identified some boats that were illegally fishing! In Alaskan waters, seabirds were found to overlap with fishing vessels and boats in high-traffic vessel corridors (Kapsar et al., 2025). This proximity to boats in high traffic areas can lead to injury. Northern fulmars (*Fulmarus glacialis*) in the North Atlantic have increased visits/attendance to fishing boats over the past 10 years, even though there is an increased risk of injury (Darby et al., 2023). Data suggest there is an energy-saving component for these birds to follow the boats and consume the fish discards even though the risk is higher rather than foraging on their own. However, this change in foraging tactics may also reflect a decrease in their natural prey.

Birds are smart! They learn to follow the fishing boats and gauge the risk versus the quality of the food they will receive and the costs of foraging on their own (Bodey et al., 2014). Northern gannets (*Morus bassanus*) learned to switch foraging tactics depending on the type of vessel and gear on the fishing boat! If the gannets saw a trawler vessel moving along, they preferred to forage on their own. If the trawler was idle/drifting, the gannets switched tactics and preferred to commute to where the vessel was. When the trawler was stopped or drifting, the crew was likely processing the previous catch so there would be a lot of discards to eat. They preferred the reverse when they encountered non-trawling vessels (Bodey et al., 2014). Scopoli shearwaters (*Calonectris diomeda*) in the south Mediterranean Sea opted to fly farther distances to be close to fishing boats and eat the fish discards rather than to forage on their own (Cianchetti-Benedetti et al., 2018). This even though the discards were of less nutritional value than consuming an entire fish. When the birds were within 1.2 m of the boat, they spent more time in the water waiting for scraps and approached the boat more often.

Avian mortality in gill nets is estimated to be up to 11,000/year along the Norwegian coast in the prior decade (Bærum et al., 2019). Their analyses indicate more severe entanglement and death in gill nets for both surface- and deeper-feeding seabirds than occurs in longline fisheries. Sea ducks suffer 100,000s deaths/year from gill nets (McGrew et al., 2022). Alaskan longline fisheries caused the mortality of over 32,000 seabirds between 1993 and 2001 (Melvin et al., 2019). In Chilean waters, over 19,000 sooty shearwaters

(*Ardenna grisea*) comprised 70% of by-catch mortality from purse seine operations (Simeone et al., 2021). The shearwaters were concentrating in areas where the Chilean anchovy and herring were being fished. Subsequently, the number of bird mortalities decreased by almost 70% between 2002 and 2015. However, this decrease was achieved by threat of penalties for catching endangered seabirds and by mitigation techniques.

It was estimated back in 2011 that approximately 160,000 seabirds are killed per year worldwide from fisheries interactions (Anderson et al., 2011). In 2013, a literature review found an estimated 400,000 birds died per year in gillnets specifically, with most mortality occurring in the Baltic and North Sea region (Žydelis et al., 2009, 2013). Unfortunately, some of the most frequently caught seabirds are albatrosses, petrels, and shearwaters (Order Procellariformes; Ryan, 2018; Anderson et al., 2011; see Box 8.2). Approximately 70% of albatrosses were threatened or endangered in the last decade, and in 2025, only 1 of the 22 species of albatross is categorized as "least concern" (IUCN, 2025). In large part, the decline in numbers is due to by-catch mortality and the fact that these birds are K-selected species and have long generation times, so recovery is slower. Black footed albatross (*Poebastria nigripes*) had significant by-catch mortality in the 1990s, which was reduced by mitigation activities (Beck et al., 2025). Unfortunately, mortality has increased again. While by-catch mortality did play a large role in the demise of some seabird species, laws and public awareness have led to changes in fishery practices and population rebounding of various seabird species.

Mitigation techniques vary between fisheries and locations. The ultimate goal is to reduce by-catch (avian mortality/injury) while preserving the target catch. Mitigation methods include visual alerts, acoustic alerts, spatiotemporal closures when target concentration is high, but bird densities are low, restriction of fishing depths such that the hooks are placed lower in the water column, and changes in fishing gear (Žydelis et al., 2013).

Box 8.2 Albatross and seabird population declines

Seabirds as a group are one of the most threatened, exhibiting continual decreases in abundance, in part due to fisheries interactions and climate change. It is estimated that between 1950 and 2010, the seabird population decreased by 70%. Albatrosses (procellariformes) as a group seem to be one of the most affected. Of the 22 species in this group, two are critically endangered, 7 are endangered, 6 are vulnerable, and 6 are "near threatened" (IUCN, 2025). Ninety percent of species are affected by by-catch, over half of the species are impacted by predators (such as felids and rodents, which prey on the birds and eggs) and other terrestrial threats, and over a third of species have suffered due to climate change and overfishing of prey. Petrels and shearwaters (the other members of the procellariformes) are primarily affected by invading species, by-catch, and effects of urbanization. Already two species of petrels have gone extinct (Dias et al., 2019).

Albatrosses are large, long-lived birds. Their young take a long time to mature to reproductive age, and their generation times are long. They live in colonies, and they can migrate large distances across the world (Votier and Sherley, 2017). Why should we care about these species? As a group, seabirds regulate plankton levels and have key roles in the functioning of marine ecosystems. Albatross and the like are largely

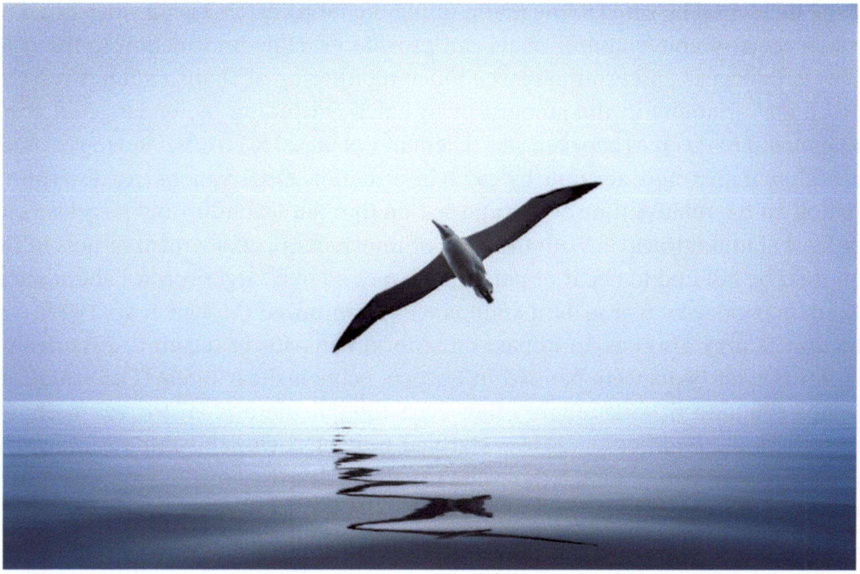
Magann/Adobe Stock Photos

responsible for significant nutrient deposition in the ocean via guano deposits (see Box 8.1). This group also contributes to climate regulation. As a result of guano decomposition, ammonia is released, and this promotes cloud formation, which increases reflectivity of solar radiation to aid cooling (Votier and Sherley, 2017). As a group, these birds are excellent sentinels of our ocean ecosystem and, by extension, human and animal health. Plus, they are sleek and beautiful birds!

Visual alerts or techniques have been tried successfully. Almeida et al. (2023) showed that a large, bird of prey-shaped "kite" (with a five-foot wingspan!) tied to the stern effectively deterred 56% of gulls (*Larus* spp.) and 72% of northern gannets (*Morus bassanus*) from approaching the fishing boats/gill nets in Portugal. Similarly, light-emitting diodes placed on the float lines of gill nets reduced avian by-catch by 84% (and 70% of marine mammal and turtle incidental catch) without affecting catch of the target species (Bielli et al., 2020). Use of streamer lines tied to the nets was also successful in scaring birds away from Alaskan longlines (Melvin et al., 2019). Other attempts to use visual deterrents were not as successful overall. In Newfoundland, Canada, high contrast banners placed at the surface of gill nets decreased avian by-catch but also decreased the target herring catch (Montevecchi et al., 2023).

Auditory deterrents ("pingers') are also being investigated. These devices have been successful in deterring marine mammals and sea turtles from nets. To aid development, McGrew et al. (2022) assessed the hearing ranges of various sea ducks, which are diving foragers, to target the correct hearing range. Other devices in use include weighted fishing hooks in longline fisheries in the north Pacific (Gilman et al., 2022). Fishing hooks were weighted to sink deeper into the water column in a tuna fishery. Avian by-catch was reduced, but so was the target tuna catch! So, this approach needs to be reworked.

Cooperation and collaboration between scientists and fisheries personnel is required to reduce the incidental by-catch while maintaining the target catch. Using video or GPS-type trackers on target seabirds and/or boats can provide valuable information to the fisheries as well as to biologists and ornithologists. Video monitoring of Danish gill net vessels documented high variability in the amount of by-catch (including the endangered common eider (*Somateria mollisima*) between sets (Glemarec et al., 2020). Thus, viewing or assessing more sets should give more accurate by-catch information. Observations can also contribute information on the relative time of day and season that the seabird(s) and target species are most or least abundant/active. With this type of information, deployment of nets in fishing sets can then be tailored to occur at particular times so that target species abundance and activity are maximized while seabird abundance is minimized (Melvin et al., 1999).

Reduction of prey also has an impact on seabird behavior in regard to fisheries operations. After trawler boats were banned in Europe, Scopoli shearwaters (*Calonectris domedea*) visited longline fisheries more often even though there is an increased chance of injury (Soriano-Redondo et al., 2016). Marbled murrelets (*Brachyramphus marmoratus*) in the Pacific Ocean had to switch their diet to krill during the breeding months due to the depletion of sardine populations (Becker and Beissinger, 2006). This step down in trophic level and nutrient density can be costly for this endangered species' reproductive success. In fact, recent data indicate that murrelets in poorer condition (potentially due to this type of diet change?) had higher concentrations of a parasite (*Leucocytozoon*) and attempted fewer or no nestings at all compared to individuals in better body condition (Michlanski et al., 2025). Added to these factors, increasing surface sea water temperatures will be a major contributing factor to reproductive decline and poorer general health (Gibson et al., 2023).

Recreational fishing also contributes to avian injury (Campbell, 2013). Between 1989 and 2012, in New Hampshire, 48% of common loon (*Gavia immer*) mortality was due to lead from ingested fishing tackle (Grade et al., 2019). An assessment of seabird injuries from a recreational fishing area showed that 30% of injuries were moderate, 46% were severe, and 24% were lethal injuries (Beron and Seco, 2021). Hook and line entanglements and hook and sinker ingestion are common in seabirds that frequent piers and fishing areas (Figure 8.6; Donnelly-Greenan, 2019; Ryan, 2018). Along the California coast and Florida's east and west coasts, brown pelicans (*Pelecanus occidentalis*) and other seabirds (usually gulls) are injured by ingestion of fish or fish parts that are still attached to the hook or sinker. Many of these are taken to local rehabilitation centers for care. The percentage of birds that get hook/sinker injuries or are entangled in fishing line varies a lot. A study in California found that brown pelicans accounted for almost 60% of injured birds (between 2001 and 2006) in northern California, while seagull injuries were seen in 16% of cases in the Los Angeles area (Dau et al., 2009). In 2019–2020, the prevalence of brown pelican injury from fishing hooks and lines was only 7% in northern Florida, and it was related to pier size and the number of perching locations (Thomas and Forys, 2022).

In South Florida, brown pelicans and seagulls are common visitors to seabird rehabilitation clinics. The prevalence of hook & sinker and line entanglement was approximately 18% in 2017 but has since decreased to less than 5% (Zaias and Acosta, unpublished data). This decrease may, in fact, be due to continual communication and education about the dangers of leaving fishing line and hooks out or tossing them back into the water. This is the primary message to relay to the public (Simmons, 2025). However, the decrease

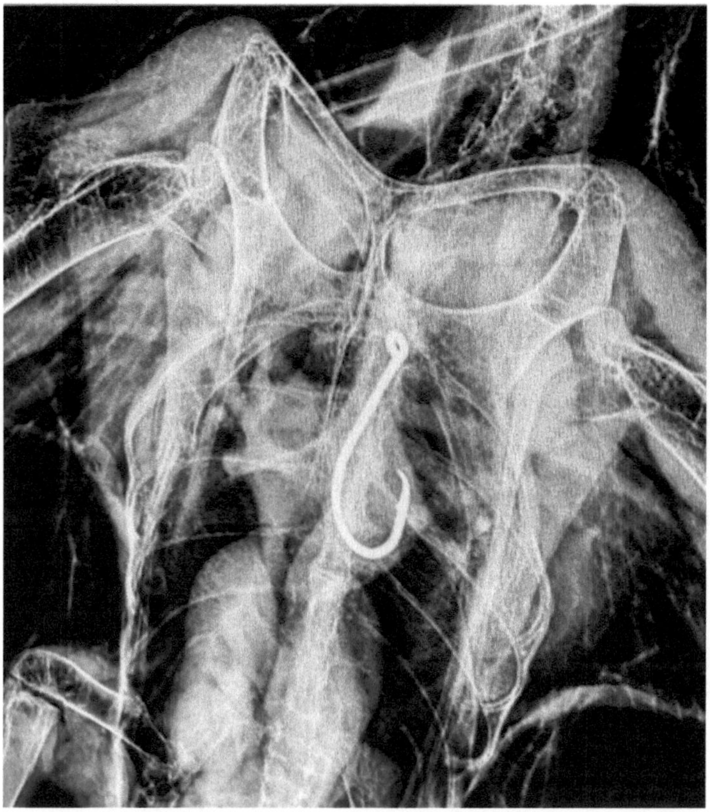

Figure 8.6 Radiograph of a pelican with a lead fishing hook ingested. *Source:* With permission of Y. Costa, Pelican Harbor Seabird Station.

in the percentage of birds entangled may also be due to a delay in finding these birds until they become weak or ill for other reasons. Unless the fishing line was observed on the animal or the bird was radiographed, the original injury/insult would not be known. Both scenarios are likely occurring. What is evident is that ingested lead hooks/sinkers will leach the lead into the bloodstream and could ultimately cause toxicity just like it does in birds hit with lead bullets (Franson et al., 2003).

Literature Cited

Adams, N., Dias, T., Skeen, H. R., et al. (2025). Genetic and morphological shifts associated with climate change in a migratory bird. *BMC Biology* 23(1):3. https://doi.org/10.1186/s12915-024-02107-5.

Al-Badri, A. M., Bargooth, A. F., Al-Jebori, J. G., et al. (2019). Identification of carbon nanotube particles in liver tissue and its effects on apoptosis of birds exposed to air pollution. *Veterinary World* 12(9):1372–1377. https://doi.org/10.14202/vetworld.2019.1372-1377.

Almeida, A., Alonso, H., Oliveira, N., et al. (2023). Using a visual deterrent to reduce seabird interactions with gillnets, *Biological Conservation* 285:110236. https://doi.org/10.1016/j.biocon.2023.110236.

Amjad, R., Ruby, T., Ali, K., et al. (2024). Exploring the effects of noise pollution on physiology and ptilochronology of birds. *PLoS One* 19(6):e0305091. https://doi.org/10.1371/journal.pone.0305091.

Anderson, O. R. J., Small, C. J., Croxall, J. P., et al. (2011). Global seabird bycatch in longline fisheries. *Endangered Species Research* 14:91–106. https://doi.org/10.3354/esr00347.

Arévalo, C., Amaya-Espinel, J. D., Henríquez, C., et al. (2022). Urban noise and surrounding city morphology influence green space occupancy by native birds in a Mediterranean-type South American metropolis. *Scientific Reports* 12(1):4471. https://doi.org/10.1038/s41598-022-08654-7.

Bærum, K. M., Anker-Nilssen, T., Christensen-Dalsgaard, S., et al. (2019). Spatial and temporal variations in seabird bycatch: Incidental bycatch in the Norwegian coastal gillnet-fishery. *PLoS One* 14(3):e0212786. https://doi.org/10.1371/journal.pone.0212786.

Barbet-Massin, M. and Jiguet, F. (2011). Back from a predicted climatic extinction of an island endemic: A future for the Corsican Nuthatch. *PLoS One* 6(3):e18228. https://doi.org/10.1371/journal.pone.0018228.

Barton, M. G., Henderson, I., Border, J. A., et al. (2023). A review of the impacts of air pollution on terrestrial birds. *Science of The Total Environment* 873:162136. https://doi.org/10.1016/j.scitotenv.2023.162136.

Barve, S., Bakley, T. D., Tringali, A., et al. (2025). Warm winters lead to increased reproductive effort, but lower reproductive success: Hidden costs of climate warming in a threatened bird. *Ornithology* 14(1):ukae053. https://doi.org/10.1093/ornithology/ukae053.

Beck, J. N., Baetscher, D. S., Tobin, C., et al. (2025). Quantifying impacts of seabird bycatch using genetic assignment: A case study of black-footed albatross in U.S. fisheries. *Biological Conservation* 303:110965. https://doi.org/10.1016/j.biocon.2025.110965.

Becker, B. H. and Beissinger, S. R. (2006). Centennial decline in the trophic level of an endangered seabird after fisheries decline. *Conservation Biology* 20(2):470–479. https://doi.org/10.1111/j.1523-1739.2006.00379.x.

Beron, M. P. and Seco, P. (2021). Fishing gear-related injuries and mortality of seabirds in coastal northern Argentina. *Marine Ornithology* 49(2):321–327. https://doi.org/10.5038/2074-1235.49.2.1439

Bielli, A., Alfaro-Shigueto, J., Doherty, P. D., et al. (2020). An illuminating idea to reduce bycatch in the Peruvian small-scale gillnet fishery. *Biological Conservation* 241:108277. https://doi.org/10.1016/j.biocon.2019.108277

Blackburn, G., Ashton, B. J., Thornton, A., et al. (2023). Cognition mediates response to anthropogenic noise in wild Western Australian magpies (*Gmynorhina tibicen dorsalis*). *Global Change Biology* 29(24):6912–6930. https://doi.org/10.1111/gcb.16975.

Blanco, G. S., Tonini, M. H., Gallo, L., et al. (2022). Tracking the exposure of a pelagic seabird to marine plastic pollution. *Marine Pollution Bulletin* 180:113767. https://doi.org/10.1016/j.marpolbul.2022.113767.

Boal, C. W. and Bibles, B. D. (2025). Weather events influence survival and recruitment of *Coereba flaveola* (Bananaquit) in the Caribbean. *Ornithology* 142(1):ukae052. https://doi.org/10.1093/ornithology/ukae052

Bodey, T. W., Jessopp, M. J., Votier, S. C., et al. (2014). Seabird movement reveals the ecological footprint of fishing vessels. *Current Biology* 24(11):R514–515. https://doi.org/10.1016/j.cub.2014.04.041.

Bonnet-Lebrun, A. S., Larsen, T., Thórarinsson, T., et al. (2022). Cold comfort: Arctic seabirds find refugia from climate change and potential competition in marginal ice zones and fjords. *Ambio* 51(2):345–354. https://doi.org/10.1007/s13280-021-01650-7.

Bosse, M., Spurgin, L.G., Laine, V. N., et al. (2017). Recent natural selection causes adaptive evolution of an avian polygenic trait. *Science* 358(6361):365–368. https://doi.org/10.1126/science.aal3298.

Both C. (2010). Flexibility of timing of avian migration to climate change masked by environmental constraints en route. *Current Biology* 20(3):243–248. https://doi.org/10.1016/j.cub.2009.11.074.

Both, C., Van Turnhout, C. A., Bijlsma, R. G., et al. (2010). Avian population consequences of climate change are most severe for long-distance migrants in seasonal habitats. *Proceedings of Biological Science* 277(1685):1259–1266. https://doi.org/10.1098/rspb.2009.1525.

Brearley, G., Rhodes, J., Bradley, A., et al. (2013). Wildlife disease prevalence in human-modified landscapes. *Biologic Reviews Cambridge Philosophical Society* 88(2):427–442. https://doi.org/10.1111/brv.12009.

Bressler, S. A., Diamant, E. S., Tingley, M. W., et al. (2020). Nests in the cities: Adaptive and non-adaptive phenotypic plasticity and convergence in an urban bird. *Proceeding Biological Science* 287(1941):20202122. https://doi.org/10.1098/rspb.2020.2122.

Brown, S. M., Harrisson, K. A., Clarke, R. H., et al. (2013). Limited population structure, genetic drift and bottlenecks characterise an endangered bird species in a dynamic, fire-prone ecosystem. *PLoS One* 8(4):e59732. https://doi.org/10.1371/journal.pone.0059732.

Burger, C., Belskii, E., Eeva, T., et al. (2012). Climate change, breeding date and nestling diet: How temperature differentially affects seasonal changes in pied flycatcher diet depending on habitat variation. *Journal of Animal Ecology* 81(4):926–936. https://doi.org/10.1111/j.1365-2656.2012.01968.x.

Campagna, L. and Toews, D. P. L. (2022). The genomics of adaptation in birds. *Current Biology* 32:R1173–R1186. https://doi.org/10.1016/j.cub.2022.07.076.

Campbell, M. (2013). *Tactical Research Fund: Reducing the Impact of Discarded Recreational Fishing Tackle on Coastal Seabirds*. Brisbane, Australia: Queensland Department of Agriculture, Fisheries and Forestry, FRDC Final Reports (2011/0). FRDC.

Chen, H., Samet, J. M., Bromberg, P. A., et al. (2021). Cardiovascular health impacts of wildfire smoke exposure. *Part Fibre Toxicology* 18(1):2. https://doi.org/10.1186/s12989-020-00394-8.

Cheung, W. W. L., Pauly, D., and Sumaila, U. R. (2025). Hope or despair revisited: Assessing progress and new challenges in global fisheries. *Fish and Fisheries* 26:257–269. https://doi.org/10.1111/faf.12877.

Cho, D. H., Lee, J. H., Jang, J. U., et al. (2025). The adaptation and fitness costs to urban noise in the calls of the tree sparrow (*Passer montanus*). *Scientific Reports* 15(1):5359. https://doi.org/10.1038/s41598-025-88287-8.

Christensen-Dalsgaard, S., Ytrehus, B., Langset, M., et al. (2022). Seabird beachcast events associated with bycatch in the Norwegian purse seine fishery. *Marine Environmental Research* 177:105625. https://doi.org/10.1016/j.marenvres.2022.105625.

Cianchetti-Benedetti, M., Dell'Omo, G., Russo, T., et al. (2018). Interactions between commercial fishing vessels and a pelagic seabird in the southern Mediterranean Sea. *BMC Ecology* 18(1):54. https://doi.org/10.1186/s12898-018-0212-x.

Cimino, M. A., Welch, H., Warzybok, P., et al. (2025). The first GPS observation of a Western Gull (*Larus occidentalis*) riding in a long-haul garbage transfer truck. *Waterbirds* 48(1):1–5. https://doi.org/10.1675/063.048.0101.

Clairbaux, M., Mathewson, P., Porter, W., et al. (2021). North Atlantic winter cyclones starve seabirds. *Current Biology* 31(17):3964–3971.e3. https://doi.org/10.1016/j.cub.2021.06.059.

Curry, C. M., Des Brisay, P. G., Rosa, P., et al. (2018). Noise source and individual physiology mediate effectiveness of bird songs adjusted to anthropogenic noise. *Scientific Reports* 8(1):3942. https://doi.org/10.1038/s41598-018-22253-5.

Cusset, F., Fort, J., Mallory, M., et al. (2019). Arctic seabirds and shrinking sea ice: Egg analyses reveal the importance of ice-derived resources. *Scientific Reports* 9:15405. https://doi.org/10.1038/s41598-019-51788-4.

Darby, J. H., Clairbaux, M., Quinn, J. L., et al. (2023). Decadal increase in vessel interactions by a scavenging pelagic seabird across the North Atlantic. *Current Biology* 33(19):4225–4231.e3. https://doi.org/10.1016/j.cub.2023.08.033.

Dau, B. K., Gilardi, K. V., Gulland, F. M., et al. (2009). Fishing gear-related injury in California marine wildlife. *Journal of Wildlife Disease* 45(2):355–362. https://doi.org/10.7589/0090-3558-45.2.355.

de Framond, L., Sharp, S. P., Duclos, K., et al. (2025). Stream noise induces song plasticity and a shift to visual signals in a riverine songbird. *Current Biology* 35(18):4570–4576.e6. https://doi.org/10.1016/j.cub.2025.07.049.

Deng, J., Zhu, Y., Luo, Y., et al. (2025). Urbanization drives biotic homogenization of the avian community in China. *Integrative Zoology* 20(1):60–72. https://doi.org/10.1111/1749-4877.12815.

Deoniziak, K. and Osiejuk, T. S. (2021). Seasonality and social factors, but not noise pollution, influence the song characteristics of two leaf warbler species. *PLoS One* 16(9):e0257074. https://doi.org/10.1371/journal.pone.0257074.

Descamps, S., Tarroux, A., Cherel, Y., et al. (2016). At-sea distribution and prey selection of Antarctic petrels and commercial krill fisheries. *PLoS One* 11(8):e0156968. https://doi.org/10.1371/journal.pone.0156968.

Dias, M. P., Martin, R., Pearmain, E. J., et al. (2019). Threats to seabirds: A global assessment. *Biological Conservation* 237:525–537. https://doi.org/10.1016/j.biocon.2019.06.033.

Divoky, G. J., Lukacs, P. M., and Druckenmiller, M. L. (2015). Effects of recent decreases in arctic sea ice on an ice-associated marine bird. *Progress in Oceanography* 136:151–161. https://doi.org/10.1016/j.pocean.2015.05.010.

Dodino, S., Lois, N. A., Riccialdelli, L., et al. (2021). Sex-specific spatial use of the winter foraging areas by Magellanic penguins and assessment of potential conflicts with fisheries during winter dispersal. *PLoS One* 16(8):e0256339. https://doi.org/10.1371/journal.pone.0256339.

Dominoni, D., Smit, J. A. H., Visser, M. E., et al. (2020). Multisensory pollution: Artificial light at night and anthropogenic noise have interactive effects on activity patterns of great tits (*Parus major*). *Environmental Pollution* 256:113314. https://doi.org/10.1016/j.envpol.2019.113314.

Doneley, B. and Xie, S. (2025). *Avian Medicine and Surgery in Practice*, 3rd Ed. CRC Press.
Donnelly-Greenan, E., Nevins, H., and Harvey, J. (2019). Entangled seabird and marine mammal reports from citizen science surveys from coastal California (1997-2017). *Marine Pollution Bulletin* 149:110557.
Duarte, R. H. L., de Oliveira Passos, M. F., Beirão, M. V., et al. (2023). Noise interferes on feeding behaviour but not on food preference of saffron finches (*Sicalis flaveola*). *Behavioral Processes* 206:104844. https://doi.org/10.1016/j.beproc.2023.104844.
Ewbank, A. C., Sacristán, C., Costa-Silva, S., et al. (2020). Postmortem findings in Magellanic penguins (*Spheniscus magellanicus*) caught in a drift gillnet. *BMC Veterinary Research* 16(1):153. https://doi.org/10.1186/s12917-020-02363-x.
Fayet, A. L., Freeman, R., Anker-Nilssen, T., et al. (2017). Ocean-wide drivers of migration strategies and their influence on population breeding performance in a declining seabird. *Current Biology* 27(24):3871–3878.e3. https://doi.org/10.1016/j.cub.2017.11.009.
Foekema, E. M. (2017). The toxic exposure of flamingos to per- and polyfluoroalkyl substances (PFAS) from firefighting foam applications in Bonaire. *Marine Pollution Bulletin* 124(1): 102–111. https://doi.org/10.1016/j.marpolbul.2017.07.017.
Francis, C. D. (2015). Vocal traits and diet explain avian sensitivities to anthropogenic noise. *Global Change Biology* 21(5):1809–1820. https://doi.org/10.1111/gcb.12862.
Frank, G. S., Betts, M. G., Kroll, A. J., et al. (2025). Distinct bird assemblages emerge after fire versus forest harvest but converge with early seral forest development. *Ecological Applications* 35(4):e70032. https://doi.org/10.1002/eap.70032.
Franson, J. C., Hansen, S. P., Creekmore, T. E., et al. (2003). Lead fishing weights and other fishing tackle in selected waterbirds. *Waterbirds* 26:345–352.
Frishkoff, L. O., Karp, D. S., Flanders, J. R., et al. (2016). Climate change and habitat conversion favour the same species. *Ecological Letters*. 19(9):1081–1090. https://doi.org/10.1111/ele.12645.
Fröhlich, A. and Ciach, M. (2019). Nocturnal noise and habitat homogeneity limit species richness of owls in an urban environment. *Environmental Science Pollution Research International* 26(17):17284–17291. https://doi.org/10.1007/s11356-019-05063-8.
Fröhlich, A., Kotowska, D., Martyka, R., et al. (2023). Allometry reveals trade-offs between Bergmann's and Allen's rules and different avian adaptive strategies for thermoregulation. *Nature Communications* 14(1):1101. https://doi.org/10.1038/s41467-023-36676-w.
Frölicher, T. L., Fischer, E. M., and Gruber, N. (2018). Marine heatwaves under global warming. *Nature* 560:360–364. https://doi.org/10.1038/s41586-018-0383-9.
García-Redondo, C., Fernández-Moure, P., Cánibe, M., et al. (2023). Burn severity and land-use legacy influence bird abundance in the Atlantic-Mediterranean biogeographic transition. *Environmental Research* 233:116510. https://doi.org/10.1016/j.envres.2023.116510.
Gibson, D., Riecke, T. V., Catlin, D. H., et al. (2023). Climate change and commercial fishing practices codetermine survival of a long-lived seabird. *Global Change Biology* 29(2):324–340. https://doi.org/10.1111/gcb.16482.
Gilman, E., Musyl, M., Wild, M., et al. (2022). Investigating weighted fishing hooks for seabird bycatch mitigation. *Scientific Reports* 12(1):2833. https://doi.org/10.1038/s41598-022-06875-4.
Glemarec, G., Kindt-Larsen, L., Lundgaard, L. S., et al. (2020). Assessing seabird bycatch in gillnet fisheries using electronic monitoring. *Biological Conservation* 243:108461. https://doi.org/10.1016/j.biocon.2020.108461.

Gosper, C. R., Watson, S. J., Fox, E., et al. (2019). Fire-mediated habitat change regulates woodland bird species and functional group occurrence. *Ecological Applications* 29(8):e01997. https://doi.org/10.1002/eap.1997.

Grade, T., Campbell, P., Cooley, T., et al. (2019). Lead poisoning from ingestion of fishing gear: A review. *Ambio* 48(9):1023–1038. https://doi.org/10.1007/s13280-019-01179-w.

Grémillet, D., Fort, J., Amélineau, F., et al. (2015). Arctic warming: Nonlinear impacts of sea-ice and glacier melt on seabird foraging. *Global Change Biology* 21(3):1116–1123. https://doi.org/10.1111/gcb.12811.

Gremillet, D., Welcker, J., Karnovsky, N., et al. (2012). Little auks buffer the impact of current Arctic climate change. *Marine Ecology Progress Series* 454:197–206. https://doi.org/10.3354/meps09590.

Grunst, M. L., Grunst, A. S., Pinxten, R., et al. (2020). Anthropogenic noise is associated with telomere length and carotenoid-based coloration in free-living nestling songbirds. *Environmental Pollution* 260:114032. https://doi.org/10.1016/j.envpol.2020.114032.

Gutowsky, S. E., Baak, J. E., Gaston, A. J., et al. (2022). Sea ice extent and phenology influence breeding of high-Arctic seabirds: 4 decades of monitoring in Nunavut, Canada. *Oecologia* 198(2):393–406. https://doi.org/10.1007/s00442-022-05117-8.

Haase, I., Hu, Z., Peng, K., et al. (2025). Climate factors and food availability shape the altitudinal migration of birds in the Xiling Snow Mountains, China. *Integrative Zoology* 20(2):376–393. https://doi.org/10.1111/1749-4877.12893.

Halfwerk, W., Holleman, L. J. M., Lessells, C. M., et al. (2010). Negative impact of traffic noise on avian reproductive success. *Journal of Applied Ecology* 48(1):210–219. https://doi.org/10.1111/j.1365-2664.2010.01914x.

Halupka, L., Arlt, D., Tolvanen, J., et al. (2023). The effect of climate change on avian offspring production: A global meta-analysis. *Proceedings of the National Academy of Science* 120(19):e2208389120. https://doi.org/10.1073/pnas.2208389120.

Halupka, L., Czyż, B., and Macias Dominguez, C. M. (2020). The effect of climate change on laying dates, clutch size and productivity of Eurasian Coots *Fulica atra*. *International Journal of Biometeorology* 64(11):1857–1863. https://doi.org/10.1007/s00484-020-01972-3.

Halupka, L. and Halupka, K. (2017). The effect of climate change on the duration of avian breeding seasons: A meta-analysis. *Proceedings of Biological Science* 284(1867):20171710. https://doi.org/10.1098/rspb.2017.1710.

Hinke, J. T., Cossio, A. M., Goebel, M. E., et al. (2017). Identifying risk: Concurrent overlap of the Antarctic krill fishery with krill-dependent predators in the Scotia Sea. *PLoS One* 12(1):e0170132. https://doi.org/10.1371/journal.pone.0170132.

Houle, C., Pelletier, F., Bélisle, M., et al. (2020). Impacts of environmental heterogeneity on natural selection in a wild bird population. *Evolution* 74(6):1142–1154. https://doi.org/10.1111/evo.13939.

Hutto, R. L. (2008). The ecological importance of severe wildfires: Some like it hot. *Ecological Applications* 18(8):1827–1834. https://doi.org/10.1890/08-0895.1.

Injaian, A. S., Gonzalez-Gomez, P. L., Taff, C. C., et al. (2019). Traffic noise exposure alters nestling physiology and telomere attrition through direct, but not maternal, effects in a free-living bird. *General Comparative Endocrinology* 276:14–21. https://doi.org/10.1016/j.ygcen.2019.02.017.

Isaksson, C. (2018). Chapter 13-Impact of urbanization on birds. In: *Bird Species*, D. T. Tietze (ed.). pp. 235–257. Fascinating Life Sciences.

Isaksson, C., Ziegler, A. K., Powell, D., et al. (2024). Transcriptome analysis of avian livers reveals different molecular changes to three urban pollutants: Soot, artificial light at night and noise. *Environmental Pollution* 358:124461. https://doi.org/10.1016/j.envpol.2024.124461.

IUCN. (2025). The IUCN Red List of Threatened Species. Version 2025-2. https://www.iucnredlist.org.

Jakubas, D., Wojczulanis-Jakubas, K., Petersen, A., et al. (2024). Decline in the West Greenland population of a zooplanktivorous seabird, the little auk *Alle alle. Scientific Reports* 14(1):20686. https://doi.org/10.1038/s41598-024-71823-3.

Jarzyna, M. A., Porter, W. F., Maurer, B. A., et al. (2015). Landscape fragmentation affects responses of avian communities to climate change. *Global Change Biology* 21(8):2942–2953. https://doi.org/10.1111/gcb.12885.

Jetz, W., Wilcove, D. S., and Dobson, A. P. (2007). Projected impacts of climate and land-use change on the global diversity of birds. *PLoS Biology* 5(6):e157. https://doi.org/10.1371/journal.pbio.0050157.

Johns, M. E., Warzybok, P., Jahncke, J., et al. (2022). Episodes of high recruitment buffer against climate-driven mass mortality events in a North Pacific seabird population. *Journal of Animal Ecology* 91(2):345–355. https://doi.org/10.1111/1365-2656.13630.

Jongsomjit, D., Lescroël, A., Schmidt, A. E., et al. (2024). Going with the floe: Sea-ice movement affects distance and destination during Adélie penguin winter movements. *Ecology* 105(2):e4196. https://doi.org/10.1002/ecy.4196.

Johnson, A. E., Barve, S., Dreiss, L., et al. (2023). Acorn woodpecker movements and social networks change with wildfire smoke. *Current Biology* 33(19):R996–R997. https://doi.org/10.1016/j.cub.2023.08.096.

Jung, H., Sherrod, A., LeBreux, S., et al. (2020). Traffic noise and responses to a simulated approaching avian predator in mixed species flocks of chickadees, titmice, and nuthatches. *Ethology* 126(6):620–629. https://doi.org/10.1111/eth.13013.

Justel-Díez, M., Delgadillo-Nuño, E., Gutiérrez-Barral, A., et al. (2023). Inputs of seabird guano alter microbial growth, community composition and the phytoplankton-bacterial interactions in a coastal system. *Environmental Microbiology* 25(6):1155–1173. https://doi.org/10.1111/1462-2920.16349.

Kapsar, K., Sullender, B. K., and Kuletz, K. J. (2025). A multiscale seasonal examination of the risk of harm to seabirds from vessels based on co-occurrence in Alaskan waters. *Conservation Biology* 20:e70115. https://doi.org/10.1111/cobi.70115.

Khaliq, I., Biber, M. E., Bowler, D., et al. (2023). Global change impacts on bird biodiversity in South Asia: Potential effects of future land-use and climate change on avian species richness in Pakistan. *PeerJ* 11:e16212. https://doi.org/10.7717/peerj.16212.

Khaliq, I., Hof, C., Prinzinger, R., et al. (2014). Global variation in thermal tolerances and vulnerability of endotherms to climate change. *Proceedings of Biological Sciences* 281(1789):20141097. https://doi.org/10.1098/rspb.2014.1097.

Kleist, N. J., Guralnick, R. P., Cruz, A., et al. (2018). Chronic anthropogenic noise disrupts glucocorticoid signaling and has multiple effects on fitness in an avian community. *Proceedings of the National Academy Sciences of the United States of America* 115(4): E648–E657. https://doi.org/10.1073/pnas.1709200115.

Knottenbelt, C. M., Bawazeer, S., Hammond, J., et al. (2012). Nicotine hair concentrations in dogs exposed to environmental tobacco smoke: A pilot study. *Journal of Small Animal Practice* 53(11):623–626. https://doi.org/10.1111/j.1748-5827.2012.01284.x.

La Sorte, F. A. and Thompson, F. R. 3rd. (2007). Poleward shifts in winter ranges of North American birds. *Ecology* 88(7):1803–1812. https://doi.org/10.1890/06-1072.1.

Lee, H. J., Shin, M. Y., and Kim, N. R. (2025). Droughts and PM2.5 air pollution in California: The roles of wildfires. *Environment International* 202:109678. https://doi.org/10.1016/j.envint.2025.109678.

Lehikoinen, A., Jaatinen, K., Vähätalo, A. V., et al. (2013). Rapid climate driven shifts in wintering distributions of three common waterbird species. *Global Change Biology* 19(7):2071–2081. https://doi.org/10.1111/gcb.12200.

Leya, M., Oh, B., Ha, S., et al. (2023). The presence of anthracosis is associated with the environmental air quality of zoo, wildlife, and companion animals in Jeollabuk-do Province, South Korea. *American Journal of Veterinary Research* 84(6):1–7. https://doi.org/10.2460/ajvr.23.01.0016.

Li, R., Tian, H., and Li, X. (2010). Climate change induced range shifts of Galliformes in China. *Integrative Zoology* 5(2):154–163. https://doi.org/10.1111/j.1749-4877.2010.00198.x.

Liu, Q., Gelok, E., Fontein, K., et al. (2022). An experimental test of chronic traffic noise exposure on parental behaviour and reproduction in zebra finches. *Biology Open* 11(4):bio059183. https://doi.org/10.1242/bio.059183.

Liu, J., Lu, Y., Zhou, F., et al. (2025). Azure-winged magpies breeding in urban areas can effectively reduce the risk of brood parasitism. *Avian Research* 16:100272. https://doi.org/10.1016/j.avrs.2025.100272.

Llacuna, S., Gorriz, A., Durfort, M., et al. (1993). Effects of air pollution on passerine birds and small mammals. *Archives of Environmental Contamination and Toxicology* 24:59–66.

Malek, I. and Haim, A. (2019). Bright artificial light at night is associated with increased body mass, poor reproductive success and compromised disease tolerance in Australian budgerigars (*Melopsittacus undulatus*). *Integrative Zoology* 14(6):589–603. https://doi.org/10.1111/1749-4877.12409.

Marquis, R. J., Whelan, C. J., and Garfinkel, M. B. (2025). Avian top-down effects on insects and their host plants under human-driven global change. *Ibis* 167(4):1089–1112. https://doi.org/10.1111/ibi.13419.

Mathiaparanam, K. J., Mulder, R. A., and Hale, R. (2024). Anthropogenic double jeopardy: Urban noise and artificial light at night interact synergistically to influence abundance. *Environmental Pollution* 363(Pt 1):125078. https://doi.org/10.1016/j.envpol.2024.125078.

Matyjasiak, P., Chacińska, P., and Książka, P. (2023). Anthropogenic noise interacts with the predation risk assessment in a free-ranging bird. *Current Zoology* 70(3):277–283. https://doi.org/10.1093/cz/zoad019.

McGinn, K., Zuckerberg, B., Jones, G. M., et al. (2025). Frequent, heterogenous fire supports a forest owl assemblage. *Ecological Applications* 35(1):e3080. https://doi.org/10.1002/eap.3080.

McGrew, K. A., Crowell, S. E., Fiely, J. L., et al. (2022). Underwater hearing in sea ducks with applications for reducing gillnet bycatch through acoustic deterrence. *Journal of Experimental Biology* 225(20):jeb243953. https://doi.org/10.1242/jeb.243953.

McKechnie, A. E. and Wolf, B. O. (2010). Climate change increases the likelihood of catastrophic avian mortality events during extreme heat waves. *Biology Letters* 6(2):253–256. https://doi.org/10.1098/rsbl.2009.0702.

McQueen, A., Klaassen, M., Glenn, J., et al. (2024). Shorebirds are shrinking and shape-shifting: Declining body size and lengthening bills in the past half-century. *Ecology Letters*,27(12):e14513. https://doi.org/10.1111/ele.14513.

Meillère, A., Buchanan, K. L., Eastwood, J. R., et al. (2024). Pre- and postnatal noise directly impairs avian development, with fitness consequences. *Science* 384(6694):475–480. https://doi.org/10.1126/science.ade5868.

Melvin, E. F., Dietrich, K. S., Suryan, R. M., et al. (2019). Lessons from seabird conservation in Alaskan longline fisheries. *Conservation Biology* 33(4):842–852. https://doi.org/10.1111/cobi.13288.

Melvin, E. F., Parrish, J.K., and Conquest, L. L. (1999). Novel tools to reduce seabird bycatch in coastal gillnet fisheries. *Conservation Biology* 13(6):1386–1397. https://doi.org/10.1046/j.1523-1739.1999.98426.x.

Michalski, F. and Peres, C. A. (2017). Gamebird responses to anthropogenic forest fragmentation and degradation in a southern Amazonian landscape. *PeerJ* 5:e3442. https://doi.org/10.7717/peerj.3442.

Michlanski, M., Dachenhaus, J., Johns, J., et al. (2025). The epidemiology of a novel *Leucocytozoon* parasite in an endangered population of marbled murrelets (*Brachyramphus marmoratus*) on the Oregon coast. *International Journal for Parasitology: Parasites and Wildlife* 27:101078. https://doi.org/10.1016/j.ijppaw.2025.101078.

Montevecchi, W. A., Lamarre, J., Rouxel, Y., et al. (2023). High-contrast banners designed to deter seabirds from gillnets reduce target fish catch. *Marine Ornithology* 51(1):115–123. https://doi.org/10.5038/2074-1235.51.1.1518.

Morelli, F., Tryjanowski, P., Ibáñez-Álamo, J. D., et al. (2023). Effects of light and noise pollution on avian communities of European cities are correlated with the species' diet. *Scientific Reports* 13(1):4361. https://doi.org/10.1038/s41598-023-31337-w.

Navarro-Herrero, L., Saldanha, S., Militão, T., et al. (2024). Use of bird-borne radar to examine shearwater interactions with legal and illegal fisheries. *Conservation Biology* 38(3):e14224. https://doi.org/10.1111/cobi.14224.

Nihei, A., Sanderfoot, O. V., LaBarbera, K., et al. (2024). Wildfire smoke impacts the body condition and capture rates of birds in California. *Ornithology* 141(4):ukae023. https://doi.org/10.1093/ornithology/ukae023.

Obomsawin, A. P., Mastromonaco, G. F., and Leonard, M. L. (2021). Chronic noise exposure has context-dependent effects on stress physiology in nestling Tree Swallows (*Tachycineta bicolor*). *General Comparative Endocrinology* 311:113834. https://doi.org/10.1016/j.ygcen.2021.113834.

O'Neil, S. T., Coates, P. S., Brussee, B. E., et al. (2020). Wildfire and the ecological niche: Diminishing habitat suitability for an indicator species within semi-arid ecosystems. *Global Change Biology* 26(11):6296–6312. https://doi.org/10.1111/gcb.15300.

Osbrink, A., Meatte, M. A., Tran, A., et al. (2021). Traffic noise inhibits cognitive performance in a songbird. *Proceedings of Biological Sciences* 288(1944):20202851. https://doi.org/10.1098/rspb.2020.2851.

Ouyang, J. Q., de Jong, M., van Grunsven, R. H. A., et al. (2017). Restless roosts: Light pollution affects behavior, sleep, and physiology in a free-living songbird. *Global Change Biology* 23(11):4987–4994. https://doi.org/10.1111/gcb.13756.

Ozkan, K., Langley, J. M., Talbott, J. W., et al. (2024). Divergent effects of short-term and continuous anthropogenic noise exposure on Western Bluebird parental care behavior. *PeerJ* 12:e18558. https://doi.org/10.7717/peerj.18558.

Passarotto, A., Morosinotto, C., and Karell, P. (2025). Experimental noise and light pollution alter prey detection in a nocturnal bird of prey. *Journal of Animal Ecology* 94(7):1398–1409. https://doi.org/10.1111/1365-2656.70062.

Piatt, J. F., Parrish, J. K., Renner, H. M., et al. (2020). Extreme mortality and reproductive failure of common murres resulting from the northeast Pacific marine heatwave of 2014-2016. *PLoS One* 15(1):e0226087. https://doi.org/10.1371/journal.pone.0226087.

Poysa, H. (2025). Climate change and nest predation affect shifts in timing and duration of breeding as well as reproductive success in a migratory species. *Journal of Avian Biology* 2025(1):e03373. https://doi.org/10.1111/jav.03373.

Qiu, M., Li, J., Gould, C. F., et al. (2025). Wildfire smoke exposure and mortality burden in the USA under climate change. *Nature* 647(8091):935–943. https://doi.org/10.1038/s41586-025-09611-w.

Radbel, J., Rebuli, M. E., Kipen, H., et al. (2024). Indoor air pollution and airway health. *Journal of Allergy Clinical Immunology* 154(4):835–846. https://doi.org/10.1016/j.jaci.2024.08.013.

Raap, T., Pinxten, R., Casasole, G., et al. (2017). Ambient anthropogenic noise but not light is associated with the ecophysiology of free-living songbird nestlings. *Scientific Reports* 7(1):2754. https://doi.org/10.1038/s41598-017-02940-5.

Renner, H. M., Piatt, J. F., Renner, M., et al. (2024). Catastrophic and persistent loss of common murres after a heatwave. *Science* 386:1272–1276.

Regos, A., Imbeau, L., Desrochers, M., et al. (2018). Hindcasting the impacts of land-use changes on bird communities with species distribution models of Bird Atlas data. *Ecological Applications* 28(7):1867–1883. https://doi.org/10.1002/eap.1784.

Revorêdo, R. A., Da Silva Santana, V. G., and Tavares-Damasceno, J. P. (2025). Wind farms and power lines: A dual threat to seabirds in Brazil. *Waterbirds* 48(2):1–12. https://doi.org/10.1675/063.048.0201.

Rey, L., Kéry, M., Sierro, A., et al. (2019). Effects of forest wildfire on inner-Alpine bird community dynamics. *PLoS One* 14(4):e0214644. https://doi.org/10.1371/journal.pone.0214644.

Ribeiro, P. V. A., Gonçalves, V. F., de Magalhães Tolentino, V. C., et al. (2022). Effects of urbanisation and pollution on the heterophil/lymphocyte ratio in birds from Brazilian Cerrado. *Environmental Science Pollution Research International* 29(26):40204–40212. https://doi.org/10.1007/s11356-022-19037-w.

Ripple, W. J., Wolf, C., Gregg, J. W., et al. (2025). Climate change threats to Earth's wild animals. *BioScience* 75(7):519–523. https://doi.org/10.1093/biosci/biaf059.

Rushing, C. S., Royle, J. A, Ziolkowski, Jr. D. J., et al. (2020). Migratory behavior and winter geography drive differential range shifts of eastern birds in response to recent climate change. *Proceedings of the National Academy of Sciences* 117(23):12897–12903. https://doi.org/10.1073/pnas.2000299117.

Ryan, P. G. (2018). Entanglement of birds in plastics and other synthetic materials. *Marine Pollution Bulletin* 135:159–164. https://doi.org/10.1016/j.marpolbul.2018.06.057.

Ryding, S., McQueen, A., Klaassen, M., et al. (2024). Long- and short-term responses to climate change in body and appendage size of diverse Australian birds. *Global Change Biology* 30(10):e17517. https://doi.org/10.1111/gcb.17517.

Saino, N., Rubolini, D., Lehikoinen, E., et al. (2009). Climate change effects on migration phenology may mismatch brood parasitic cuckoos and their hosts. *Biological Letters* 5(4):539–541. https://doi.org/10.1098/rsbl.2009.0312.

Salmon, P., Nilsson, J., Watson, H., et al. (2017). Selective disappearance of great tits with short telomeres in urban areas. *Proceedings of the Royal Society London* 284:20171349. https://doi.org/10.1098/rspb.2017.1349.

Samset, B. H., Zhou, C., Fuglestvedt, J. S. et al. (2023). Steady global surface warming from 1973 to 2022 but increased warming rate after 1990. *Communications Earth & Environment* 4:400. https://doi.org/10.1038/s43247-023-01061-4.

Sanderfoot, O. V. and Holloway, T. (2017). Air pollution impacts on avian species via inhalation exposure and associated outcomes. *Environmental Research Letters* 12:083002. https://doi.org/10.1088/1748-9326/aa8051.

Santos, E. G., Herter, J. V., Wiederhecker, H. C., et al. (2025). Health stress in birds increase with urbanization in a large tropical city. *EcoHealth* 22:233–243. https://doi.org/10.1007/s10393-025-01708-y.

Saunders, S. P., Piper, W., Farr, M. T., et al. (2021). Interrelated impacts of climate and land-use change on a widespread waterbird. *Journal of Animal Ecology* 90(5):1165–1176. https://doi.org/10.1111/1365-2656.13444.

Sauve, D., Friesen, V. L., Hatch, S. A., et al. (2023). Shifting environmental predictors of phenotypes under climate change: a case study of growth in high latitude seabirds. *Journal of Avian Biology* 2023 (5–6):e03062. https://doi.org/10.1111/jav.03062.

Senzaki, M., Ando, H., and Kadoya, T. (2024). Noise pollution alters the diet composition of invertebrate consumers both in and beyond a noise-exposed grassland ecosystem. *Ecology Letters* 27(1):e14323. https://doi.org/10.1111/ele.14323.

Senzaki, M., Kadoya, T., and Francis, C. D. (2020). Direct and indirect effects of noise pollution alter biological communities in and near noise-exposed environments. *Proceedings of Biological Science* 287(1923):20200176. https://doi.org/10.1098/rspb.2020.0176.

Scarrow, R. (2021). Coastal guano transformed Andean agriculture. *Nature Plants* 7:1525. https://doi.org/10.1038/s41477-021-01055-0.

Simeone, A., Anguita, C., Daigre, M., et al. (2021). Spatial and temporal patterns of beached seabirds along the Chilean coast: Linking mortalities with commercial fisheries. *Biological Conservation* 256:109026. https://doi.org/10.1016/j.biocon.2021.109026.

Simmons, B. A. (2025). Angler perceptions of pelican entanglement reveal opportunities for seabird conservation on fishing piers in Tampa Bay. *PLoS One* 20(3):e0320424. https://doi.org/10.1371/journal.pone.0320424.

Smith, V. A., McBrearty, A. R., Watson, D. G., et al. (2017). Hair nicotine concentration measurement in cats and its relationship to owner-reported environmental tobacco smoke exposure. *Journal of Small Animal Practice* 58(1):3–9. https://doi.org/10.1111/jsap.12616. PMID: 28094859.

Soriano-Redondo, A., Cortés, V., Reyes-González, J. M., et al. (2016). Relative abundance and distribution of fisheries influence risk of seabird bycatch. *Scientific Reports* 6:37373. https://doi.org/10.1038/srep37373.

Sousa-Lima, L. V., Saggioro, E. M., Dorneles, P. R., et al. (2025). Fire on the ground: Wildfires impacts on soil health and biodiversity – A review. *Chemosphere* 388:144686. https://doi.org/10.1016/j.chemosphere.2025.144686.

Srinivasan, U. and Wilcove, D. S. (2021). Interactive impacts of climate change and land-use change on the demography of montane birds. *Ecology* 102(1):e03223. https://doi.org/10.1002/ecy.3223.

Templeton, C. N., Zollinger, S. A., and Brumm, H. (2016). Traffic noise drowns out great tit alarm calls. *Current Biology* 26(22):R1173–R1174. https://doi.org/10.1016/j.cub.2016.09.058.

Thomas, F. L. and Forys, E. A. (2022). The role of fishing piers in brown pelican (*Pelecanus occidentalis*) entanglement. *Animals* 12:2352. https://doi.org/10.3390/ani12182352.

Tyrrell, E. A., Coates, P. S., Prochazka, B. G., et al. (2023). Wildfire immediately reduces nest and adult survival of greater sage-grouse. *Scientific Reports* 13(1):10970. https://doi.org/10.1038/s41598-023-32937-2.

van de Pol, M., Vindenes, Y., Saether, B. E., et al. (2010). Effects of climate change and variability on population dynamics in a long-lived shorebird. *Ecology* 91(4):1192–1204. https://doi.org/10.1890/09-0410.1.

van Gils, J. A., Lisovski, S., Lok, T., et al. (2016). Body shrinkage due to Arctic warming reduces red knot fitness in tropical wintering range. *Science* 352(6287):819–821. https://doi.org/10.1126/science.aad6351.

Vega, M. L., Fransson, T., and Kullberg, C. (2021). The effects of four decades of climate change on the breeding ecology of an avian sentinel species across a 1,500-km latitudinal gradient are stronger at high latitudes. *Ecology and Evolution* 11(11):6233–6247. https://doi.org/10.1002/ece3.7459.

Viljur, M. L., Abella, S. R., Adámek, M., et al. (2022). The effect of natural disturbances on forest biodiversity: An ecological synthesis. *Biological Reviews of the Cambridge Philosophical Society* 97(5):1930–1947. https://doi.org/10.1111/brv.12876.

Votier, S. C. and Sherley, R. B. (2017). Seabirds. *Current Biology* 27:R431–R510.

Voskamp, A., Hof, C., Biber, M. F., et al. (2022). Projected climate change impacts on the phylogenetic diversity of the world's terrestrial birds: More than species numbers. *Proceedings of Biological Sciences* 289(1979):20212184. https://doi.org/10.1098/rspb.2021.2184.

Wang, K., Shen D., Dai, P., et al. (2023). Particulate matter in poultry house on poultry respiratory disease: A systematic review. *Poultry Science* 102:102556. https://doi.org/10.1016/j.psj.2023.102556.

Wei, J., Xu, F., Cole, E. F., et al. (2024). Spatially heterogeneous shifts in vegetation phenology induced by climate change threaten the integrity of the avian migration network. *Global Change Biology* 30(1):e17148. https://doi.org/10.1111/gcb.17148.

Wheeler, M., Ton, R., Brandl, H. B., et al. (2025). Reduced parental brood visit rate in wild zebra finches (*Taeniopygia castanotis*) is correlated with high maximum daily temperature. *Journal of Avian Biology* 2025(1):e03152. https://doi.org/10.111/jav.03152.

Williams, S. E. and de la Fuente, A. (2021). Long-term changes in populations of rainforest birds in the Australia Wet Tropics bioregion: A climate-driven biodiversity emergency. *PLoS One* 16(12):e0254307. https://doi.org/10.1371/journal.pone.0254307.

Williams, J. B., Munoz-Garcia, A., and Champagne, A. (2012). Climate change and cutaneous water loss of birds. *Journal of Experimental Biology* 215(7):1053–1060. https://doi.org/10.1242/jeb.054395.

Wilson, A. A., Ditmer, M. A., Barber, J. R., et al. (2021). Artificial night light and anthropogenic noise interact to influence bird abundance over a continental scale. *Global Change Biology* 27(17):3987–4004. https://doi.org/10.1111/gcb.15663.

Yang, D., Yang, A., Yang, J., et al. (2021). Unprecedented migratory bird die-off: A citizen-based analysis on the spatiotemporal patterns of mass mortality events in the Western United States. *GeoHealth* 5(4):e2021GH000395. https://doi.org/10.1029/2021GH000395.

Zhou, W., Wen, Z., Sun, B., et al. (2025). Global analysis links ambient fine particulate matter to bacterial antimicrobial resistance based on 110,000 + genomes. *Environment International* 202:109696. https://doi.org/10.1016/j.envint.2025.109696.

Zhu, B. R., Verhoeven, M. A., Velasco, N., et al. (2022). Current breeding distributions and predicted range shifts under climate change in two subspecies of Black-tailed Godwits in Asia. *Global Change Biology* 28(18):5416–5426. https://doi.org/10.1111/gcb.16308.

Ziegler, A. K., Watson, H., Hegemann, A., et al. (2021). Exposure to artificial light at night alters innate immune response in wild great tit nestlings. *Journal of Experimental Biology* 224(10):jeb239350. https://doi.org/10.1242/jeb.239350.

Žydelis, R., Bellebaum, J., Österblom, H., et al. (2009). Bycatch in gillnet fisheries – an overlooked threat to waterbird populations. *Biological Conservation* 142:1269–1281.

Žydelis, R., Small, C., and French, G. (2013). The incidental catch of seabirds in gillnet fisheries: A global review. *Biological Conservation* 162:76–88. https://doi.org/10.1016/j.biocon.2013.04.002.

9

Biologic and Chemical Anthropogenic Stressors

In this day and age, environmental contamination and pollutants are a fact of life. So what can we, avian health advocates, realistically do about them? There are no quick ways to slow or reverse the effects of contaminants that are present now; however, there is a lot we can do that will incrementally (slowly!) help in the future. But why discuss them again? To properly evaluate the health effects of contaminants and pollution, we need to understand a little detail about how the toxins/contaminants are managed in the body. How does the body metabolize and excrete toxins? Ingestion of foreign substances, such as plastics? We need to know this to understand on an individual level how to medically treat intoxication. And we need to know this to manage and conserve populations that are exposed chronically to these agents.

A *toxin* is a poisonous substance produced by a living organism (e.g., toxins from phytoplankton). A *toxicant* is a poisonous or harmful substance that is usually produced by nonbiologic sources and is usually related to industrial processes or synthetic substances. Many toxicants (contaminants and pollutants) are *xenobiotics*; that is, they are *foreign* to the body. The liver is responsible for detoxifying xenobiotics and other agents. Generally, the liver structurally modifies the xenobiotic chemically, usually rendering it less toxic. Then the liver conjugates the chemical to other molecules to facilitate its excretion out of the body via urine or feces. The liver's ability to metabolize and detoxify agents is determined by the presence and number of hepatic enzymes responsible for these functions. There are too many families and types of enzymes to discuss in detail here; however, quantification of these enzymes and/or mRNA upregulation of the genes (gene expression) to produce these enzymes (e.g., CYP1A) make good biomarkers of xenobiotic exposure. For example, CYP1A enzymes are involved in the detoxification of xenobiotics. Therefore, they would be expected to increase with exposure to toxins or other xenobiotics.

In the environment, many contaminants are taken in by plankton and invertebrates lower in the food chain. As larger and larger predators consume them, the amount of contaminants will *bioaccumulate* or be *biomagnified* within them. That is, the amount of contamination will accumulate and become greater in individuals as you move up the food chain. Thus, top predators will be consuming prey with a high and accumulating level of contaminants. *Bioavailability* refers to the amount of contaminants in the body that is available for binding and exerting cellular effects. Bioavailability is not equivalent to bioaccumulation. Bioavailability depends on the contaminant characteristics (hydrophilic or lipophilic, size, charge, etc.) and host features such as age, sex, health status, and reproduction. As a general rule, hydrophilic (water-soluble) contaminants will be largely bioavailable from the bloodstream, but hydrophobic (non-soluble in water) contaminants may settle in fatty tissues and be "unavailable".

Toxins

Harmful Algal Blooms

Harmful algal blooms, or HAB, are population explosions of various algae, phytoplankton, or cyanobacteria that produce a harmful effect on other species when they reach a critical population density. One way the blooms are harmful is by producing a toxin. These toxins are often by-products of metabolic activity and are referred to as *bioactive secondary metabolites*. It is believed that toxin production evolved in phytoplankton as a predator defense mechanism (Chakraborty et al., 2019). In fact, there are data showing active avoidance of toxin-laden bivalves by gulls, which is consistent with that hypothesis (Kvitek and Bretz, 2005). Toxins can also poison prey resources affecting seabird health and populations.

The other method to cause harm is simply by interfering with normal activities. High densities of phytoplankton/bacteria prevent light from penetrating deeper into the water, thus preventing photosynthesis and resulting in decreased dissolved oxygen levels. Bioactive compounds (other than toxins) can be produced by plankton at different stages of the bloom. Some diatom species produce an oily substance that can affect plumage and cause strandings (Ben-Gigirey et al., 2021). Some dinoflagellate species release a proteinaceous fluid/foam that can cause feather damage, resulting in reduced flight, foraging, and death (Ben-Gigirey et al., 2021). These bioactive compounds, however, do not bioaccumulate.

Since phytoplankton and cyanobacteria reside at or near the surface of the water, any animal frequenting the air/water interface (e.g., to breathe or eat) or diving will come in contact with any toxin produced. Wind-driven aerosolization of toxin-laden surface waters can occur and has been documented to result in toxin-induced respiratory signs in people up to a few miles away from the coast in red tide-prone areas (e.g., brevetoxin; Fleming et al., 2011). Similarly, cyanotoxins have been found aerosolized in outdoor and indoor air samples (Morris et al., 2025). In addition, higher trophic level predators (sea birds, turtles, and marine mammals) become exposed when consuming fish or invertebrates that have accumulated the toxin. Thus, HAB toxins can affect every level of the food chain.

Toxin-producing HAB species likely have been present and causing die-offs back to the 1800s. Descriptions of large fish kills have been documented in areas that would have been likely to have these blooms. Descriptions in the scientific literature of abnormal neurologic behaviors, such as loss of equilibrium, twisting, and hematologic abnormalities, have been documented in large fish mortality events. Although a cause was not identified, these likely reflected a HAB event.

By 2006, a HAB event had been documented throughout *every* coastal area of the USA. HAB events have been reported as increasing in frequency over the past 30–40 years. This increase is partially due to increased vigilance and research; however, it is known that increased eutrophication of the coastal waters is responsible for increases of certain HAB species (Lan et al., 2024). HAB events have caused acute mortality in marine mammals, marine birds, turtles, fish, and humans. However, information on HAB effects on seabirds (and birds in general) is less well represented in the literature than effects on marine mammals (Bean et al., 2024). Although acute intoxication episodes and mortalities are often studied, other questions, such as the effects of chronic exposure to low levels of toxin, remain unanswered.

Table 9.1 lists the best-known phytoplankton and bacterial species and their toxins that have caused significant illness and/or disease in *both* humans and birds. There are many types of algae that produce toxins in freshwater and other marine phytoplankton species that produce toxins, but for simplicity, we will restrict discussion to marine HAB events that have affected both birds and humans. Understanding the type of toxin each species produces and its physiologic effects is necessary to formulate treatment plans for affected individuals.

Domoic Acid

Domoic acid (DA) is the toxin produced by a diatom (genus *Pseudo-nitzschia*) when it blooms to high densities. Shellfish and other invertebrates take up toxin through ingestion/filtration, which results in the accumulation of high levels of domoic acid. Animals and humans become exposed by consuming prey with accumulated domoic acid. In human intoxications, gastrointestinal signs, such as nausea, vomiting, and diarrhea, are observed within 24 hours. In severe exposure, neurologic symptoms, such as amnesia (short-term memory loss) and dizziness, can be observed within 48 hours. This is rarely fatal in humans. The toxin's mechanism of action is as a glutamate (a neurotransmitter) agonist. It binds where glutamate binds and results in uncontrolled calcium influx into the neuron resulting in cell death. Detailed studies indicate that the preferred binding area of DA is in the hippocampus, which is the region that is responsible for memory (Scallet and Ye, 1997). Neuronal cell death in this area results in temporary memory loss; thus, in humans, the syndrome is termed Amnesic Shellfish poisoning.

Toxicity from DA was first discovered in 1987 in Canada when people died or became ill or died from consuming contaminated mussels (Wright et al., 1989). In 1991, various brown pelicans (*Pelecanus occidentalis*) and Brandt's cormorants (*Urile penicillatus*) stranded with clinical signs consistent with a neurotoxin (inability to raise their head, convulsions/seizures, and/or ataxia, dizziness, disorientation, which turned out to be DA; Rattner et al., 2022).

Table 9.1 Select toxin-producing HAB and bacterial species associated with human disease syndromes and avian epizootics.

Species	Toxin name	Human syndrome/common name
Karenia brevis	Brevetoxin	Neurotoxic shellfish poisoning/Red Tide
Pseudo-nitzschia	Domoic Acid	Amnesic shellfish poisoning
Alexandrium *Gymnodinium*	Saxitoxin	Paralytic shellfish poisoning
Cyanobacteria	Microcystin	Hepatotoxic, carcinogenic
Clostridium botulinum	Botulinum	Botulism

Upon postmortem, DA was found in their stomachs and within the anchovies they consumed. In general, intoxicated birds present to rehabilitation facilities in good body condition, showing neurologic signs, or are found dead. Since then, numerous epizootics due to DA alone and DA with another HAB toxin have resulted in the death of thousands of birds and other species along the US west coast and elsewhere (Gibble et al., 2021). In addition to exposure of coastal birds, two pelagic sea bird species were found to contain levels of DA in their blood, indicating that the exposure potential extends far beyond the shoreline (Soliño et al., 2019). DA intoxication may be best known as the cause of the recurrent pinniped mortalities off the coast of California.

Domoic acid is a hydrophilic (water-loving) toxin. As such, it does not accumulate in fatty tissues. Hydrophilic toxins circulate, bind their targets, and then are cleared from the body relatively rapidly via urine and feces. Therefore, treatment to prevent toxin binding isn't usually successful unless provided very early on after exposure. Treatment includes fluids, supportive care, and medical control of seizures if present.

Saxitoxin

Paralytic shellfish poisoning is the human disease syndrome caused by intoxication with saxitoxin, which is produced by dinoflagellates in the *Alexandrium* and *Gymnodinium* genera. Humans become intoxicated by eating contaminated shellfish and fish. The clinical signs come on rapidly and are primarily neurologic (tingling, numbness, and ataxia). In severe exposure, intoxication can be life threatening causing respiratory arrest and death. The mechanism of action of saxitoxin is to bind the sodium voltage-gated channels and block neuronal firing in peripheral nerves. This effectively paralyzes the diaphragmatic muscle, which is innervated by peripheral nerves, thus resulting in respiratory arrest. If treatment, which is supportive care and fluids, is successful, recovery is complete.

In a review of HAB events in Canada between 1988 and 2017, the presence of saxitoxin as well as other HAB toxins resulted in numerous closures of shellfish harvesting to prevent human exposure (McKenzie et al., 2021). In birds, saxitoxin has been the cause of various epizootics. In 2008–2012, the Kittlitz's murrelet (*Brachyramphus brevirostris*) in Alaska suffered high nestling loss and reproductive failure after saxitoxin was found in the sand lance fish fed to the nestlings (Shearn-Boschsler et al., 2014). This was a huge loss for this endangered species. Arctic terns (*Sterna paradisaea*) in Alaska suffered high mortality in 2019 due to saxitoxin poisoning. After examination of tern nests, the prey fish regurgitate contained saxitoxin, thus directly tying DA to this die off (Van Hemert et al., 2022). In 2014–2017, fulmars and shearwaters died in an epizootic due to saxitoxin in the Bering and Chukchi seas (Van Hemert et al., 2020). Marine shorelines are not the only locations affected. Saxitoxin caused an epizootic including marine mammals and more than 500 seabirds in the St Lawrence Estuary in 2008 (Starr et al., 2017).

Just as often, saxitoxin and another agent or toxin are involved in epizootics. In 2015/2016 common murres (*Uria aalge*) suffered a large-scale epizootic in Alaska due to saxitoxin and domoic acid (Van Hemert et al., 2020). While both toxins were found in intoxicated/dead birds, they were also found in nonexposed birds. This suggests that neither toxin was likely the sole cause of death, but that both may have contributed to reduced fitness, which left the birds vulnerable to other disease or impairment. Similarly, seabirds in Portugal in 2020 were intoxicated/died from HAB, but this time it was saxitoxin and microcystin (Soliño et al., 2025). Other studies investigated saxitoxin's effect on seabirds by evaluating if there were any behavior changes in captive birds dosed with the toxin (Smith et al., 2025). Using common murres, they dosed the animals with saxitoxin and found that exposed birds had a decreased fish intake over the week of observation (relative to controls). So, while the saxitoxin was not fatal, it resulted in decreased food consumption, which could make the birds vulnerable to an additional stressor or infection.

Saxitoxin is a hydrophilic toxin and, as such, stays in circulation until cleared via urine or feces. It does not partition into the fat. Because of the physiologic adaptations for diving (especially peripheral vasoconstriction), the toxin may concentrate in the heart, brain, and other vital organs resulting in death.

Brevetoxin

Neurotoxic shellfish poisoning is the human syndrome caused by intoxication from brevetoxin, which is produced by a dinoflagellate known as *Karenia brevis*. These blooms are commonly referred to as "red tides" because the affected water area appears reddish to brown in color (Figure 9.1). *K. brevis* is a common resident along the Gulf coast of Florida and blooms occur frequently. Many red tides over the past several decades have resulted in epizootics of marine mammals (dolphins and manatees), sea turtles, and sea birds (Pierce and Henry, 2008). In human intoxications, clinical signs include gastrointestinal (diarrhea, vomiting, and cramps), neurologic (ataxia and dizziness), and respiratory (nasal congestion, coughing, and increased airway resistance) signs. Ingestion is the route of exposure for gastrointestinal and neurologic symptoms. Inhalation is the route for the respiratory effects. In 2007, the NE Florida CDC documented a cluster of upper respiratory illness among beach workers related to a red tide event. This suggests a mode of exposure to more pelagic species or inland bird species depending on which direction the wind is blowing.

Since the 1970s, there have been numerous documented epizootics involving brevetoxin and seabirds. Lesser scaup (*Aythya affinis*) and double-crested cormorants (*Nannopterum auritum*) fell victim to brevetoxicosis in 1973–1974 (Forrester et al., 1977). Between 1995 and 1999 and then again in 2005–2006, hundreds of shore and seabirds were either found

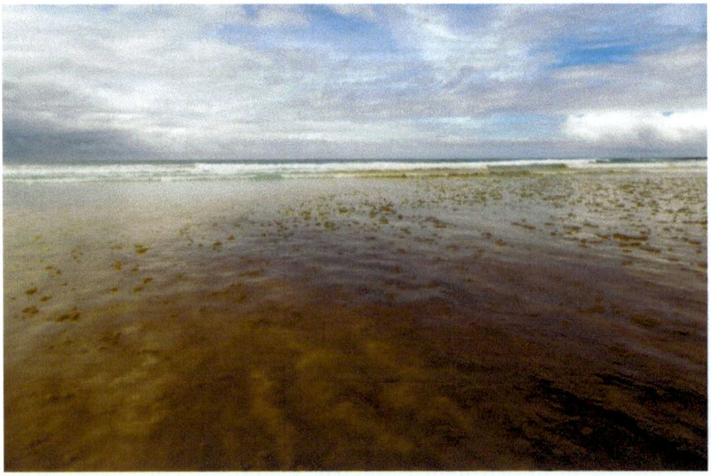

Buteo/Adobe Stock Photos

Figure 9.1 "Red tide" – note the brownish/reddish discoloration of water from the bloom of *K. brevis* dinoflagellate in a HAB.

dead or alive with neurologic signs of disorientation, ataxia, inability to stand, and/or seizures (Fauquier et al., 2013). Seventy percent of the birds and 12 of the 19 species had brevetoxin in their system. No other lesions were found suggesting that brevetoxin was the likely cause of death.

Brevetoxin is a hydrophilic neurotoxin. Similar to the other toxins discussed, animals that were stranded due to intoxication were in good body condition but presented with neurologic signs or were found dead. Immunohistochemical studies on exposed dolphins and in rat animal models showed that brevetoxin is taken up by lymphocytes and exerts an immunomodulatory effect (Bossart et al., 1998). Other studies, including experiments using purified brevetoxin, showed decreased immunologic function suggesting an immune modulatory effect as well (Brammer-Robins et al., 2022; Zaias et al., 2011; Walsh et al., 2005, 2010). Brevetoxin has been shown to accumulate in seagrass also (Flewelling et al., 2005)! This presents the potential for delayed ingestional exposure of toxin by shorebirds as they forage in shallow grassy areas even after the peak bloom occurs. What we do not know is the extent or longevity of the immunologic compromise from intoxication, nor the effect of chronic exposure to low doses of toxin.

Cyanotoxins

Cyanobacteria are another group of HAB-producing species that are more common in freshwater and estuarine areas. Cyanobacteria are autotrophic gram-negative bacteria. They are present in aquatic and terrestrial environments and can tolerate a wide range of environmental conditions (e.g., low and high temperatures and pH). These bacteria are well adapted to environmental changes, including anthropogenic changes. Given their ability to adapt, it is believed that increasing temperatures will favor cyanobacterial growth more so than other photoautrophs (photosynthesizers; Morris et al., 2025). Not all cyanobacteria produce toxins. Production of toxin is likely a method of defense from predation and/or a response to changes in the environment.

There are various types of toxins produced by the different cyanobacterial species. The routes of exposure to cyanotoxins include ingestion, inhalation, and maternal transfer. Ingestional exposure can result from cyanotoxins on vegetation or prey consumed and in water uptake near waste and effluent from cities and industry. In addition, cyanotoxins and bacteria can be aerosolized and inhaled. The molecules of toxin can adhere to particulate matter on dry land or can adhere to bubbles or water molecules, aerosolize, and be carried afar by winds. Maternal transfer in birds can occur during egg formation or passed during maternal feeding of nestlings in altricial species. For the sake of brevity, we will focus on the cyanotoxins that are common to human and avian intoxication and are the most well-known.

Arguably, the best-known cyanotoxins are the microcystins. These toxins grow well with increasing nitrogen and phosphorus in eutrophication. They have documented hepatoxicity, multiorgan failure, and are considered tumor promoters because of their ability to cause DNA damage, disrupt signaling pathways in the cells, and cause abnormal cell proliferation (Rajput et al., 2024). Their toxic effects relate to the increase in reactive oxygen species, inflammation, and inhibition of protein phosphatases, all of which can contribute to dysfunction and apoptosis of the cell.

Anatoxin-a is another cyanotoxin. It functions as a mimic of acetylcholine, which stimulates neurotransmitters. However, it cannot be degraded by enzymes as would normally occur to turn off/control stimulation. Therefore, the result is continual overstimulation, which can result in paralysis, asphyxiation, abnormal muscle contractions, and death of the individual (Morris et al., 2025). Similar in function to anatoxin-a (but different in structure) is guanitoxin. This is an organophosphate molecule which acts to prevent acetylcholine from being degraded, thus resulting in continual stimulation just as anatoxin.

Cyanobacteria also produce neurotoxic amino acids such as BMAA (β-Methylamino-L-alanine). BMAA can biomagnify in the food chain, accumulate in the brain, cause protein misfolding, excitotoxicity, and damage motor neurons. In laboratory studies, BMAA has caused increased oxidative stress, which can lead to apoptosis, inflammation, and induce epigenetic changes in the cell (Morris et al., 2025). Multiorgan (intestine, kidney, and liver) failure due to BMAA has been demonstrated (Wang et al., 2025). In addition, it is believed that aerosolized BMAA may be linked to neurodegenerative diseases in humans, including amyotrophic lateral sclerosis (ALS), Parkinson's disease, and potentially Alzheimer's disease (Morris et al., 2025)! This is very scary! Another cyanoneurotoxin, aetokthonotoxin, causes degenerative neurologic injury resulting in a disease called avian vacuolar myelinopathy in eagles and other raptors who consume contaminated prey (Breinlinger et al., 2021).

Microcystin is the dominant cyanotoxin type in Chesapeake Bay (Rattner et al., 2022). Twenty years of research (2000–2022) has revealed wildlife, including avian, mortality associated with microcystins, which were found to be at levels very close to human safety limits. An epizootic of birds was found to be caused by a microcystin bloom in 2012 near Chesapeake Bay (Foss et al., 2018). Microcystin was the cause of death in white Pelicans (*Pelecanus erythrorhynchos*), Dalmatian pelicans (*Pelecanus crispus*) in Greece, multiple species in Argentina, ducks in Japan, various avian species in Danish Lakes, and was one of multiple cyanotoxin types responsible for a lesser flamingo (*Phoeniconaias minor*) die-off in the East African rift valley lakes (McCain et al., 2020; Papadimitriou et al., 2018; Metcalf et al., 2013; Mancini et al., 2010; Matsunaga et al., 1999; Henriksen et al., 1997).

In summary, the vast majority of HAB, cyanotoxins, and bacterial toxins are neurotoxins that are rapidly cleared from the bloodstream. Animals strand in good body condition but show clinical signs or are found dead. This indicates a rapid effect of toxin activity. As the toxin binds to channels or receptors on neurons, the neurons either malfunction or die leading to respiratory paralysis or massive cell death. Once bound, it isn't clear that the toxin can be unbound, and neurons can be restored to normal function. Unless the animal is treated immediately after exposure to these toxins, it is very difficult to prevent toxin binding and action. Thus, recovery from intoxication is largely based on how much of the toxin was internalized and timely supportive care.

Botulism

The disease botulism is caused by the toxin botulinum, which is produced by the bacterial species *Clostridium botulinum*. Botulinum toxin is critical for the bacteria's successful invasion of the host. Production of botulinum is well known as a cause of mass mortality events involving waterbirds, such as ducks, sea gulls, pelicans, and other waterbirds (Gutiérrez-Arnal and Marin, 2024). Birds become affected by ingestion of the toxin in decomposing or contaminated food or water (Uzal et al., 2024). The toxin binds to motor nerve endings resulting in some measure of paralysis. Clinical signs are usually paralysis, weakness, inability to fly, and/or sudden death. As with other intoxications, affected animals are in good general body condition. *C. botulinum* favors warm, nutrient rich, and low oxygen (often stagnant) water bodies. They produce spores that can remain dormant until conditions are more favorable for recrudescence (Uzal et al., 2024). These spores can be transferred to other sites by unaffected carrier birds. Treatment of affected birds includes supportive care primarily, but antitoxin is effective if given early in infection. However, the antitoxin is not readily available in large enough quantities to save a mass die-off. Scavengers can become affected if they consume prey killed by botulism; however, it appears that vultures may be "resistant" to the effects of the toxin to some degree (Gutiérrez-Arnal and Marin, 2024; Uzal et al., 2024; Callaway, 2014).

In the early 1900s, mass die-offs of birds were related to *C. botulinum* and linked to farming and water management practices, which presumably caused excessive growth of the bacteria and toxin production (Jessup, 2023). Management to reduce potential botulism events includes control of water bodies, water flow, and nutrient run-off; identification and mapping of areas prone to botulism; active surveillance of outbreaks; and removal and incineration of carcasses containing botulinum toxin (Gutiérrez-Arnal and Marin, 2024).

Organic Contaminants

Persistent organic pollutants (POPs) are the large, carbon-based contaminant molecules that include organochlorines and organohalogenated compounds, such as pesticides, industrial waste compounds, and the like. (For simplicity, I will refer to all forms as POP.) At room temperatures, they are volatile liquids or vapors. There is a relatively long anecdotal history of POP causing reproductive and other negative health effects in wild animals. With the industrial explosion, more and more POP gained access to the water, bays, oceans, and soils. It wasn't until the 1980s that new diagnostic techniques permitted better quantification and identification of these compounds.

The problem with POP in general is that they have a long residence time in the environment because of their high molecular weight (large compounds), their chemical stability (they do not decompose), and their resistance to metabolic degradation in animals. POP can adsorb onto particles and settle into the sediment, soil, or stay in the water column. When ingested by animals, POP can *biomagnify* up the food chain. As each trophic level preys on the one below, their POP content becomes additive so that the higher trophic level prey bioaccumulate more POP than the lower-level prey. For many avian species that feed at a high trophic level, the POP burden can be very high. They are present in essentially all natural or synthetic compounds, and if in the volatile state, they can cause direct (carcinogenic, mutagenic, and/or teratogenic) or indirect effects on animals (Mangotra and Singh, 2023).

POPs are lipophilic compounds; that is, they are soluble in fat and can deposit and reside in fatty tissues like subcutaneous tissue, liver, and lipid storage molecules. Here they can accumulate freely. Recall that when stored in fatty tissues, they are *not* bioavailable. Bioavailable compounds are able to bind to cells and tissues, be distributed in the bloodstream, and be integrated into metabolic processes. It is when POPs are bioavailable that they cause trouble.

POPs are known endocrine disrupters. They can agonize or antagonize hormone binding to negatively affect various aspects of reproduction and/or immune function (Galligan et al., 2019). The extent of impact of POP depends on the individual animal – its age, whether it is growing, migrating, or ill. These life phases require a lot of energy. Often this energy is ultimately derived from fat catabolism. When fat is catabolized, the POP is released into the bloodstream, becomes bioavailable, and can exert direct toxic effects in animals.

While some large organic molecules are naturally produced, most of the POP that have wreaked havoc in the animal kingdom are anthropogenic in origin. Industrial plant effluent along the coasts, pesticides, flame retardants, etc., are all anthropogenic in origin. These have markedly increased in the marine and terrestrial environment since WWII. Studies evaluating POP levels over time have shown some decreases in total POP body burdens worldwide (Lewis et al., 2022). The advent of more sophisticated chemical techniques allowed scientists to understand their effects in more detail.

There are various samples ("diagnostic matrices") that can be obtained from birds to evaluate POP burden. The definitive sample is blood or tissue. Other matrices must be validated against blood for accurate interpretation. Studies on the comparability of diagnostic matrices to evaluate POP levels (e.g., feathers and preen oil vs. traditional blood and organs/tissues) show inconsistent results. Some studies showed good relationships between the less invasive feather and preen oil levels with blood or organ levels (Gray et al., 2024; Cao et al., 2024; Eulaers et al., 2013; but other studies did not (for example, Acampora et al., 2018). Eggshell thickness has been proposed as an indication of increases POP levels, in this case, DDT. Burger et al. (1995) measured eggshell thickness in several seabirds and noted increased thickness for two decades 1970–1990 after the DDT ban. Similarly, in Norway, peregrine falcons (*Falco peregrinus*) eggshell thickness also increased after the DDT ban (Nygard et al., 2019).

All categories of POP (PCB, DDE/DDT pesticides, flame retardants, etc.) have been found worldwide in bird tissues and the environment (Padayachee et al., 2023). The ever-increasing literature on POP in birds shows a wide range of data with some contradictory results. However, there are a few consistent findings. Legacy contaminants (e.g., contaminants, such as DDT, produced long ago before we understood their toxicological effects), despite their ban decades ago, persist in the environment and are still taken up by birds (for example, see Lewis et al., 2022; Sonne et al., 2020). The data indicate that those levels are decreased relative to before the ban though, which is good (Hidalgo et al., 2021; Braune et al., 2005) Diet and trophic level are the major determinants of POP levels in birds (for example, Hong et al., 2014; Rudolph et al., 2016; Lu et al., 2023a; Mo et al., 2018; except see Corsolini et al., 2017). Offshore and pelagic foragers generally have lower POP levels than inshore/coastal foraging species (for example, Nzabanita et al., 2024), and resident populations have greater levels than migratory populations (Mo et al., 2018; Hong et al., 2014). There were no consistent differences in overall POP concentrations between the sexes nor between ages (chick vs. adult). There may be exceptions to these.

POP levels are related to urbanization. Urbanization led to increased POP concentrations in soil and blood (corrected for body mass and/or volume) of little penguins (*Eudyptula minor*) in Tasmania (Wells et al., 2024). Their eggs had approximately four times the concentration of POP than the soil or parental blood samples, and molting birds had lower POP levels than non-molting birds. These findings are consistent with depuration (offloading) of POP from females into eggs and into feathers. Finally, they found that increased POP levels in urbanized areas resulted in lower total protein and hematocrit levels in females suggesting a potential impact on their health. As would be expected, increased urbanization creates more waste. Landfills and garbage dumps are hotspots for foraging birds to accumulate POP across the world! Especially worrisome are "e-waste" sites where computers and related equipment are dumped (for example, Cao et al., 2024; Mo et al., 2018; Tongue et al., 2019). Perhaps even more concerning is the exposure to infectious and/or zoonotic pathogens that may also be acquired at the dump site (Sangkachai et al., 2024) and subsequent transfer of these in the course of normal foraging, movements, or migration (Grant et al., 2024).

Clearly POP have a detrimental effect on *populations* of animals (Sonne et al., 2020; Dietz et al., 2019). Immunologic compromise due to POP exposure has been documented in glaucus gulls (*Larus hyperboreus*), herring gulls (*Larus smithsonianus*), and Caspian terns (*Hydroprogne caspia*; Sagerup et al., 2000; Grasman et al., 1996). As in other animals, reduced immunity can permit overgrowth of parasites (e.g., helminths); although this aspect requires additional evaluation (Schwantes, 2023). Exposure to a mixture of POP led to suppression of a T cell response and a decreased ability to mount an antibody response when stimulated (Grasman et al., 1996). These reductions in immune cell function could result in increased infection or disease from other agents.

Maternal transfer of contaminants to offspring has been documented in birds as well as mammals. However, in birds, the opportunity for the actual transfer is reduced/consolidated to ≤ 24 hours versus the longer gestation and lactation periods in mammals. While birds do not have the abundance of fat stores that mammals do, female birds can have organic contaminants stored in the liver, which can transfer to the egg during development. Verreault et al. (2006) and Knudtzon et al. (2021) demonstrate maternal transfer of POPs to developing glaucous and herring gull eggs, respectively. This phenomenon has also been documented in other avian species (Bargar et al., 2001). In the wild, unless the egg-laying date is known, it is more difficult to confirm exactly what POP congeners and how much of them are directly from maternal contribution. After egg laying, effects of the environment, food provisioning, habitat, and parental brooding can contribute POP to the developing egg.

Experimental studies have shown physiologic effects of POP on chicks from POP containing eggs persisting in subsequent generation's chicks. Fernie et al. (2003) demonstrated that nestling American kestrel (*Falco sparverius*) chicks of the F2 generation of parents that were exposed to POP had altered growth rates and hormone values. Female Bermuda petrels (*Pterodroma cahow*) with higher contaminant levels laid eggs that had a lower probability of hatching (Campioni et al., 2024). Extrapolating these data to wild populations, these potential effects could lead to decreased reproductive success.

Consider the population effect of losing a significant number of animals, including an entire year's class of chicks. For a population close to extinction, this could be a devastating loss. High contaminant levels in chicks and eggs, coupled with compromised immune and endocrine systems, may put these animals at increased risk from an infectious agent and/or extinction (Schnelle et al., 2025). If presented with a metabolically challenging environmental condition (e.g., persistently cold-water temperatures, decrease prey abundance, and HAB event), the population survival and/or recovery could be irreversibly damaged.

Oil Spills

Oil spills from drilling rigs and cargo ships have caused several huge mortality events in marine animals and other coastal species (Figure 9.2). In 1989, the Exxon Valdez oil spill totaled 11 million gallons of crude oil in Prince William Sound in Alaska. More recently,

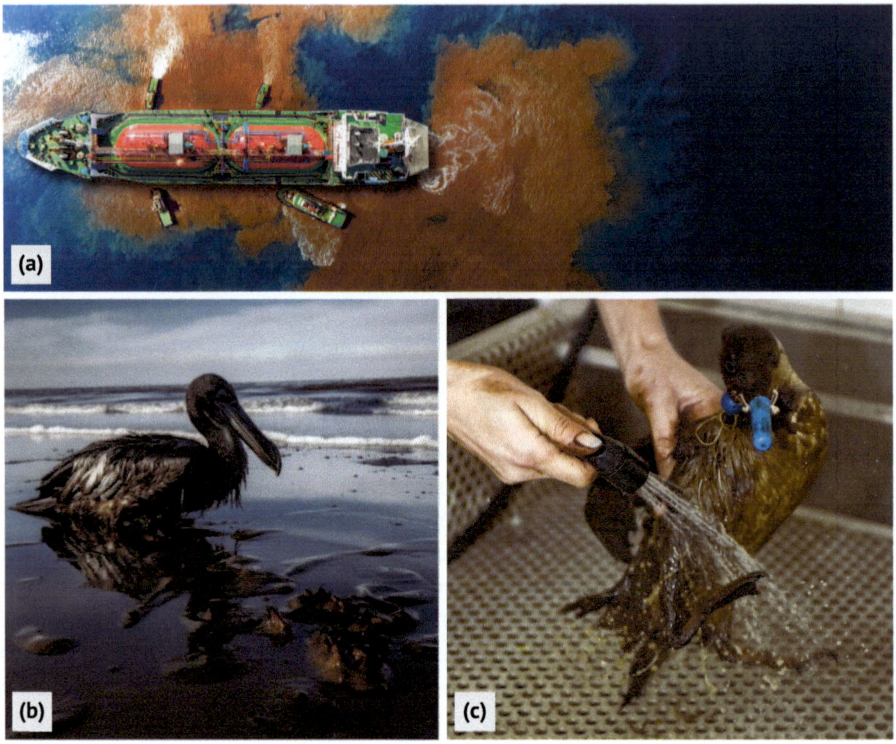

Yellow Boat/Adobe Stock Photos

Jouni/Adobe Stock Photos

Corepics VOF/Shutterstock

Figure 9.2 Oil spill from a large oil tanker (a), an oiled seabird (b), and cleaning off oil from a seabird (c).

the Deepwater Horizon (DWH) oil spill resulted in 210 million gallons of oil dumped into the Gulf of Mexico between 2010 and 2014! This spill resulted in a huge increase of polycyclic aromatic hydrocarbons (a form of POP) in the water, which affected all species from plankton to marine mammals. Even deep-sea corals were affected! Approximately 800,000 coastal birds and 200,000 pelagic birds died in the acute phase of the spill. More were affected in the days, months and years afterward. In total, well over a million birds died, representing 93 species.

Petroleum (oil) contains thousands of organic and inorganic components, 98% of which are aromatic hydrocarbons (Ziccardi, 2023). There are two main types of aromatic hydrocarbons – monocyclic and polycyclic aromatics. Monocyclic aromatics are the most acutely toxic compounds. They are readily bioavailable in the body because they are water soluble (hydrophilic). In the water, they are not often found in high concentrations due to their volatility (Ziccardi, 2023). These compounds, which include benzene, toluene, and xylene, have been linked with carcinogenesis, organ damage, and death. Polycyclic aromatics, on the other hand, are insoluble in water (lipophilic) and can bioaccumulate. Like monocyclics, these aromatics have also been linked to carcinogenesis and reproductive failure.

A multitude of experimental studies have been conducted on the effects of crude oil, oil dispersants, etc. on birds. Experimental investigations on the pathophysiology of oil intoxication indicate alterations in amino acid and fatty acid metabolism, increases in liver,

GI, and kidney enzymes, alterations in electrolytes, cardiotoxicity, immunology, reduced reproductive success, embryotoxicity, and behavioral changes that could impact survival (examples include Horak et al., 2017; King et al., 2021; Goodchild et al., 2020b; Dorr et al., 2019; Dean et al., 2017; Harr et al., 2017b). Evidence of anemia and ultrastructural damage of RBC were observed in sea birds experimentally and naturally exposed to oil (Fallon et al., 2018; Harr et al., 2017a). Upregulation of genes related to cellular proliferation and liver regeneration was seen in Seaside sparrows (*Ammospiza maritima*) exposed during the DWH spill (Bonisoli-Alquati et al., 2020). Experimental exposure of zebra finch (*Taeniopygia guttata*) eggs to oil on their surface found altered embryonic heart and metabolic rates, which could lead to failures in hatching or survival during the nestling stage (Goodchild et al., 2020a). Oil exposure led to reproductive decrease and behavioral changes that included cessation of breeding, disruption of pair bonds, and nest abandonment in various species (Fry et al., 1986; Butler et al., 1988). These are a few examples. There are many more studies.

The effects of oil on feathers (Figure 9.2) are clear – the feather structure is disrupted, and the barbules clump together, eliminating the seamless boundary that helps prevent heat loss and permits proper flight. Washing off the oil from the feathers allows proper realignment of the barbules. Sandpipers exposed to oil had reduced ability to take flight into the air from the ground (Maggini et al., 2017a, b). This could cause an increased chance of predation because they cannot escape fast enough. Investigation of the residue from the remediation practice of "burning" the oil off the sediment indicated that this residue was equally, if not worse, for the feathers than the oil itself (Fritt-Rasmussen et al., 2016). Despite the prevalence of acute studies, we know very little about chronic sublethal effects of oil exposure to birds (Moreau et al., 2022). Data from marine mammals (bottlenose dolphins, *Tursiops truncatus*), many years post-DWH spill, show that reproductive and respiratory impairment persist (Lane et al., 2015). Is the same true for oiled long-lived birds?

Treatment of individual animals is possible. The response of the public and rehabilitation centers to wash off the oil-soaked feathers was largely productive acutely; however, the long-term effects on these animals are unknown. Birds in rehabilitation or zoos that have suffered high exposure to POP/oil will be managed and likely survive. Individuals who may have a compromised immune system would not be good candidates for release. They can be managed using medical therapy, provision of antibiotics and immunoglobulins, and constant vigilance for infection. Consistent nutritive support and disease treatment would allow weight gain, return to health, and release of eligible individuals.

Heavy Metals

Heavy metals are naturally occurring in the earth's crust and enter the environment via erosion and weathering processes. Anthropogenic industrial activities, refineries, power plants, and agriculture have greatly increased the quantity of heavy metals in our environment. In trace amounts, many heavy metals are essential to animal biological processes as cofactors for many enzymatic reactions. However, small increases in these essential metals can become toxic. They can impact cellular integrity, cause DNA damage that can lead to carcinogenesis, and create reactive oxygen species that can wreak havoc in normal cell functioning (Rehman et al., 2018). A review of heavy metals in seabirds indicated that mercury (Hg), cadmium, and lead (Pb) were the three most common metals seen, although more than 10 metals have been identified in birds (Ma et al., 2022). Heavy metal concentrations were elevated in wedge-billed woodcreepers (*Glyphorynchus spirutus*) in protected areas of the Amazon; however, they were near oil and gold extraction sites (Loera et al., 2024). Heavy metals can be measured in various tissues including organs, blood, muscle, uropygial gland oil, and feathers (Varaglya et al., 2022). As with other contaminants, the less invasive feather and preen oil samples should be validated against blood or organ values.

Lead is one of the most common heavy metals which negatively impacts health. Lead exposure is mainly via lead shot/bullets, inhalation, ingestion of contaminated food and water, and incidental/accidental ingestion of lead fishing tackle, sinkers, and hooks. A 35-year (1983–2019) review of published data on raptors in Europe found that scavenger species had the greatest levels of lead and were the most at risk of lead poisoning (Monclús et al., 2020). These high levels coincided with hunting seasons and thus bullets were the most likely culprits. Bald eagles in rehabilitation had similar prevalence (90%) of blood lead concentrations as wild bald eagles (McTee et al., 2023). The levels were greater than background lead levels. The researchers concluded that these eagles live with these lead levels chronically. In birds, lead and other metals can be deposited into developing eggs by females (Dauwe et al., 2005). In mammals, lead can cross the placenta negatively affecting the fetus and fetal development (Rahman and Singh, 2019).

In the body, lead accumulates in the bones/skeletal system, kidney, liver, heart, and brain. Toxicity affects the neurologic, hepatic, renal, hematopoietic, endocrine, and reproductive systems. Specifically, lead results in increased oxidative stress, immune changes that lead to decreased cell-mediated immunity, decreased growth, body weight, and reproductive success (Schwantes, 2023; Vallverdú-Coll et al., 2019; Williams et al., 2018; Mateo et al., 2003; De Francisco et al., 2003; Burger and Gotchfeld, 2000). In nestling herring gulls (*L. smithsonianus*), experimental lead exposure caused behavioral changes (such as reduced locomotion, poor balance, and reduced food begging) that led to decreased growth and survival (Burger and Gochfeld, 2000). In New Hampshire, Grade et al. (2019) identified a 48% mortality in adult loons (*Gavia immer*) from ingestion of fishing tackle containing lead.

Mercury can exist in nature in three forms; however, it is the organic methylmercury form that is the most widespread environmental toxicant. Ubiquitous in nature, methylmercury is taken in via ingestion and is absorbed by the gastrointestinal tract. Methylmercury is lipid soluble so can partition into subcutaneous fat and reside in the liver fat depots. The majority of the mercury accumulates in the kidneys, liver, and neurologic tissues and abnormal signs are consistent with nephro-, gastrointestinal, and neuro-toxicities (Whitney and Cristol, 2017). Excretion of mercury is via feces, urine, maternal transfer to eggs, or through feather loss during molting (Beccardi et al., 2025; Ackerman et al., 2016, 2017).

Several studies have shown the various health effects of mercury in birds. Mercury exposure in wild albatrosses and experimentally in zebra finches (*T. castanotis*) resulted in decreased reproductive success (Mills et al., 2020; Varian-Ramos et al., 2014). Immunologic function, measured by B cell proliferation and immune response to an antigen, also decreased with experimental mercury exposure in zebra finches (Lewis et al., 2013). As with POPs, methylmercury is present at greater concentrations in higher trophic level birds consistent with biomagnification (Carrasco, 2025; Sayers et al., 2023; Mills et al., 2020).

Mercury levels in common terns (*Sterna hirundo*) were correlated with death during the early nestling period, decreased growth, and survival (Bertram et al., 2025). There appear to be species differences in the amount of mercury passed into eggs; however, the first laid egg of the clutch often has the greatest level (per mg egg weight) than subsequent eggs (Hartman et al., 2024; Ackerman et al., 2016, 2017). A few studies on seabirds have shown increasing parasite loads with increasing metal levels (Schwantes, 2023). There are many more studies in the scientific literature.

Metallothioneins are metal-binding proteins that regulate the availability, distribution, and transport of heavy metal levels within cells (Vignesh and Deepe, 2017). These proteins are present in all animals and plants, even bacteria, which speaks to the pervasiveness of heavy metals in the environment over evolutionary time and their effects on cellular processes. The upregulation (increase) of the mRNA message, gene expression, and increased amounts of metallothioneins in the body can be used as sensitive indicators (*biomarkers*) of heavy metal increase or intoxication.

Microplastics

Microplastics (MPs) are small particles of plastic ranging from 1 nm (10^{-9} m) to 5 mm (10^{-3} m) in size. Larger pieces of plastics end up in the oceans due to terrestrial runoff, runoff from agriculture/farms, sewage sludge used as fertilizer on soil, wastewater treatment plants, and garbage from urbanization in general. Larger plastic items undergo chemical and physical degradation (at a very, very, slow rate) to smaller particles. The potential effects of plastics on birds include entanglement (which we will review in the next chapter), increased nest detection and predation (because the plastics may be more easily visible to predators), affect ectoparasite load in the nest, and have a direct health impact on the nestlings (Mansfield et al., 2024). Although the full extent of the physiologic effects of ingested MP is unclear, it is now abundantly clear that birds and all animals, including humans, have MP in their/our bodies (Cui et al., 2025). A retrospective assessment of plastic in norther fulmars (*Fulmaris glacialis*) in Svalbard in the far northern Atlantic Ocean found that already in 1997, 91% of the birds had internalized plastic, and on average, there were 10 plastic items in each individual (Collard et al., 2022)! In humans, MPs have been associated with coronary cholesterol plaques, found in the placenta in females, and caused respiratory toxicity in mice (Cui et al., 2025; Li et al., 2025; Wang et al., 2025). Some plastics have hazardous additives which may or may not degrade in the environment (Turner and Filella, 2021). Sadly, from the Antarctic to the Arctic, plastics are ubiquitous from the air down to the sediments (Kibria, 2024). And the presence of marine protected areas (MPAs) does not prevent plastic uptake or accumulation (Lavers and Bond, 2024).

All birds are affected. Seabirds have high rates of interactions with and ingestion of plastics and other debris in the oceans (Figure 9.3). The plastic can be within the prey they consume, they can mistake a piece of plastic for a prey item, or they can get tangled and die (drown) from fishing lines. While the jury is still out on the full effects of MP and smaller pieces (such as nanoplastics, 1 nanometer = 10^{-9} m), birds with internalized plastics have been seen with grossly irritated or torn GIT/ stomachs, plastic stuck in their GIT and/or obstructing passage of food, and emaciation from starvation while their stomachs are full of plastics (presumably which caused them to feel full and they stopped foraging;

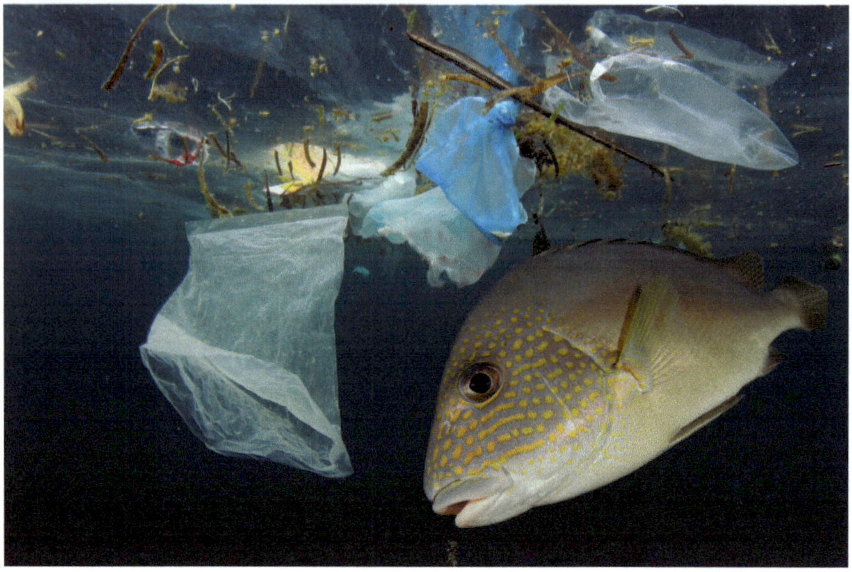

Rich Carey/Shutterstock.com

Figure 9.3 Plastics in the ocean.

Kibria, 2024; Puskic et al., 2024; Hoang and Mitten, 2022). In fact, a new disease syndrome called "plasticosis" has been defined wherein ingested plastic causes fibrosis (scarring) and inflammation in the stomach resulting in decreased feeding (Charlton-Howard et al., 2023). Plastics have also been found in blood, uropygial (preen) gland oils, lung, feathers, feces, and other tissues (Tokunaga et al., 2023; Vanstreels et al., 2023). MP (10^{-6} m) appears to be the most common plastic size internalized in birds (Zhao et al., 2016; Deoniziak et al., 2022).

Histopathology and molecular studies of tissues and blood show altered metabolism, vascular leakage (e.g., leaking out of vessels, which makes the blood-brain-barrier open to crossing), heart and/or lung injury, increased apoptosis, increased reactive oxygen species due to cellular stress, and disruption of microflora from MP exposure (de Jersey et al., 2025; Cunha et al., 2022; Zhang et al., 2022b; Yin et al., 2022, 2023; Lu et al., 2023b). One study showed that MPs were associated with a decrease in the (good) commensal bacteria of the gut and an increase in the zoonotic, pathogenic, and/or antibiotic-resistant bacteria ("bad") species (Fackelmann et al., 2023).

Plastics of varying shapes and sizes have been seen in the nests of many species (Nguyen et al., 2025; Lato et al., 2021). The plastic debris consists of fiber, fragments, and strings which can cause entanglement of the nestlings in the nest. Of the marine debris found in seabird nests, 90% or more were plastic (Brandão et al., 2011; Vanstreels et al., 2021). What makes this worse is that the plastics are likely carrying toxins, contaminants, and bacteria which get stuck on them (Colabuono et al., 2010; Navarro et al., 2023; Matos et al., 2023). Plastics particles can also carry metals and other elements. High concentrations of plastics were positively associated with increased concentrations of chlorine, iron, lead, manganese, and rubidium in feathers of Laysan Albatross (*Phoebastria immutabilis*; Lavers et al., 2025; Lavers and Bond, 2016). In the nest, these other agents are transferred to the nestlings or to conspecifics via fecal droppings (Martín-Vélez et al., 2024; Turner and Filella, 2021; Thaysen et al., 2020; Teuten et al., 2009).

The presence of microbes on plastics is interesting in terms of its infectability. Meng et al. (2022) determined that avian influenza virus can survive on plastic for up to two weeks in their experimental setting. This observation indicates that the onset of effects or infections from influenza virus may occur at a later time than the actual date of bacterial transfer of the plastic. Zhang et al. (2022a) found that plastics can increase the bioavailability of zoonotic protozoans such as *Giardia, Toxoplasma,* and *Cryptosporidium*. Anything that adheres to debris or plastic can be transferred to other sites and individuals by feces, body fluids, and feathers. Plastics and their associated toxins or infectious agents can also accumulate in bird colonies due to regurgitation and defecation of plastic particles in the colony area. When they fly or migrate, birds thus become unwitting vectors of infectious agents and/or contaminants.

Data suggest that nanoplastics and nanoparticles can pass across the blood brain barrier into the brain and other organs. Their smaller size permits them entry into the peripheral circulation. Data from mice indicate nanoplastics in the brain caused depression and cognitive disorders (da Costa Araújo and Malafaia, 2021). Given that nanoparticles are frequently used in biomedical research as a vehicle to deliver treatment agents, it seems logical to assume nanoplastics can pass anywhere in the body (Singh et al., 2023).

Terrestrial birds, of course, are not immune to plastic ingestion. Top predators (e.g., raptors) and scavenger species (e.g., vultures) have been found with plastic in their systems (Cunha et al., 2022; Carlin et al., 2020; Wang et al., 2021; Houston et al., 2007). Scavenger bird species foraging at garbage dumps increases the likelihood of ingesting plastics there and subsequently transferring them elsewhere. Similar to acquisition of POP at landfills, all plastic debris with their adhered contaminants, infectious agents, etc. can be found at landfills and garbage dumps! As urbanization spreads into new areas and impinges on avian habitat, birds may be more likely to visit garbage dumps for food. Data on smaller terrestrial species are scarcer than for seabirds, but we are still discovering the impact of MP in them.

Clinical Pharmaceuticals

The presence of pharmaceutical agents in water, sediment, and soil is a stunning problem aquatic and terrestrial organisms face. Clinical pharmaceuticals are medicines (and other therapeutics) developed for use in treatment and management of diseases in the medical and veterinary realm. They encompass a broad range of substances of synthetic or biological origin used to diagnose, treat, mitigate, prevent disease, or promote well-being (Bean et al., 2024). They are substances able to stimulate, depress, or replace physiological functioning in a biological system. This implies that the underlying mechanism by which the drug functions must be present for a physiological effect to occur. This definition could be extended to pesticides and their kind; however, this discussion will be limited to pharmaceuticals used in human or veterinary medicine. In addition, human skin care and other cosmetic products are not included.

The main pharmaceuticals in the environment are medications used to treat disease in humans and agriculture animals, mainly livestock and poultry. Sources include waste effluents from treatment plants, aquaculture, hospitals, drug manufacturers, farm/crop runoff, livestock treatments that include topical administration or dips (e.g., parasiticides), veterinary clinic disposal, and home medication disposal. Over the years, the major categories of pharmaceuticals found in the environment are antibiotics, hormones, antidepressants, nonsteroidal anti-inflammatories, followed by cardiovascular drugs, cancer drugs, and even opioid analgesics (Mezzelani and Regoli, 2022)! Pharmaceuticals were first identified in the water in early 1990 (Mezzelani and Regoli, 2022). By 2010, over 160 active pharmaceuticals or their bioactive ingredients/metabolites have been identified from water bodies. In the 2020s, that number increased to over 300 compounds! (To my horror, fentanyl, the powerful opioid, was found in bottlenose dolphins from the Gulf of Mexico (Ocampos et al., 2024)! I am not sure if that is a testament to pollution or to the illegal drug trade! But I digress.)

The persistence of a given pharmaceutical agent in the environment varies with their chemical makeup, solubility, and environmental conditions (e.g., temperature and acidity). Some drugs may get completely eliminated and others may get chemically transformed. When they are active, they target metabolic, enzymatic, or cell signaling pathways (Mezzelani and Regoli, 2022). These pathways are likely the most evolutionarily conserved. In the environment however, animals are usually exposed to mixtures of various pharmaceuticals, and the activity of the mixtures is hard to predict. In the water or soil, these pharmaceuticals will be taken up by algae, invertebrates, and fish, can bioaccumulate in them, and kill or otherwise negatively affect them (Świacka et al., 2022).

One of the first mainstream wildlife events that brought the issue of the negative impact of pharmaceuticals in the environment was the increasing mortality of old world vultures in Asia due to the nonsteroidal anti-inflammatory drug (NSAID) diclofenac (Bean et al., 2024). By the early 2000s, the population of vultures had decreased by 90%! It was ultimately discovered that the vultures accumulated diclofenac from consuming carcasses of cattle to which it was administered. The vultures died from liver and kidney failure secondary to toxicity from the diclofenac. Since that discovery, the manufacture of this medication was banned, and safer NSAIDs were substituted for veterinary use. However, it opened our eyes to this problem. Many of those vulture species are still threatened or endangered. Recent studies have revealed that NSAIDS (the cyclooxygenase inhibitors) decrease calcium availability in females leading to eggshell thinning (de Solla et al., 2023).

Other direct effects of ingesting certain pharmaceuticals are clear. Scavengers foraging on the carcass of an animal that was euthanized by pentobarbital (or similar agent) can also die (Herrero-Villar et al., 2024). Oral mycosis (fungi in the oral cavity) developed in an avian scavenger who fed on a carcass that was given antibiotics recently before death (Pitarch et al., 2017). The antibiotic killed the resident bacteria in the oral cavity, which permitted the fungus to grow and cause disease.

Other than direct toxicity to birds, pharmaceuticals in the environment can accumulate in invertebrate prey species, thus affecting non-scavenging birds as well. The specific impact (behavioral and mortality) the drug has on the invertebrate is not always clear. Burket et al. (2023) demonstrated that in an urban freshwater location in Texas, levels of sertraline (a human antidepressant) were present in mussels (bivalves) in concentrations orders of magnitude higher than in fish from the same water body. This highlights the potential magnification effect that at least some bivalves can achieve, so any avian predator eating the mussel will get a whopping load of drug.

Perhaps the negative consequence of greatest concern regarding pharmaceuticals in the environment is increased potential for development and spread of antimicrobial resistant (AMR) bacteria. Numerous classes of antibiotics have been found in the environment. AMR bacteria develop due to exposure of microorganisms to subinhibitory concentrations of an antibiotic. The bacteria that are sensitive to antibiotic exposure will die, leaving the other bacteria that are resistant to that antibiotic to survive and reproduce. In addition, bacteria can pass "antibiotic resistance genes" horizontally to other bacteria. This may give receiving bacteria a survival advantage because they will not be susceptible to a particular antibiotic. Before the extent of the environmental pharmaceutical situation was front line, we (humans) were already dealing with an influx of AMR bacteria that are harder and harder to treat. Wider spread environmental contamination with antibiotics just exacerbates this problem.

How do we manage the environmental pharmaceutical problem? We need to be *ecopharmacovigilant*. This concept was promulgated by Shore et al. (2014). Basically, we need to actively be vigilant to assess what is out there in the environment, especially the environments of bird species/populations that are threatened or endangered. Birds of prey and scavengers may make good sentinels to sample. Raptors also range over large distances and can spread AMR bacteria far and wide (Bean et al., 2024; Porrero et al., 2013). We can assess critical avian areas for pharmaceutical presence. Alternatively, we can evaluate the presence of pharmaceutical active ingredients in untreated sewage to understand what to expect regionally (Osena et al., 2025). Assessment of the amounts of pharmaceuticals in invertebrates and fish (for example) would also be prudent to understand the potential risk to human health if those fish were eaten. This approach was utilized by Rehage et al. (2025). They captured red drum fish from nine estuaries along Florida's coast. The fish's plasma concentration of a pharmaceutical was compared to 33 and 100% of the human therapeutic plasma level. They found values in the fish that were close to 33% of the human level, suggesting more risk for humans to experience the drug's effect.

The Big Picture

We have learned over the years that the environment, infectious agents, and/or host factors interact to produce the negative health effects seen in the vast majority of epizootics impacting free-ranging/wild avian populations. While not every causative factor is known, retrospective analyses often demonstrate the involvement of at least two of the three factors. We know much about the acute/short-term effects of many of the contaminants, but we know very little about the long-term or chronic effects of sublethal and/or repeated exposure. There is likely an immune suppression resulting from the environmental, contaminant, and/or infectious insult. Whether immune suppression is acute or chronic is not always clear. However, multiple insults (infectious agent, toxin, etc.) can overwhelm the body and result in worsening health and/or death. Given increasing sea surface temperature and global warming in general, emerging infectious diseases are predicted to increase and expand out of their usual ranges. There are ample data indicating birds (especially migratory species) can transfer contaminants and diseases far distances (Grant et al., 2024). In these new areas, the animals may be naïve immunologically ("sitting ducks" as they say) to these infectious agents. If impaired by effects of organic contaminants or other agents, the birds may succumb to the new disease more quickly and intensely, possibly resulting in more epizootics, increasing the loss of biodiversity, and more extinctions in the future. What can we do about this?

Literature Cited

Acampora, H., White, P., Lyashevska, O., et al. (2018). Contrasting congener profiles for persistent organic pollutants and PAH monitoring in European storm petrels (*Hydrobates pelagicus*) breeding in Ireland: a preen oil versus feathers approach. *Environmental Science & Pollution Research International* 25(17):16933–16944. https://doi.org/10.1007/s11356-018-1844-2.

Ackerman, J. T., Eagles-Smith, C. A., Herzog, M. P., et al. (2016). Maternal transfer of contaminants in birds: Mercury and selenium concentrations in parents and their eggs. *Environmental Pollution* 210:145–154. https://doi.org/10.1016/j.envpol.2015.12.016.

Ackerman, J. T., Hartman, C. A., and Herzog, M. P. (2017). Maternal transfer of mercury to songbird eggs. *Environmental Pollution* 230:463–468. https://doi.org/10.1016/j.envpol.2017.06.099.

Bargar, T. A., Scott, G. I., and Cobb, G. P. (2001). Maternal transfer of contaminants: Case study of the excretion of three polychlorinated biphenyl congeners and technical grade endosulfan into eggs by white leghorn chickens (*Gallus domesticus*). *Environmental Toxicology and Chemistry* 20:61–67. https://doi.org/10.1002/etc.5620200106.

Bean, T. G., Chadwick, E. A., Herrero-Villar, M., et al. (2024). Do pharmaceuticals in the environment pose a risk to wildlife? *Environmental Toxicology and Chemistry* 43(3):595–610. https://doi.org/10.1002/etc.5528.

Beccardi, M., Bertram, J., Bouwhuis, S., et al. (2025). Experimental evidence for maternal offloading of mercury pollution via reproduction. *Environmental Pollution* 385:127121. https://doi.org/10.1016/j.envpol.2025.127121.

Ben-Gigirey, B., Soliño, L., Bravo, I., et al. (2021). Paralytic and amnesic shellfish toxins impacts on seabirds, analyses and management. *Toxins* 13(7):454. https://doi.org/10.3390/toxins13070454.

Bertram, J., Bichet, C., Moiron, M., et al. (2025). Mercury levels in chicks of a long-lived seabird – parental effects and links with growth and survival. *Environmental Research* 285:122283. https://doi.org/10.1016/j.envres.2025.122283.

Bonisoli-Alquati, A., Xu, W., Stouffer, P. C., et al. (2020). Transcriptome analysis indicates a broad range of toxic effects of Deepwater Horizon oil on Seaside Sparrows. *Science of the Total Environment* 720:137583. https://doi.org/10.1016/j.scitotenv.2020.137583.

Bossart, G. D., Baden, D. G., Ewing, R. Y., et al. (1998). Brevetoxicosis in Manatees (*Trichechus manatus latirostris*) from the 1996 epizootic: Gross, histologic, and immunohistochemical features. *Toxicologic Pathology* 26:276–282.

Brammer-Robbins, E., Costa, K. A., Bowden, J. A., et al. (2022). Putative high-level toxicity pathways based on evidence of brevetoxin immunotoxicity in marine fauna. *Aquatic Toxicology* 252:106298. https://doi.org/10.1016/j.aquatox.2022.106298.

Brandão, M. L., Braga, K. M., and Luque, J. L. (2011). Marine debris ingestion by Magellanic penguins, *Spheniscus magellanicus* (Aves: Sphenisciformes), from the Brazilian coastal zone. *Marine Pollution Bulletin* 62(10):2246–2249. https://doi.org/10.1016/j.marpolbul.2011.07.016.

Braune, B. M., Outridge, P. M., Fisk, A. T., et al. (2005). Persistent organic pollutants and mercury in marine biota of the Canadian Arctic: An overview of spatial and temporal trends. *Science of the Total Environment* 351-352:4–56. https://doi.org/10.1016/j.scitotenv.2004.10.034.

Breinlinger, S., Phillips, T. J., Haram, B. N., et al. (2021). Hunting the eagle killer: A cyanobacterial neurotoxin causes vacuolar myelinopathy. *Science* 371(6536):eaax9050. https://doi.org/10.1126/science.aax9050.

Burger, J. and Gochfeld, M. (2000). Effects of lead on birds (Laridae): A review of laboratory and field studies. *Journal of Toxicology & Environmental Health B Critical Reviews* 3(2):59–78. https://doi.org/10.1080/109374000281096.

Burger, J., Viscido, K., and Gochfeld, M. (1995). Eggshell thickness in marine birds in the New York Bight – 1970s to 1990s. *Archive of Environmental Contaminants and Toxicology* 29:187–191.

Burket, S. R., Sims, J. L., Dorman, R., et al. (2023). Bioaccumulation kinetics of model pharmaceuticals in the freshwater unionid pond mussel, *Sagittunio subrostratus. Environmental Toxicology and Chemistry* 42(6):1183–1189. https://doi.org/10.1002/etc.5590.

Butler, R. G., Harfenist, A., Leighton, F., et al. (1988). Impact of sublethal oil and emulsion exposure on the reproductive success of Leach's storm-petrels: short- and long-term effects. *Journal of Applied Ecology* 25(1):125–143. https://doi.org/10.2307/2403614.

Callaway, E. (2014). Microbes help vultures eat rotting meat. *Nature* 16345. https://doi.org/10.1038/nature.

Campioni, L., Oró-Nolla, B., Granadeiro, J. P., et al. (2024). Exposure of an endangered seabird species to persistent organic pollutants: Assessing levels in blood and link with reproductive parameters. *Science of the Total Environment* 930:172814. https://doi.org/10.1016/j.scitotenv.2024.172814.

Cao, X., Wu, X., Lu, R., et al. (2024). Persistent organic pollutants in feathers of various terrestrial and aquatic bird species: Interspecies difference and source apportionment. *Journal of Hazardous Materials* 474:134810. https://doi.org/10.1016/j.jhazmat.2024.134810.

Carlin, J., Craig, C., Little, S., et al. (2020). Microplastic accumulation in the gastrointestinal tracts in birds of prey in central Florida. *Environmental Pollution* 264:114633. https://doi.org/10.1016/j.envpol.2020.114633.

Carrasco, N. (2025). Mercury exposure and potential health risks to Antarctic seabirds: A synthesis. *Science of the Total Environment* 996:180137. https://doi.org/10.1016/j.scitotenv.2025.180137.

Chakraborty, S., Pancic, M., Andersen, K. H., et al. (2019). The cost of toxin production in phytoplankton: The case of PST producing dinoflagellates. *The ISME Journal* 13:64–75. https://doi.org/10.1038/s41396-018-0250-6.

Charlton-Howard, H. S., Bond, A. L., Rivers-Auty, J., et al. (2023). 'Plasticosis': Characterizing macro- and microplastic-associated fibrosis in seabird tissues. *Journal of Hazardous Materials* 450:131090. https://doi.org/10.1016/j.jhazmat.2023.131090.

Colabuono, F. I., Taniguchi, S., and Montone, R. C. (2010). Polychlorinated biphenyls and organochlorine pesticides in plastics ingested by seabirds. *Marine Pollution Bulletin* 60(4):630–634. https://doi.org/10.1016/j.marpolbul.2010.01.018.

Collard, F., Bangjord, G., Herzke, D., et al. (2022). Plastic burdens in northern fulmars from Svalbard: Looking back 25 years. *Marine Pollution Bulletin* 185(Pt B):114333. https://doi.org/10.1016/j.marpolbul.2022.114333.

Corsolini, S., Ademollo, N., Martellini, T., et al. (2017). Legacy persistent organic pollutants including PBDEs in the trophic web of the Ross Sea (Antarctica). *Chemosphere* 185:699–708. https://doi.org/10.1016/j.chemosphere.2017.07.054.

Cui, C., Guo, Z., Liu, Y., et al. (2025). Tissue-specific distribution of microplastics in human blood and carotid plaques: A paired sample analysis. *Environment International* 203:109743. https://doi.org/10.1016/j.envint.2025.109743.

Cunha, W. A., Freitas, Í. N., Gomes, L. A. S., et al. (2022). From carrion-eaters to plastic material plunderers: Toxicological impacts of plastic ingestion on black vultures, *Coragyps atratus* (Cathartiformes: Cathartidae). *Journal of Hazardous Materials* 424(Pt D):127753. https://doi.org/10.1016/j.jhazmat.2021.127753.

da Costa Araújo, A. P. and Malafaia, G. (2021). Microplastic ingestion induces behavioral disorders in mice: A preliminary study on the trophic transfer effects via tadpoles and fish. *Journal of Hazardous Materials* 401:123263. https://doi.org/10.1016/j.jhazmat.2020.123263.

Dauwe, T., Janssens, E., Bervoets, L., et al. (2005). Heavy-metal concentrations in female laying great tits (*Parus major*) and their clutches. *Archives of Environment Contaminant and Toxicology* 49:249–256. https://doi.org/10.1007/s00244-003-0209-z.

Dean, K. M., Bursian, S. J., Cacela, D., et al. (2017). Changes in white cell estimates and plasma chemistry measurements following oral or external dosing of double-crested cormorants, *Phalacocorax auritus*, with artificially weathered MC252 oil. *Ecotoxicology and Environment Safety* 146:40–51. https://doi.org/10.1016/j.ecoenv.2017.08.007.

De Francisco, N., Ruiz Troya, J. D., and Agüera, E. I. (2003). Lead and lead toxicity in domestic and free-living birds. *Avian Pathology* 32(1):3–13. https://doi.org/10.1080/0307945021000070660.

de Jersey, A. M., Lavers, J. L., Bond, A. L., et al. (2025). Seabirds in crisis: Plastic ingestion induces proteomic signatures of multiorgan failure and neurodegeneration. *Science Advances* 11(11):eads0834. https://doi.org/10.1126/sciadv.ads0834.

Deoniziak, K., Cichowska, A., Niedźwiecki, S., et al. (2022). Thrushes (Aves: Passeriformes) as indicators of microplastic pollution in terrestrial environments. *Science of the Total Environment* 853:158621. https://doi.org/10.1016/j.scitotenv.2022.158621.

de Solla, S. R., King, L. E., and Gilroy, E. A. M. (2023). Environmental exposure to non-steroidal anti-inflammatory drugs and potential contribution to eggshell thinning in birds. *Environment International* 171:107638. https://doi.org/10.1016/j.envint.2022.107638.

Dietz, R., Letcher, R. J., Desforges, J.-P., et al. (2019). Current state of knowledge on biological effects from contaminants on arctic wildlife and fish. *Science of the Total Environment* 696:133792. https://doi.org/10.1016/j.scitotenv.2019.133792.

Dorr, B. S., Hanson-Dorr, K. C., Assadi-Porter, F. M., et al. (2019). Effects of repeated sublethal external exposure to deep water horizon oil on the avian metabolome. *Scientific Reports* 9(1):371. https://doi.org/10.1038/s41598-018-36688-3.

Eulaers, I., Jaspers, V. L., Bustnes, J. O., et al. (2013). Ecological and spatial factors drive intra- and interspecific variation in exposure of subarctic predatory bird nestlings to persistent organic pollutants. *Environment International* 57-58:25–33. https://doi.org/10.1016/j.envint.2013.03.009.

Fackelmann, G., Pham, C. K., Rodríguez, Y., et al. (2023). Current levels of microplastic pollution impact wild seabird gut microbiomes. *Nature Ecology Evolution* 7(5):698–706. https://doi.org/10.1038/s41559-023-02013-z.

Fallon, J. A., Smith, E. P., Schoch, N., et al. (2018). Hematological indices of injury to lightly oiled birds from the Deepwater Horizon oil spill. *Environmental Toxicology and Chemistry* 37(2):451–461. https://doi.org/10.1002/etc.3983.

Fauquier, D. A., Flewelling, L. J., Maucher, J. M., et al. (2013). Brevetoxicosis in seabirds naturally exposed to *Karenia brevis* blooms along the central west coast of Florida. *Journal of Wildlife Diseases* 49(2):246–260. https://doi.org/10.7589/2011-09-270.

Fernie, K., Bortolotti, G., Drouillard, K., et al. (2003). Developmental toxicity of *in ovo* exposure to polychlorinated biphenyls: II. Effects of maternal or paternal exposure on second-generation nestling American kestrels. *Environmental Toxicity and Chemistry* 22:2688–2694. https://doi.org/10.1897/02.551.

Fleming, L. E., Kirkpatrick, B., Backer, L. C., et al. (2011). Review of red tide and human health effects. *Harmful Algae* 10(2):224–233. https://doi.org/10.1016/j.hal.2010.08.006.

Flewelling, L. J., Naar, J. P., Abbott, J. P., et al. (2005). Red tides and marine mammal mortalities. *Nature* 435:755–756. https://doi.org/10.1038/nature435755a.

Forrester, D., Gaskin, J., White, F., et al. (1977). An epizootic of waterfowl associated with a red tide episode in Florida. *Journal of Wildlife Diseases* 13:160–167.

Foss, A. J., Miles, C. O., Samdal, I. A., et al. (2018). Analysis of free and metabolized microcystins in samples following a bird mortality event. *Harmful Algae* 80:117–129. https://doi.org/10.1016/j.hal.2018.10.006.

Fritt-Rasmussen, J., Linnebjerg, J. F., Sørensen, M. X., et al. (2016). Effects of oil and oil burn residues on seabird feathers. *Marine Pollution Bulletin* 109(1):446–452. https://doi.org/10.1016/j.marpolbul.2016.05.029.

Fry, D. M., Swenson, J., Addiego, L. A., et al. (1986). Reduced reproduction of wedge-tailed shearwaters exposed to weathered Santa Barbara crude oil. *Archives of Environmental Contamination and Toxicology* 15:453–463.

Galligan, T. M., Balmer, B. C., Schwacke, L. H., et al. (2019). Examining the relationships between blubber steroid hormones and persistent organic pollutants in common bottlenose dolphins. *Environmental Pollution* 249:982–991. https://doi.org/10.1016/j.envpol.2019.03.083.

Gibble, C. M., Kudela, R. M., Knowles, S., et al. (2021). Domoic acid and saxitoxin in seabirds in the United States between 2007 and 2018. *Harmful Algae* 103:101981. https://doi.org/10.1016/j.hal.2021.101981.

Goodchild, C. G., Grisham, K., Belden, J. B., et al. (2020a). Effects of sublethal application of Deepwater Horizon oil to bird eggs on embryonic heart and metabolic rate. *Conservation Biology* 34(5):1262–1270. https://doi.org/10.1111/cobi.13539.

Goodchild, C. G., Love, A. C., Krall, J. B., et al. (2020b). Weathered Mississippi Canyon 252 crude oil ingestion alters cytokine signaling, lowers heterophil:lymphocyte ratio, and induces sickness behavior in zebra finches (*Taeniopygia guttata*). *Environmental Pollution* 267:115302. https://doi.org/10.1016/j.envpol.2020.115302.

Grade, T., Campbell, P., Cooley, T., et al. (2019). Lead poisoning from ingestion of fishing gear: A review. *Ambio* 48(9):1023–1038. https://doi.org/10.1007/s13280-019-01179-w.

Grant, M. L., Bond, A. L., Reichman, S. M., et al. (2024). Seabird transported contaminants are dispersed in island ecosystems. *Chemosphere* 361:142483. https://doi.org/10.1016/j.chemosphere.2024.142483.

Grasman, K. A., Fox, G. A., Scanlon, P. F., et al. (1996). Organochlorine-associated immunosuppression in prefledgling Caspian terns and herring gulls from the Great Lakes: An ecoepidemiological study. *Environmental Health Perspective* 104 (Suppl 4):829–842. https://doi.org/10.1289/ehp.96104s4829.

Gray, F. E., Derous, D., and Bize, P. (2024). Is minimally invasive sampling the future of persistent organic pollutant (POP) research in birds? A meta-analysis on tissue comparisons. *Chemosphere* 362:142591. https://doi.org/10.1016/j.chemosphere.2024.142591.

Gutiérrez-Arnal, J. and Marín, C. (2024). The latent threat in wild birds: *Clostridium botulinum. Veterinary Science* 11(1):36. https://doi.org/10.3390/vetsci11010036.

Harr, K. E., Cunningham, F. L., Pritsos, C. A., et al. (2017a). Weathered MC252 crude oil-induced anemia and abnormal erythroid morphology in double-crested cormorants (*Phalacrocorax auritus*) with light microscopic and ultrastructural description of Heinz bodies. *Ecotoxicology and Environmental Safety* 146:29–39. https://doi.org/10.1016/j.ecoenv.2017.07.030.

Harr, K. E., Reavill, D. R., Bursian, S. J., et al. (2017b). Organ weights and histopathology of double-crested cormorants (*Phalacrocorax auritus*) dosed orally or dermally with artificially weathered Mississippi Canyon 252 crude oil. *Ecotoxicology and Environmental Safety* 146:52–61. https://doi.org/10.1016/j.ecoenv.2017.07.011.

Hartman, C. A., Ackerman, J. T., Cooney, B., et al. (2024). Egg mercury concentration and egg size varies with position in the laying sequence in two songbird species. *Environmental Toxicology & Chemistry* 43(8):1844–1854. https://doi.org/10.1002/etc.5900.

Henriksen, P., Carmichael, W. W., An, J., et al. (1997). Detection of an anatoxin-a(s)-like anticholinesterase in natural blooms and cultures of cyanobacteria/blue-green algae from Danish lakes and in the stomach contents of poisoned birds. *Toxicon* 35(6):901–913. https://doi.org/10.1016/s0041-0101(96)00190-0.

Herrero-Villar, M., Taggart, M. A., and Mateo, R. (2024). Pharmaceuticals in avian scavengers and other birds of prey: A toxicological perspective to improve risk assessments. *Science of the Total Environment* 948:174425. https://doi.org/10.1016/j.scitotenv.2024.174425.

Hidalgo, C. M., Mora, M. A., Sericano, J. L., et al. (2021). Persistent organic pollutants in eggs from south Texas Aplomado falcons. *Environmental Pollution* 268(Pt B):115685. https://doi.org/10.1016/j.envpol.2020.115685.

Hoang, T. C. and Mitten, S. (2022). Microplastic accumulation in the gastrointestinal tracts of nestling and adult migratory birds. *Science of the Total Environment* 838(Pt 1):155827. https://doi.org/10.1016/j.scitotenv.2022.155827.

Hong, S. H., Shim, W. J., Han, G. M., et al. (2014). Levels and profiles of persistent organic pollutants in resident and migratory birds from an urbanized coastal region of South Korea. *Science of the Total Environment* 470-471:1463–1470. https://doi.org/10.1016/j.scitotenv.2013.07.089.

Horak, K. E., Bursian, S. J., Ellis, C. K., et al. (2017). Toxic effects of orally ingested oil from the Deepwater Horizon spill on laughing gulls. *Ecotoxicology and Environmental Safety* 146:83–90. https://doi.org/10.1016/j.ecoenv.2017.07.018.

Houston, D. C., Mee, A., McGrady, M., et al. (2007). Why do condors and vultures eat junk? The implications for conservation. *Journal of Raptor Research* 41:235–238.

Jessup, D. A. (2023). Waterfowl diseases. In: *Wildlife Disease and Health in Conservation*, D. A. Jessup and R. W. Radcliffe (eds.), pp. 293–308. Johns Hopkins University Press.

Kibria, G. (2024). Contamination of coastal and marine bird species with plastics: Global analysis and synthesis. *Marine Pollution Bulletin* 206:116687. https://doi.org/10.1016/j.marpolbul.2024.116687.

King, M. D., Elliott, J. E., and Williams, T. D. (2021). Effects of petroleum exposure on birds: A review. *Science of the Total Environment* 755:142834. https://doi.org/10.1016/j.scitotenv.2020.142834.

Knudtzon, N. C., Thorstensen, H., Ruus, A., et al. (2021). Maternal transfer and occurrence of siloxanes, chlorinated paraffins, metals, PFAS and legacy POPs in herring gulls (*Larus argentatus*) of different urban influences. *Environment International* 152:106478. https://doi.org/10.1016/j.envint.2021.106478.

Kvitek, R. and Bretz, C. (2005). Shorebird foraging behavior, diet, and abundance vary with harmful algal bloom toxin concentrations in invertebrate prey. *Marine Ecology Progress Series* 293:303–309. https://doi.org/10.3354/meps293303.

Lan, J., Pengfei Liu, X. H., and Shanshan, Z. (2024). Harmful algal blooms in eutrophic marine environments: Causes, monitoring, and treatment. *Water* 16(7):2525. https://doi.org/10.3390/w16172525.

Lane, S. M., Smith, C. R., Mitchell, J., et al. (2015). Reproductive outcome and survival of common bottlenose dolphins sampled in Barataria Bay, Louisiana, USA, following the Deepwater Horizon oil spill. *Proceedings of the Royal Society B: Biological Sciences* 282(1818):20151944. https://doi.org/10.1098/rspb.2015.1944.

Lato, K. A., Thorne, L. H., Fuirst, M., et al. (2021). Microplastic abundance in gull nests in relation to urbanization. *Marine Pollution Bulletin* 164:112058. https://doi.org/10.1016/j.marpolbul.2021.112058.

Lavers, J. L. and Bond, A. L. (2016). Ingested plastic as a route for trace metals in Laysan Albatross (*Phoebastria immutabilis*) and Bonin Petrel (*Pterodroma hypoleuca*) from Midway Atoll. *Marine Pollution Bulletin* 110(1):493–500. https://doi.org/10.1016/j.marpolbul.2016.06.001.

Lavers, J. L. and Bond, A. L. (2024). Beyond the surface: Seabirds and plastics as indicators in a large, remote marine protected area. *Marine Pollution Bulletin* 116574. https://doi.org/10.1016/j.marpolbul.2024.116574.

Lavers, J. L., Howell, N. R., Bond, A. L., et al. (2025). Elemental analysis by neutron activation analysis and synchrotron x-ray fluorescence microscopy of ocean plastics ingested by pelagic seabirds. *Journal of Hazardous Materials* 494:138528. https://doi.org/10.1016/j.jhazmat.2025.138528.

Lewis, C. A., Cristol, D. A., Swaddle, J. P., et al. (2013). Decreased immune response in zebra finches exposed to sublethal doses of mercury. *Archives of Environmental Contaminants Toxicology* 64:327–336. https://doi.org/10.1007/s00244-012-9830-z.

Lewis, P. J., Lashko, A., Chiaradia, A., et al. (2022). New and legacy persistent organic pollutants (POPs) in breeding seabirds from the East Antarctic. *Environmental Pollution* 309:119734. https://doi.org/10.1016/j.envpol.2022.119734.

Li, Y., Zhang, X., Sun, J., et al. (2025). Inhalable microplastics of different shapes disrupt airway epithelial homeostasis: A comparative study of fibers and irregular particles. *Environment International* 203:109736. https://doi.org/10.1016/j.envint.2025.109736.

Loera, Y., Gruppi, C., Swing, K., et al. (2024). Heavy metal contamination in birds from protected regions in the Amazon. *Environmental Toxicology and Chemistry* 43(12):2601–2607. https://doi.org/10.1002/etc.5984.

Lu, R., Cao, X., Zheng, X., et al. (2023a). Biomagnification and elimination effects of persistent organic pollutants in a typical wetland food web from South China. *Journal of Hazardous Materials* 457:131733. https://doi.org/10.1016/j.jhazmat.2023.131733.

Lu, H., Yin, K., Su, H., et al. (2023b). Polystyrene microplastics induce autophagy and apoptosis in birds lungs via PTEN/PI3K/AKT/mTOR. *Environmental Toxicology* 38(1):78–89. https://doi.org/10.1002/tox.23663.

Ma, Y., Choi, C.-Y., Thomas, A., et al. (2022). Review of contaminant levels and effects in shorebirds: Knowledge gaps and conservation priorities. *Ecotoxicology and Environmental Safety* 242:113868. https://doi.org/10.1016/j.ecoenv.2022.113868.

Maggini, I., Kennedy, L. V., Bursian, S. J., et al. (2017a). Toxicological and thermoregulatory effects of feather contamination with artificially weathered MC 252 oil in western sandpipers (*Calidris mauri*). *Ecotoxicology and Environmental Safety* 146:118–128. https://doi.org/10.1016/j.ecoenv.2017.04.025.

Maggini, I., Kennedy, L. V., Macmillan, A., et al. (2017b). Light oiling of feathers increases flight energy expenditure in a migratory shorebird. *Journal of Experimental Biology* 220 (Pt 13):2372–2379. https://doi.org/10.1242/jeb.158220.

Mancini, M., Rodriguez, C., Bagnis, G., et al. (2010). Cianobacterial bloom and animal mass mortality in a reservoir from Central Argentina. *Brazilian Journal of Biology* 70(3 Suppl):841–845. https://doi.org/10.1590/s1519-69842010000400015.

Mangotra, A. and Singh, S. K. (2023). Volatile organic compounds: A threat to the environment and health hazards to living organisms – A review. *Journal of Biotechnology* 382:51–69. https://doi.org/10.1016/j.jbiotec.2023.12.013.

Mansfield, I., Reynolds, S. J., Lynch, I., et al. (2024). Birds as bioindicators of plastic pollution in terrestrial and freshwater environments: A 30-year review. *Environmental Pollution* 348:123790. https://doi.org/10.1016/j.envpol.2024.123790.

Martín-Vélez, V., Cano-Povedano, J., Cañuelo-Jurado, B., et al. (2024). Leakage of plastics and other debris from landfills to a highly protected lake by wintering gulls. *Waste Management* 177:13–23. https://doi.org/10.1016/j.wasman.2024.01.034.

Mateo, R., Beyer, W. N., Spann, J., et al. (2003). Relationship between oxidative stress, pathology, and behavioral signs of lead poisoning in mallards. *Journal of Toxicology and Environmental Health, Part A* 66(14):1371–1389. https://doi.org/10.1080/15287390306390.

Matos, D. M., Ramos, J. A., Brandão, A. L. C., et al. (2023). Microplastics ingestion and endocrine disrupting chemicals (EDCs) by breeding seabirds in the east tropical Atlantic: Associations with trophic and foraging proxies (δ^{15}N and δ^{13}C). *Science of the Total Environment* 912:168664. https://doi.org/10.1016/j.scitotenv.2023.168664.

Matsunaga, H., Harada, K. I., Senma, M., et al. (1999). Possible cause of unnatural mass death of wild birds in a pond in Nishinomiya, Japan: Sudden appearance of toxic cyanobacteria. *Natural Toxins* 7(2):81–84. https://doi.org/10.1002/(sici)1522-7189(199903/04)7:2<81::aid-nt44>3.0.CO;2-0.

McCain, S., Sim, R. R., Howerth, E. W., et al. (2020). Myonecrosis and death due to presumed microcystin toxicosis in American white pelicans (*Pelecanus erythrorhyncos*). *Zoo Wildlife Medicine* 51(2):407–415. https://doi.org/10.1638/2019-0117.

McKenzie, C. H., Bates, S. S., Martin, J. L., et al. (2021). Three decades of Canadian marine harmful algal events: Phytoplankton and phycotoxins of concern to human and ecosystem health. *Harmful Algae* 102:101852. https://doi.org/10.1016/j.hal.2020.101852.

McTee, M., Kean, B., Pons, A., et al. (2023). The seasonal threat of lead exposure in bald eagles. *Science of the Total Environment* 889:164256. https://doi.org/10.1016/j.scitotenv.2023.164256.

Meng, J., Zhang, Q., Ma, M., et al. (2022). Persistence of avian influenza virus (H9N2) on plastic surface. *Science of the Total Environment* 834:155355. https://doi.org/10.1016/j.scitotenv.2022.155355.

Metcalf, J. S., Banack, S. A., Kotut, K., et al. (2013). Amino acid neurotoxins in feathers of the Lesser Flamingo, *Phoeniconaias minor. Chemosphere* 90(2):835–839. https://doi.org/10.1016/j.chemosphere.2012.09094.

Mezzelani, M. and Regoli, F. (2022). The biological effects of pharmaceuticals in the marine environment. *Annual Reviews Marine Science* 14:105–128. https://doi.org/10.1146/annurev-marine-040821-075606.

Mills, W. F., Bustamante, P., McGill, R. A. R., et al. (2020). Mercury exposure in an endangered seabird: Long-term changes and relationships with trophic ecology and breeding success. *Proceedings of the Royal Society B: Biological Sciences* 287:20202683. https://doi.org/10.1098/rspb.2020.2683.

Mo, L., Zheng, X., Sun, Y., et al. (2018). Selection of passerine birds as bio-sentinel of persistent organic pollutants in terrestrial environment. *Science of the Total Environment* 633:1237–1244. https://doi.org/10.1016/j.scitotenv.2018.03.311.

Monclús, L., Shore, R. F., and Krone, O. (2020). Lead contamination in raptors in Europe: A systematic review and meta-analysis. *Science of the Total Environment* 748:141437. https://doi.org/10.1016/j.scitotenv.2020.141437.

Moreau, J., Rabdeau, J., Badenhausser, I., et al. (2022). Pesticide impacts on avian species with special reference to farmland birds: A review. *Environmental Monitoring Assessment* 194(10):790. https://doi.org/10.1007/s10661-022-10394-0.

Morris, Z. J., Stommel, E. W., and Metcalf, J. S. (2025). Airborne cyanobacterial toxins and their links to neurodegenerative diseases. *Molecules* 30(11):2320. https://doi.org/10.3390/molecules30112320.

Navarro, A., Luzardo, O. P., Gómez, M., et al. (2023). Microplastics ingestion and chemical pollutants in seabirds of Gran Canaria (Canary Islands, Spain). *Marine Pollution Bulletin* 186:114434. https://doi.org/10.1016/j.marpolbul.2022.114434.

Nguyen, D., Nguyen, M. K., Pham, M. T., et al. (2025). Plastic debris in bird nests: Sources, ecological impacts, and bioindicator potential for monitoring microplastic pollution. *Environmental Geochemistry and Health* 47(10):405. https://doi.org/10.1007/s10653-025-02688-2.

Nygard, T., Sandercock, B. K., Reinsborg, T., et al. (2019). Population recovery of Peregrine Falcons in central Norway in the 4 decades since the DDT-ban. *Ecotoxicology* 28(10):1160–1168. https://doi.org/10.1007/s10646-019-02111-4.

Nzabanita, D., Shen, H., Grist, S., et al. (2024). Exposure to persistent organic pollutants in Australian waterbirds. *Environmental Toxicology and Chemistry* 43(4):736–747. https://doi.org/10.1002/etc.5804.

Ocampos, A. I., Guinn, M. A., Elliott, J., et al. (2024). Pharmaceuticals in the blubber of live free-swimming common bottlenose dolphins (*Tursiops truncatus*). *iScience* 27:111507. https://doi.org/10.1016/j.isci.2024.111507.

Osena, G., Fick, J., Flach, C. F., et al. (2025). Evaluating wastewater surveillance for estimating pharmaceutical use. *Environment International* 204:109807. https://doi.org/10.1016/j.envint.2025.109807.

Padayachee, K., Reynolds, C., Mateo, R., et al. (2023). A global review of the temporal and spatial patterns of DDT and dieldrin monitoring in raptors. *Science of the Total Environment* 858(Pt 1):159734. https://doi.org/10.1016/j.scitotenv.2022.159734.

Papadimitriou, T., Katsiapi, M., Vlachopoulos, K., et al. (2018). Cyanotoxins as the "common suspects" for the Dalmatian pelican (*Pelecanus crispus*) deaths in a Mediterranean reconstructed reservoir. *Environmental Pollution* 234:779–787. https://doi.org/10.1016/j.envpol.2017.12.022.

Pierce, R. H. and Henry, M. S. (2008). Harmful algal toxins of the Florida red tide (*Karenia brevis*): Natural chemical stressors in south Florida coastal ecosystems. *Ecotoxicology* 17:623–631. https://doi.org/10.1007/s10646-008-0241-x.

Pitarch, A., Gil, C., and Blanco, G. (2017). Oral mycoses in avian scavengers exposed to antibiotics from livestock farming. *Science of the Total Environment* 605–606:139–146. https://doi.org/10.1016/j.scitotenv.2017.06.144.

Porrero, M. C., Mentaberre, G., Sánchez, S., et al. (2013). Methicillin resistant *Staphylococcus aureus* (MRSA) carriage in different free-living wild animal species in Spain. *Veterinary Journal* 198(1):127–130. https://doi.org/10.1016/j.tvjl.2013.06.004.

Puskic, P. S., Slocombe, R., Ploeg, R., et al. (2024). Exploring the pathology of liver, kidney, muscle, and stomach of fledgling seabirds associated with plastic ingestion. *Journal of Hazardous Materials* 465:133306. https://doi.org/10.1016/j.jhazmat.2023.133306.

Rajput, S., Jain, D., Dash, N., et al. (2024). Role of cyanotoxins in the development and promotion of cancer. *Toxicology Reports* 101798. https://doi.org/10.1016/j.toxrep.2024.101798.

Rahman, Z. and Singh, V. P. (2019). The relative impact of toxic heavy metals (THMs) (arsenic (As), cadmium (Cd), chromium (Cr)(VI), mercury (Hg), and lead (Pb)) on the total environment: An overview. *Environmental Monitoring Assessment* 191(7):419. https://doi.org/10.1007/s10661-019-7528-7.

Rattner, B. A., Wazniak, C. E., Lankton, J. S., et al. (2022). Review of harmful algal bloom effects on birds with implications for avian wildlife in the Chesapeake Bay region. *Harmful Algae* 120:102319. https://doi.org/10.1016/j.hal.2022.102319.

Rehman, K., Fatima, F., Waheed, I., et al. (2018). Prevalence of exposure of heavy metals and their impact on health consequences. *Journal of Cellular Biochemistry* 119(1):157–184.

Rehage, J. S., Castillo, N. A., Distrubell, A., et al. (2025). A multi-estuary assessment of pharmaceutical exposure and risk of pharmacological effects in a recreational fishery. *Environmental Toxicology and Chemistry* 44(10):2832–2847. https://doi.org/10.1093/etojnl/vgaf125.

Rudolph, I., Chiang, G., Galbán-Malagón, C., et al. (2016). Persistent organic pollutants and porphyrins biomarkers in penguin faeces from Kopaitic Island and Antarctic Peninsula. *Science of the Total Environment*. 573:1390–1396. https://doi.org/10.1016/j.scitotenv.2016.07.091.

Sagerup, K., Henriksen, E. O., Skorping, A., et al. (2000). Intensity of parasitic nematodes increases with organochlorine levels in the glaucous gull. *Journal of Applied Ecology* 37(3):532–539. https://doi.org/10.1046/j.1365-2664.2000.00521.x.

Sangkachai, N., Gummow, B., Hayakijkosol, O., et al. (2024). A review of risk factors at the human-animal-environmental interface of garbage dumps that are driving current and emerging zoonotic diseases. *One Health* 19:100915. https://doi.org/10.1016/j.onehlt.2024.100915.

Sayers, 2nd., C. J., Evers, D. C., Ruiz-Gutierrez, V., et al. (2023). Mercury in Neotropical birds: A synthesis and prospectus on 13 years of exposure data. *Ecotoxicology* 32(8):1096–1123. https://doi.org/10.1007/s10646-023-02706-y.

Schwantes, U. (2023). Impact of anthropogenous environmental factors on the marine ecosystem of trophically transmitted helminths and hosting seabirds: Focus on N Atlantic, North Sea, Baltic and the Arctic seas. *Helminthologia* 60(4):300–326. https://doi.org/10.247/helm-2023-0034.

Scallet, A. C. and Ye, X. (1997). Excitotoxic mechanisms of neurodegeneration in transmissible spongiform encephalopathies. *Annals of the New York Academy of Sciences* 825:194–205. https://doi.org/10.1111/j.1749-6632.1997.tb48429.x.

Schnelle, A., Peter, M., Müller, C., et al. (2025). A comprehensive assessment of contaminant exposure in an endangered tern population. *Environmental Research* 285(Pt 3):122444.

Shearn-Bochsler, V., Lance, E. W., Corcoran, R., et al. (2014). Fatal paralytic shellfish poisoning in Kittlitz's Murrelet (*Brachyramphus brevirostris*) nestlings, Alaska, USA. *Journal of Wildlife Diseases* 50(4):933–937. https://doi.org/10.7589/2013-11-296.

Singh, N., Shi, S., and Goel, S. (2023). Ultrasmall silica nanoparticles in translational biomedical research: Overview and outlook. *Advances in Drug Delivery Reviews* 192:114638. https://doi.org/10.1016/j.addr.2022.114638.

Shore, R. F., Taggart, M. A., Smits, J., et al. (2014). Detection and drivers of exposure and effects of pharmaceuticals in higher vertebrates. *Philosophical Transactions of the Royal Society B: Biological Sciences* 369(1656):20130570. https://doi.org/10.1098/rstb.2013.0570.

Smith, M. M., Dusek, R. J., Hollmen, T., et al. (2025). Paralytic shellfish toxins and seabirds: Evaluating sublethal effects, behavioral responses, and ecological implications of saxitoxin ingestion by common murres (*Uria aalge*). *Harmful Algae* 148:102919. https://doi.org/10.1016/j.hal.2025.102919.

Soliño, L., Ferrer-Obiol, J., Navarro-Herrero, L., et al. (2019). Are pelagic seabirds exposed to amnesic shellfish poisoning toxins? *Harmful Algae* 84:172–180. https://doi.org/10.1016/j.hal.2019.03.014.

Soliño, L., Turner, A. D., Ben-Gigirey, B., et al. (2025). Investigation into paralytic shellfish toxins and Microcystins in seabirds from Portugal. *Toxins (Basel)* 17(3):135. https://doi.org/10.3390/toxins17030135.

Sonne, C., Siebert, U., Gonnsen, K., et al. (2020). Health effects from contaminant exposure in Baltic Sea birds and marine mammals: A review. *Environment International* 139:105725. https://doi.org/10.1016/j.envint.2020.105725.

Starr, M., Lair, S., Michaud, S., et al. (2017). Multispecies mass mortality of marine fauna linked to a toxic dinoflagellate bloom. *PLoS One* 12(5):e0176299. https://doi.org/10.1371/journal.pone.0176299.

Świacka, K., Maculewicz, J., Kowalska, D., et al. (2022). Presence of pharmaceuticals and their metabolites in wild-living aquatic organisms – Current state of knowledge. *Journal of Hazardous Materials* 424(Pt A):127350. https://doi.org/10.1016/j.jhazmat.2021.127350.

Teuten, E. L., Saquing, J. M., Knappe, D. R., et al. (2009). Transport and release of chemicals from plastics to the environment and to wildlife. *Philosophical Transactions of the Royal Society London B: Biological Sciences* 364(1526):2027–2045. https://doi.org/10.1098/rstb.2008.0284.

Thaysen, C., Sorais, M., Verreault, J., et al. (2020). Bidirectional transfer of halogenated flame retardants between the gastrointestinal tract and ingested plastics in urban-adapted ring-billed gulls. *Science of the Total Environment* 730:138887. https://doi.org/10.1016/j.scitotenv.2020.138887.

Tokunaga, Y., Okochi, H., Tani, Y., et al. (2023). Airborne microplastics detected in the lungs of wild birds in Japan. *Chemosphere* 321:138032. https://doi.org/10.1016/j.chemosphere.2023.138032.

Tongue, A. D. W., Reynolds, S. J., Fernie, K. J., et al. (2019). Flame retardant concentrations and profiles in wild birds associated with landfill: A critical review. *Environmental Pollution* 248:646–658. https://doi.org/10.1016/j.envpol.2019.01.103.

Turner, A. and Filella, M. (2021). Hazardous metal additives in plastics and their environmental impacts. *Environment International* 156:106622. https://doi.org/10.1016/j.envint.2021.106622.

Uzal, F. A., Henderson, E., and Asin, J. (2024). Botulism in fish: A review. *Journal of Veterinary Diagnostic Investigation* 36(3):312–318. https://doi.org/10.1177/10406387241236725.

Vallverdú-Coll, N., Mateo, R., Mougeot, F., et al. (2019). Review Immunotoxic effects of lead on birds. *Science of the Total Environment* 689(1):505–515. https://doi.org/10.1016/j.scitotenv.2019.06.251.

Van Hemert, C., Harley, J. R., Baluss, G., et al. (2022). Paralytic shellfish toxins associated with Arctic Tern mortalities in Alaska. *Harmful Algae* 117:102270. https://doi.org/10.1016/j.hal.2022.102270.

Van Hemert, C., Schoen, S. K., Litaker, R. W., et al. (2020). Algal toxins in Alaskan seabirds: Evaluating the role of saxitoxin and domoic acid in a large-scale die-off of Common Murres. *Harmful Algae* 92:101730. https://doi.org/10.1016/j.hal.2019.101730.

Vanstreels, R. E. T., Gallo, L., Serafini, P. P., et al. (2021). Ingestion of plastics and other debris by coastal and pelagic birds along the coast of Espírito Santo, Eastern Brazil. *Marine Pollution Bulletin* 173(Pt B):113046. https://doi.org/10.1016/j.marpolbul.2021.113046.

Vanstreels, R. E. T., Piccinin, I. N. L., Maraschin, M., et al. (2023). Phthalate esters (plasticizers) in the uropygial gland and their relationship to plastics ingestion in seabird along the cost of Espirito Santo, Eastern Brazil. *Journal of Zoo and Wildlife Medicine* 53(4):733–743. https://doi.org/10.1638/2022-0053.

Varaglya, D., Jethva, B., and Pandya, D. (2022). Feather heavy metal contamination in various species of waterbirds from Asia: A review. *Environmental Monitoring Assessment* 194:26. https://doi.org/10.1007/s10661-021-09678-8.

Varian-Ramos, C. W., Swaddle, J. P., and Cristol, D. A. (2014). Mercury reduces avian reproductive success and imposes selection: An experimental study with adult- or lifetime-exposure in zebra finch. *PLoS One* 9(4):E95674. https://doi.org/10.1371/journal.pone.0095674.

Verreault, J., Villa, R. A., Gabrielsen, G., et al. (2006). Maternal transfer of organohalogen contaminants and metabolites to eggs of arctic-breeding glaucous gulls. *Environmental Pollution* 144:1050–1053. https://doi.org/10.1016/j.envpol.2005.10.055.

Vignesh, K. S. and Deepe, Jr, G. S. (2017). Metallothioneins: Emerging modulators in Immunity and infection. *International Journal of Molecular Sciences* 18:2197.

Walsh, C. J., Leggett, S. R., Carter, B. J., et al. (2010). Effects of brevetoxin exposure on the immune system of loggerhead sea turtles. *Aquatic Toxicology* 97:293–303.

Walsh, C. J., Luer, C. A., and Noyes, D. R. (2005). Effects of environmental stressors on lymphocyte proliferation in Florida manatees, *Trichechus manatus latirostris. Veterinary Immunology and Immunopathology* 103:247–256.

Wang, P., Li, G., Shou, H., et al. (2025). Microplastic abundance in placental chorionic villi detected by pyrolysis-gas chromatography/mass spectrometry in cases of spontaneous miscarriage during early pregnancy. *EBioMedicine* 120:105918. https://doi.org/10.1016/j.ebiom.2025.105918.

Wang, L., Nabi, G., Yin, L., et al. (2021). Birds and plastic pollution: Recent advances. *Avian Research* 12(1):59. https://doi.org/10.1186/s40657-021-00293-2.

Wells, M. R., Coggan, T. L., Stevenson, G., et al. (2024). Per- and polyfluoroalkyl substances (PFAS) in little penguins and associations with urbanisation and health parameters. *Science of the Total Environment* 912:169084. https://doi.org/10.1016/j.scitotenv.2023.169084.

Whitney, M. C. and Cristol, D. A. (2017). Impacts of sublethal mercury exposure on birds: A detailed review. In: *Reviews of Environmental Contamination and Toxicology*, P. de Voogt (eds.), vol. 244. Cham: Springer. https://doi.org/10.1007/398_2017_4.

Williams, R. J., Holladay, S. D., Williams, S. M., et al. (2018). Environmental lead and wild birds: A review. *Reviews of Environmental Contaminants and Toxicology* 245:157–180. https://doi.org/10.1007/398_2017_9.

Wright, J. L. C., Boyd, R. K., Freitas, A. D., et al. (1989). Identification of domoic acid, a neuroexcitatory amino acid, in toxic mussels from eastern Prince Edward Island. *Canadian Journal of Chemistry* 67(3):481–490.

Yin, K., Wang, D., Zhang, Y., et al. (2023). Dose-effect of polystyrene microplastics on digestive toxicity in chickens (*Gallus gallus*): Multi-omics reveals critical role of gut-liver axis. *Journal of Advanced Research* 52:3–18. https://doi.org/10.1016/j.jare.2022.10.015.

Yin, K., Wang, D., Zhao, H., et al. (2022). Polystyrene microplastics up-regulates liver glutamine and glutamate synthesis and promotes autophagy-dependent ferroptosis and apoptosis in the cerebellum through the liver-brain axis. *Environmental Pollution* 307:119449. https://doi.org/10.1016/j.envpol.2022.119449.

Zaias, J., Fleming, L. E., Baden, D. G., et al. (2011). Repeated exposure to aerosolized Brevetoxin-3 induces prolonged airway hyper-responsiveness and lung inflammation in sheep. *Inhalation Toxicology* 23(4):205–211.

Zhang, E., Kim, M., Rueda, L., et al. (2022a). Association of zoonotic protozoan parasites with microplastics in seawater and implications for human and wildlife health. *Scientific Reports* 12:6532. https://doi.org/10.1038/s41598-022-10485-5.

Zhang, Y., Wang, D., Yin, K., et al. (2022b). Endoplasmic reticulum stress-controlled autophagic pathway promotes polystyrene microplastics-induced myocardial dysplasia in birds. *Environmental Pollution* 311:119963. https://doi.org/10.1016/j.envpol.2022.119963.

Zhao, S., Zhu, L., and Li, D. (2016). Microscopic anthropogenic litter in terrestrial birds from Shanghai, China: Not only plastics but also natural fibers. *Science of the Total Environment* 550:1110–1115. https://doi.org/10.1016/j.scitotenv.2016.01.112.

Ziccardi, M. (2023). Oil spills and their management. In: *Wildlife Disease and Health in Conservation*, D. A. Jessup and R. W. Radcliffe (eds.), pp. 69–89. Johns Hopkins University Press.

10

High Impact Avian Infectious Diseases – the Past and Future Outlook

Introduction

Various epizootics have caused massive die-offs of birds in the past two centuries, most of which impacted agricultural poultry farms. These epizootics have been due to infectious agents such as viruses and bacteria and noninfectious factors such as toxins and toxicants (Jessup, 2023). We covered toxins and contaminants in the last chapter. Let's (briefly) review major infectious outbreaks of the past and discuss the potential for these and other infectious agents to cause future outbreaks, how we can mitigate or manage them, and how they could impact wild and captive avian health and populations. Box 10.1 contains a glossary of often-used terms describing diseases.

Box 10.1 Glossary of commonly used terms to describe diseases

Amplifying/amplifier host – an organism that permits a pathogen (e.g., parasite and virus) to replicate in them, increasing their numbers for transmission to other hosts.
Carrier – an organism that harbors a pathogen but does not exhibit any signs of disease but can pass the organism to others.
Dead end host – an organism that is unable to transmit a pathogen to others, thereby preventing completion of the pathogen's life cycle.
Definitive host – an organism in which the pathogen sexually matures and can reproduce.
Fomite – a physical object that is likely to carry an infection from one place to another.
Intermediate host – an organism that harbors a pathogen during its development but before reaching sexual maturity.
Pathogenicity – the ability of a pathogen/agent to cause disease.
Reservoir/reservoir host – an organism that harbors a pathogen and serves as a source of infection to others.
Shedder – an organism that excretes (sheds) a pathogen into the environment. They may or may not show clinical signs.
Virulence – the severity or harmfulness of a disease.
Zoonosis – a disease or pathogen that is able to move from an animal into a human and cause disease.

Viruses

Avian Influenza Virus

Avian influenza A (AIV) is an RNA virus in the *Orthomyxoviridae* family. There are four types of influenza viruses – A, B, C, and D. Type A viruses infect birds. Types A–C are known to infect humans. Influenza type A viruses include the "avian" and "swine" flus and are the only AIV group known to produce *pandemics* in humans. The influenza virus contains neuraminidase (N) and hemagglutinin (H) proteins on its surface. Neuraminidase proteins help degrade the mucous in the respiratory tract, allowing the virus to get close to the respiratory epithelial cells. Hemagglutinin proteins on the influenza virus envelope bind to respiratory epithelial cells via sialic acid receptors. This binding stimulates engulfment into the cells, which permits viral replication (Ramey, 2023). There are approximately 18 H subtypes and 11 N subtypes. Depending on the combination of these proteins, the virus may be more or less *virulent* (severity of disease). For example, one type of H1N1 (aka, swine flu) is thought to be endemic in humans and is a known cause of the seasonal flu in people. Different subtypes of this virus come about by recombination and reassortment of antigens on the viral surface, which is one reason why annual revaccination is important.

The avian, swine, and human flu types belong to the same genus. Thus, crossover and recombination among these strains is likely permitting the virus to survive in any of those species (making it a zoonotic pathogen). The influenza virus does not have RNA polymerase proofreading activity, and this favors faster genetic change and evolution of mutations (Ramey, 2023). In humans, clinical signs of the flu include upper respiratory signs (nasal congestion, infection) and/or lower respiratory infection (pneumonia, etc.). Vaccination is recommended annually to mitigate the extent of disease manifestation should one get exposed to the virus.

In birds, the H5 and H7 types are known to be highly pathogenic (HP) to domestic poultry and are referred to as highly pathogenic avian influenza viruses (HPAIV). Other H types are considered to be low pathogenic (LP) and are referred to as low pathogenic avian influenza viruses (LPAIV). In the 1960s–1970s, wild waterfowl of the duck, geese, and shorebird families, were identified as the reservoir hosts for a wide range of influenza types (Philippa, 2008). These viruses were able to spill over and infect domestic poultry. In 1996, an HP H5N1 strain in geese in Guangdong, China, spread to cause massive loss of poultry and caused major human illness and death throughout East Asia. In 2002, a related strain of influenza killed many captive and wild aquatic birds in Hong Kong. Then in 2005, over 6,000 wild birds (including geese, gulls, and other species) were killed by an HP strain in Qinghai Lake, China (Philippa, 2008). In 2014–2015, in the United States and Canada, over 50 million birds (mostly poultry) died in a flu epidemic caused by a variant strain originating in China. These losses included direct death from the virus and depopulation of exposed flocks to mitigate additional spread. The eradication costs and the economic burden posed by these losses amounted to millions of dollars! Subsequently, the outbreak in North America starting in the early 2020s has impacted more than 81 million poultry including commercial and backyard flocks. Wild birds worldwide have also been severely impacted, especially colonial seabirds, birds of prey, and scavengers (the latter two feeding on infected animals/carcasses; Kuiken et al., 2025; Puryear and Runstadler, 2024). Antibody levels for AIV exposure in seabirds increased in prevalence between 2022 and 2023 in the Northwest Atlantic Ocean (McLaughlin et al., 2025). HPAI cases in seabirds along the Atlantic, North Sea, and Baltic coasts were significantly increased in 2024 (EFSA, 2024). Similarly, antibodies against AIV were found in 70% of bald eagles in the Midwest United States in 2023, which was significantly increased over those measured in 2012 (Rayment et al., 2025).

Wild birds (many species, but especially waterbirds, ducks, etc.) are known carriers of AIV, may be asymptomatic shedders of the virus, and were the source of the HPAIV spread from Asia out to all parts of the world. Meta-analysis of data suggests that migratory species disperse the virus along migration pathways but that resident birds drive local transmission (Qiu et al., 2025). Data also suggest that in Europe, HPAI may be endemic in resident birds also driving local spread (Pohlmann et al., 2022). Once in the new area, the virus infects other conspecifics and spills over into other species (e.g., humans, mammals, and other bird species). Spillover from wild waterfowl to poultry farms has been well documented (Cullen et al., 2025). Based on HPAIV strain analyses, mammal (fur seals, *Arctocephalus australis*) to avian (seabird species) transmission appears to have occurred in Uruguay (Tomás et al., 2024). Transmission is likely also from bird to marine mammal.

Bird species are differentially affected by the virus. Captive juvenile and adult mallards (*Anas platyrhynchos*) followed for 15 months showed variability in natural AIV infection frequency, HPAIV subtype, and humoral immune responses (Tolf et al., 2013). Antibodies passed from female yellow-legged gulls (*Larus michahellis*) to their eggs decreased over the nestling stage (Lamb et al., 2024). The differential antibody changes are likely due to environmental presence and exposure to AIV. HPAIV-induced mortality in Peruvian pelicans (*Pelecanus thagus*) was severe, up to 40% of their population, but HPAI mortality in Canadian herring gulls (*Larus argentatus*) was less than 10%, and the disease was self-limiting (Leguia et al., 2023; Taylor et al., 2023). LP strains are thought to be endemic in waterbirds, and smaller die-offs occur sporadically (Philippa, 2008). In poultry, LP virus strains can cause mild to severe respiratory signs, excessive lacrimation (tearing), decreased egg production, and signs of generalized lethargy (including ruffled feathers, depression, and decreased food and water intake). Disease in poultry from HPAIV strains includes more severe signs, including cyanosis (blueish skin/mucosa color due to poor circulation), hemorrhage, change in iris color, neurologic signs, and mortality (Puryear and Runstadler, 2024; Philippa, 2008).

AIV can remain viable in the environment for several weeks to months and be stuck onto particles that can become aerosolized (Ramey, 2023; Ramey et al., 2020; Philippa, 2008). Virus inactivation can occur by using detergents to break the virus's outer lipid layer and/or exposure to high temperatures. Management of outbreaks includes active surveillance, disinfection, vaccination, and control of human and animal movements into areas of outbreaks. Vaccination may not always prevent infection because of the genetic reassortment; however, it does reduce the extent and severity of disease. Vaccination of poultry appeared to be successful in reducing HPAIV and produced good immune responses in China (Liu et al., 2023); however, it is not used in all countries. In the United States, it is only conditionally approved for poultry (Puryear and Runstadler, 2024). After almost 10% of endangered California condors died from HPAIV infection, the United States obtained urgent approval to give vaccinations to these birds in captive breeding to stem the mortality related to influenza (Kozlov, 2023). Antibody persistence against AIV lasted for seven years in Flamingos (*Phoenicopterus ruber*) in a zoo in Barcelona (Fernández-Bellon et al., 2016). Another anti-AIV vaccine trialed in Switzerland also showed high antibody response in chickens which lasted a year in almost 98% of individuals (Stettler et al., 2025). No side effects were observed from this vaccine in chickens or in other bird species in two Switzerland zoos that also received it. These studies suggest that vaccination and revaccination are a good option. AIV is a reportable disease in the United States. Positive evidence of the presence of AIV requires reporting to US governmental and veterinary authorities.

Newcastle Disease Virus

Newcastle disease (ND) virus is an RNA virus of the family *Paramyxoviridae*. There are nine types of avian viruses in this family; however, APMV-1 (Avian paramyxovirus type -1) is the type that causes ND and the epizootics. ND (aka APMV-1 or more recently reclassified as Avian orthoavulavirus -1; Ul-Rahman et al., 2022) is one of the most economically important diseases of poultry worldwide and is highly pathogenic (spreads easily) in domestic chickens. For simplicity, we will refer to it as ND virus, NDV. NDV is global in its distribution and appears capable of infecting all species of birds and some vertebrates including various mammals and humans (Ul-Rahman et al., 2022; Leighton and Heckert, 2007).

The first worldwide occurrence of an NDV epizootic in domestic chickens was between the mid-1920s and early 1960s (Leighton and Heckert, 2007). This was followed by another worldwide epizootic from 1969 to 1973 and then again in Europe in the 1990s. In 1949–1951, a domestic chicken die-off occurred in Scotland and Ireland. The source of the NDV was confirmed to be from infected cormorant entrails that were fed to the chickens. Interestingly, cormorants are the only wild bird species in which NDV has caused large-scale mortality (Leighton and Heckert, 2007). Other notable mortality events have been traced back to psittacines in the international pet bird trade and in pigeons that lived in a grain storage loft on a farm. Since the mid-1950s, serologic evidence of NDV has been found worldwide (Arctic to Antarctic), especially in free-living waterfowl. Small poultry flocks are thought to be primary reservoirs of NDV around the world (Leighton and Heckert, 2007).

Affected susceptible birds usually show neurologic clinical signs including ataxia, weakness, and/or paralysis, if not acute death. Other clinical signs may be present in the respiratory, gastrointestinal, or renal systems. The virus can be shed from and/or reside in feces, body fluids, eggs, and muscle/tissues. The virus is very stable outside of the host and can survive for long periods of time in the environment. NDV is highly infectious and can be easily transmitted via bird-to-bird contact as well as via fomites. Most manifestations of disease are inapparent or subclinical, and birds can mount an immune response against the virus, but viral shedding can still persist for a very long time (Leighton and Heckert, 2007).

NDV is zoonotic and considered a human pathogen of minor importance; however, its presence is reportable to governmental and veterinary authorities (as is AIV). Vaccination is an important aspect of protection from the disease in poultry flocks as well as in zoos and captive breeding programs, especially if they involve endangered species or species of concern. Imported birds to the United States are screened for NDV. If positive, they are prohibited from entry into the United States, although this could be circumvented by the illegal trade industry. There does not appear to be significant wild population concerns with this agent.

Arboviruses

Arboviruses are viruses that are spread from host to host by arthropods. The arthropod vectors (various mosquito species, ticks, sand flies, etc.) permit replication of virus within them, which then gets passed on to the next host via a bite for a blood meal (Figure 10.1). The arbovirus group includes several families which are the source of avian (and human) diseases. Birds are also amplifying hosts for many of these viruses, which means that viruses can replicate in them producing a robust viremia (infectious viral particles circulate in high numbers in the blood). This facilitates viral uptake into the arthropod host during a blood meal. Transmission of virus between insects and birds is contingent on various environmental, host, and other factors that favor close proximity to each other (e.g., cooccur at the same time of day, specific location [canopy vs. ground; urban vs. rural] and time of year; McLean and Urbico, 2007). Areas where birds (or humans) congregate are very fruitful for insect vectors and the virus to flourish. And as humans move into and invade more rural areas and increasingly concentrate in urban areas, they are more likely to come into contact with an insect vector during the warmer and/or wetter times of the year.

Flaviviruses (recently renamed Orthoflaviviruses) are enveloped viruses belonging to the arbovirus family. Birds are critical natural hosts for several of these viruses, which are known to cause human and/or avian illnesses. Table 10.1 summarizes the primary arboviruses and other arthropod-transmitted diseases that contribute to significant avian and human morbidity and/or mortality. The best known and studied flavivirus is the West Nile virus (WNV).

WNV has the broadest host and vector distribution range than other flaviviruses (Jessup, 2023). Wild birds are the primary hosts, and the virus cycles between them and mosquitos of the *Culex* genus. In the wild bird host, the virus replicates to produce a viremia (level of

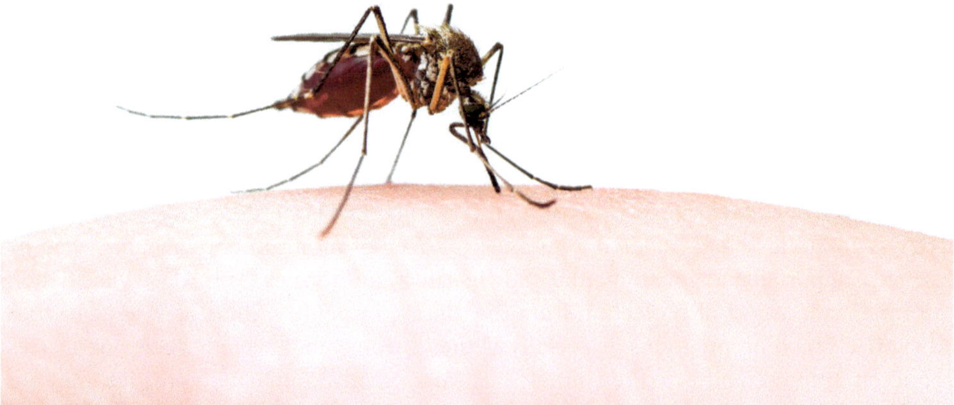

Nechaevkon/Adobe Stock Photos

Figure 10.1 *Culex* mosquito.

Table 10.1 Arthropod transmitted diseases of significance to birds and humans.

Disease name/vector	Microbe	Arthropod
Japanese encephalitis virus	*Orthoflavivirus japonicum*	Mosquito (*Culex tritaeniorhynchus*)
St. Louis encephalitis virus	*Orthoflavivirus louisense*	Mosquito (*Culex tarsalis; Culex pipiense quinquefasciatus*)
West Nile virus	*Orthoflavivirus nilense*	Mosquito (*Culex* spp.)
Usutu encephalitis virus[a]	*Orthoflavivirus usutuense*	Mosquito (*Culex pipiens*)[b]
Western encephalitis virus	*Alphavirus western*	Mosquito (*C. tarsalis*)
Eastern encephalitis virus	*Alphavirus eastern*	mosquito (*Culiseta melanura*)
Malaria	*Plasmodium* spp.	Mosquito (*Anopheles* spp.)
Lyme disease	*Borrelia burgdorferi*	Tick (*Ixodes* spp.)
Tick-borne encephalitis virus	*Orthoflavivirus* spp.	Tick (*Ixodes* spp.)

Source: Adapted from McLean and Ubico (2007).
a. Emerging virus of concern.
b. Primary vector. Spp. = species.

circulating infectious virus particles), which is then picked up and transferred to another host by mosquito bites. Humans and other animals are thought to be "dead end" hosts; that is, they get disease but do not permit viral replication. Apparently, other than domestic geese, domestic birds do not produce a productive WNV viremia and as such are also considered dead-end hosts (Jessup, 2023).

WNV is endemic in Africa and Asia (Eastern hemisphere) but arrived in the United States in 1999 in New York City. The strain that arrived in the United States was a very virulent strain. Corvids were hit the hardest as the virus caused an epizootic in the local birds and caused disease in people (Caffrey et al., 2005). The epizootic expanded in range possibly due to the movement of infected crows. Although the percentage of birds with antibodies against WNV was under 40%, the mortality rate was above 70% (McLean and Ubico, 2007). By 2004, the range had expanded across the continental United States, resulting in approximately 47,000 avian and 650 (out of greater than 16,000 cases) human deaths (George et al., 2015; McLean and Ubico, 2007)! By 2006, the WNV was present in Canada and down into Mexico, the Caribbean, Puerto Rico, and Central America. The virus was able to be maintained in the southern United States during the winters and spread via migratory birds. The infection route paralleled the migration pathways in the United States. Transmission of WNV other than via the *Culex* mosquitos includes transovarian passage (vertical) and possibly by ticks within whom the virus has been shown to survive a long time (McLean and Ubico, 2007). The virus can also spread by direct contact with contaminated oral and cloacal fluids (in which the virus is shed).

The pathogenicity and virulence of WNV vary across avian species. Infection with WNV has led to decreased survivorship in approximately 47% of terrestrial bird species between 1992 and 2007 (George et al., 2015). In addition to cases observed in wild birds, an outbreak of WNV in a captive colony of owls showed a distinct difference in pathogenicity. Northern owl species had 100% mortality; owl species with a southerly distribution had no mortality, and owls with a wide North American breeding range had intermediate mortality (Gancz et al., 2004). Domestic poultry appear to be a heterogenous group relative to morbidity and viremia level; very young chickens and domestic geese show clinical signs and produce a strong viremia, while adult chickens and turkeys develop a very low viremia (McLean and Ubico, 2007). As of 2015, we know that there is a long and lengthy list of avian species affected by WNV; in humans, there are long-term neurologic sequelae to infection, and the virus can be transmitted by additional routes in humans, including via blood transfusion, organ transplant, and breast milk (McNamara, 2015).

Usutu virus (USUV) is a virus closely related to WNV. It often co-circulates with WNV and can be found in some infections with WNV because they share the same vector-bird cycle (*C. pipiens* is the primary vector; Nelson and Ploss, 2024). USUV can also use other mosquito species in its transmission cycles. USUV seropositivity has been found in many birds and mammals and has been known to cause disease in humans. The main avian reservoirs are Eurasian blackbirds and Great gray owls who have suffered morbidity and mortality from infection. In 2015–2016, over 400 blackbirds were killed by USUV. In these years, the mosquito population had increased from 1000 (in the previous year) to 4000, which likely was the underlying cause of the outbreak (Rijks et al., 2016). While human disease from USUV is thought to be less virulent than from other flaviviruses, USUV is considered an "emerging pathogen of concern" because it is known to produce neurologic disorders in humans and can cause increasing avian mortality (Laratta et al., 2025).

The *togaviridae* family includes the Western equine encephalitis (WEE) and the Eastern equine encephalitis (EEE) viruses. WEE was first isolated from sick horses in the western United States and Canada in 1930, and there have been many outbreaks with numerous deaths of horses and humans since then. *C. tarsalis* is the primary mosquito vector, and passerines are the primary vertebrate vector. The WEE life cycle is more complex than that of WNV. There are different intermediate mosquito and small mammal vectors involved initially in the spring until *C. tarsalis* emerges in June/July, and then it takes over as the major vector. At this time, infection leads to viral amplification and transmission in *C. tarsalis* for the rest of the summer (McLean and Ubico, 2007). EEE also has likely been around since the 1930s–1940s, and its range is the eastern United States. EEE is less common than WEE, but more pathogenic, affecting both exotic and native avian species.

Disease in birds caused by arboviruses produces generalized signs, signs related to the central nervous system or acute death. Clinical signs, if present, occur after viremia. Neutralizing antibody is produced. The virus is carried throughout the body in the blood or lymphatic system and can infect any organ in the body (McLean and Urbico, 2007). By and large, the avian epizootics caused by arboviruses likely have not significantly impacted avian population levels to date. The major impact of birds is their role as hosts that permit arboviral replication and spread the virus, which can affect humans, other mammals, any threatened or endangered species, and/or immunodeficient individuals.

The threat of WNV and other arboviruses to impact wild bird populations is real. LaDeau et al. (2007) showed from a 26-year bird breeding survey that seven species of birds suffered population declines since WNV arrival in 1999. Global warming, urbanization, land use changes, concentration of water bodies and wetlands, and avian congregations in high numbers all contribute to the likelihood of continued impact and spread of arboviruses. Mosquito populations (primarily from the *Culex* and *Aedes* genera) have already and will likely continue to undergo niche expansions with global warming, which will result in exposure to new, possibly naïve, host species. As Flaviviruses have high mutation capability, new strains are likely to emerge (Nelson and Ploss, 2024). Retrospective data on *Anopheles* mosquito levels between 1898–2016 showed that its range spread to higher elevations (6.5 m/year) and expansion poleward (4.7 km/year; Carlson et al., 2023). A study aiming to predict mosquito abundance with increasing global temperatures modeled the potential heat tolerance levels of eight mosquito species that are known transmitters of zoonotic diseases (Couper et al., 2024). Their conclusion was that heat stress would be greatest in the sub tropics but that the mosquitos would be able to survive the heat due to behavioral thermoregulation (Couper et al., 2024). Thus, increasing heat may not get to a point to be lethal for the mosquitos and likely would permit mosquito range to move into higher latitudes (Couper et al., 2024; Saarman et al., 2025). Management and mitigation of arbovirus infection morbidity and mortality ideally involves a combination of arthropod control (e.g., mosquito-proof caging/netting to keep mosquitos out), husbandry practices (to remove potential arthropod/mosquito breeding areas), and vaccination.

Herpesviruses

Herpesviruses (HV) are DNA viruses within a lipid outer envelope. Several HV have been identified as the cause of disease in various avian species worldwide. HV are unique in their ability to establish latent infections wherein there are no clinical signs or viral replication, but the virus remains in the body. Due to any of various host (e.g., immunosuppression) or environmental factors, the virus can recrudesce (actively start replication) and produce disease. The lipid envelope makes HV sensitive to cleaning and disinfection. Viral transmission can be via ingestion, inhalation, or direct contact. Virus can be found in feather follicles, mucosa, saliva, conjunctiva and tears, crop milk, and feces (Kaleta and Docherty, 2007). Infected individuals may or may not show clinical signs of disease and still be latently infected. There are several well-known avian HV diseases in aviculture, poultry farming, and the wild. These include, in order of outbreak severity, duck viral enteritis (aka, duck plague), Marek's disease of chickens, and Pacheco's disease in parrots. Avian-specific herpesviruses are not known to infect mammals (although there are many mammal-specific HV).

Duck viral enteritis, also known as Duck Plague, is a disease primarily affecting domestic ducks but is a concern for wild waterfowl as well due to its highly contagious nature. Outbreaks of this virus have resulted in the decimation of naïve flocks of ducks, and decreased egg production and fertility, which had a great economic impact on those areas that rely on ducks for food (Hansen and Gough, 2007). In 1967, an outbreak of duck viral enteritis in the United States resulted in the death of 42,000 mallards! While other members of the family Anatidae (duck, geese, and swans) are susceptible to the disease, there appears to be species variability in susceptibility and virulence in wild waterfowl species (Hansen and Gough, 2007).

Transmission of duck viral enteritis is via direct contact of infected to uninfected individuals or via contact with contaminated environment/water body. Inhalation, ingestion, cloacal, and vertical transmission of the virus have also been shown (Hansen and Gough, 2007). Survivors of the initial infection become persistent carriers and shedders of the virus. Clinical signs of disease vary from focal ulcerations under the tongue to rapid, acute death. Vaccination is successful in producing lifelong immunity. The effects of viral outbreaks on wild populations are unclear; however, the potential harmful impact on endangered and/or sensitive species exists.

Marek's disease is a highly contagious disease in chickens that results in neoplasia (lymphosarcoma) and immunosuppression. Infected birds can be carriers and shedders of the virus for life. Virus is shed via dander from feather follicles and is transmitted by inhalation. Immunity from maternal antibodies or vaccination will not prevent disease infection but can decrease viral shedding load and can prevent tumor formation (Kaleta and Docherty, 2007). Virus interferes with T-cell immunity, ultimately resulting in immunosuppression. Naïve and/or unvaccinated flocks may suffer a >80% mortality rate if infected with Marek's disease virus. These epizootics caused substantial poultry losses prior to the development of a vaccine (Kaleta and Docherty, 2007).

Pacheco's disease affects psittacines (parrots) the most of all species, although south and central American parrot species coevolved with and are hosts for some of these serotypes. This virus is highly infectious, and infected birds usually die acutely without preceding clinical signs. It is transmitted via contact and inhalation of infected feces, body fluids, or secretions. Asymptomatic carriers may serve as viral reservoirs. Surviving parrots can harbor the virus latently, have no clinical signs, but still shed the virus periodically. The highly infectious nature of this virus puts large collections, flocks, and zoos at risk of widespread infection and/or mortality. Thus, all new parrots should be tested for the virus before introduction to a new flock. Vaccination and use of the anti-viral drug Acyclovir have been variably successful in reducing the amount of virus shed and transmission of the disease. (Kaleta and Docherty, 2007; Doneley and Xie, 2025).

Circovirus

Circoviruses are small non-enveloped DNA viruses. They are the causative agent of Psittacine beak and feather disease (PBFD). PBFD has been documented in wild parrots, is endemic in wild psittacines in Australia, and is an important disease in captive and pet parrots, although new World species appear to be less affected (Doneley and Xie, 2025; Pare and Robert, 2007). Adult immunocompetent birds usually clear the infection; however, young birds are especially vulnerable. Virus is passed in feces, crop secretions, in feather dander, and is thought to be vertically transmitted through the egg (Pare and Robert, 2007). Viral particles are very stable in the environment and resistant to degradation. In general, infection with the PBFD virus is often subclinical or latent, but can cause feather abnormalities and/or immunosuppression. Dystrophic feather abnormalities and/or beak deformities (specifically in cockatoos) are suggestive of PBFD. Thus, this disease can potentially be detected in the wild by careful observation and then confirmed by viral assay of feces or feathers. New psittacines to a captive collection should be quarantined and tested before entry.

Coronavirus

Coronaviruses warrant discussion if not simply because of the potential for zoonoses and pandemic. The main avian coronaviruses are in the gamma-coronavirus genus, but some bird species are reservoirs for delta-coronaviruses (which include COVID-19). Gamma-coronaviruses are known to be worldwide in distribution; they are found in wild and domestic waterfowl and in wild birds (Guo et al., 2024). In fact, geese were involved in a major mortality event in Canada in 2017 from a coronavirus (Guo et al., 2024). Birds have also been found to be positive for the coronavirus of human fame (Vestal-Laborde et al., 2025). Most of these positive species are waterbirds (Charadriiformes, Anseriformes) that tend to congregate in large numbers in areas in close proximity to urban areas. Surveillance is clearly needed to guard against a resurgence of the coronavirus that infects humans and for new emerging coronavirus types that may jump to infect humans.

Poxvirus

Poxvirus (or Avipox) has been associated with decreased production of poultry, resulting in huge economic losses. It is a widespread virus present in over 300 bird species (Giotis and Skinner, 2019). Pox virus can be transmitted by direct contact, ingestion, inhalation, and via insect vectors. Disease is characterized by firm nodules on the non-feathered areas of skin or these can be mucosal lesions inside the body; this latter form of the disease is more virulent. Infected animals may become immunosuppressed, leaving them vulnerable to secondary infection/disease which can lead to mortality (Qiu et al., 2025). Control of poxviral infections is by vaccination and good hygiene. Birds transported or traded should be tested for the presence of poxvirus. While not a primary agent of major epizootics in birds, poxvirus can leave bird populations susceptible to other agents which do cause epizootics due to the immunosuppressive effects.

Bacteria

Several bacterial species have been responsible for major epizootics in wild and captive birds (including poultry). A few bacterial species are primary pathogens (e.g., *Pasteurella multocida, Salmonella*, *Vibrio*, and *Mycoplasma*) and have been responsible for avian outbreaks of high mortality. The majority of other bacteria are secondary pathogens that opportunistically invade, infect, and ultimately may cause mortality. The vast majority of bacterial species are able to infect multiple avian and non-avian animals including humans making these zoonotic agents. A novel, emerging opportunistic bacterium, *Ornithobacterium rhinotrachaele*, has recently come on the scene causing illness, decreased egg production, and decreased meat quality in chickens (El-Ghany, 2021). It appears that this bacterium prefers to work in concert with other bacterial pathogens to magnify disease. A few notable bacteria will be briefly discussed below.

"Avian cholera" is caused by infection with *P. multocida*, an infectious gram-negative bacterium. These bacteria are distributed worldwide and prefer moist areas and wetlands. Large congregations of waterfowl have suffered and continue to experience large epizootics due to infection with *P. multocida* (Samuel et al., 2007). Transmission is via bird-to-bird contact, aerosolization, and fecal-oral. Migratory birds have spread the disease along their flyways. Dead and decomposing birds that died from *P. multocida* also contribute to the spread of the bacterial disease. Avian cholera was found to be the cause of a severe population decrease of the endangered Amsterdam albatross (*Diomedea amsterdamensis*) between 2000 and 2013 and in 2013–2017 in the yellow-nosed albatross (*Thalassarche carteri*) on Amsterdam Island in the South Indian Ocean (Jaeger et al., 2018, 2020). Other seabird species on the island are also suffering decreased reproductive success and population declines from this disease. As the climate warms, wetlands shrink, agriculture and farming spread, and birds will likely be in more concentrated aggregations. These factors enhance the spread of bacteria and disease.

Salmonellosis is an enteric disease caused by *Salmonella* species (a gram-negative bacterium). *Salmonella* species are worldwide in distribution. Infection severity depends on serotype and host species, which present as an asymptomatic carrier state, acute enteritis or septicemia, or have a chronic infection (Daoust and Prescott, 2007). The distribution of *Salmonella* parallels that of humans and other animals. Increased amounts of untreated sewage from human or livestock waste favor *Salmonella* presence. In fact, there is a relationship between the prevalence of *Salmonella* from the intestines of wild birds and the proximity of their habitat to humans or livestock (Daoust and Prescott, 2007). Birds acquire *Salmonella* from the environment including from landfills (Malekian et al., 2021). Unfortunately, a heavily populated bird feeder (and the ground below it) can be a rich *Salmonella* environment. In humans, *Salmonella* is a leading cause of food-borne illness and gastrointestinal disease.

Chlamydia psittaci is a bacterial disease of birds which causes ornithosis or psittacosis in humans. Birds are primary hosts for *Chlamydia*, which is worldwide in distribution. It is particularly common in captive/pet parrots, much more so than in wild parrots (Stokes et al., 2021). It can infect a wide variety of avian species. Infections can be overt, subclinical, or latent with a carrier state. Overt clinical signs may include conjunctivitis, respiratory disease, and lethargy. Immunity in birds is short-lived, and susceptible birds can be repeatedly infected (Doneley and Xie, 2025). Humans are most susceptible to psittacosis when they are immunocompromised.

Mycoplasmosis is a disease caused by the bacterial species *Mycoplasma gallisepticum*. *Mycoplasma* are very small bacteria in the class Mollicutes that lack a cell wall. The lack of cell walls makes them resistant to many antibiotics. Disease is usually respiratory in nature involving the lungs, parabronchi, and/or sinuses and can also cause immune suppression (Yadav et al., 2022). In poultry, it is an economically important disease as it leads to decreased weight, egg production, hatchability, and production. In 1994, it was observed that *Mycoplasma* caused conjunctivitis in house finches (*Haemorhous mexicanus*) in Maryland, United States. Within four years, the bacteria had spread throughout North America and caused the death of millions of additional house finches (Staley and Bonneand, 2015)! Now *M. gallisepticum* is believed to be endemic in many areas, and the finches have evolved immune resistance and tolerance to it.

There are other bacterial species that infect and can cause disease in birds, but they are usually secondary invaders. There are also various fungal species that contribute to disease, but they are also usually secondary invaders. Control of bacterial and fungal invasion includes good hygiene, husbandry, personal protective equipment (PPE), medications, and/or vaccinations (for captive or pet birds). Clearly captive populations and pet birds can be managed more easily than wild bird populations due to veterinary involvement and treatment. What about wild populations? In a world of increasing heat, urbanization which often includes increasing density of humans (and pets) and waste, new or altered environments/niches, and spread of pathogen ranges due to global warming, we will be challenged in how to respond (Braga and Vierira, 2025). We know that various viruses and bacteria can be found in terrestrial passerines as well as in seabirds. Microbial species are abundant in migrating bird species, but zoonotic agents are more prevalent in resident species, especially waterfowl (Qiu et al., 2025; Williams et al., 2023). Increased temperature and nutrients from waste provide ripe environments for bacterial growth and spread especially latitudinally. Geographical spread of viruses, bacteria, and other agents may result in exposure of naïve populations and/or contribute to immune compromise placing many populations at risk. Will we know if this happens *before* witnessing high avian mortality? What can we do?

Protozoa

The primary protozoan pathogen in birds is *Plasmodium* species, which is responsible for the disease malaria. *Plasmodium* is an intraerythrocytic apicomplexan parasite in the Haemosproidia group (which includes other species that infect birds). There are many species of *Plasmodium* that can cause malaria disease (Paez et al., 2022). *Plasmodium* species are transmitted by *Culex* and other genera of mosquitos. Mosquitos ingest *Plasmodium* gametocytes from an infected bird at a blood meal. Replication of the parasite occurs inside the mosquito to form sporozoites, which then invade the mosquito's salivary glands. At its next blood meal, the sporozoites pass to a new bird host. In this host, they invade RBC, undergo asexual reproduction to form gametocytes, which can then infect a new mosquito and the cycle continues. Avian hosts may be infected for life (Atkinson, 2023). If humans are bitten, the gametocytes infect RBC, reproduce, form parasitemia within two weeks, and can destroy RBC resulting in anemia (low RBC count). Other reproductive stages can lodge in capillary cells and cause obstructions (infarcts), which can result in death depending on their location (Atkinson, 2023).

Protozoans have severely impacted wild populations of birds. *Plasmodium* invaded the Hawaiian Islands and severely impacted native Honeycreeper bird species (Atkinson, 2023). Mortality was extremely high as approximately 80% RBC in individuals were destroyed in some cases. The more resistant and surviving birds of the acute infection became reservoirs of the *Plasmodium*. By 2012, the honeycreeper populations decreased by almost 90% and the remaining individuals moved up to the higher elevations of the mountains. Mosquitos like warmer temperatures and with global warming, it is anticipated that the mosquito's range will climb further up to higher elevations of the mountains. (So, will the honeycreepers be safe up there?)

A 26-year study (1996–2021) on blue tits (*Cyanistes caerulens*) in Northern Europe documents an increase in prevalence of malaria parasites (*Plasmodium, Haemoproteus*, and *Leucocytozoon*) during this time (Theodosopoulos et al., 2025). The greatest increase was a doubling in prevalence of *Haemoproteus* (46–92%) and its vector, a biting midge in the *Culicoides* genera. Penguins appear to be uniquely susceptible to malaria and infection with *Plasmodium* is a significant disease especially in captive situations (Ings and Denk, 2022). The prevalence of infection in captive animals is higher than in wild penguins. Affected penguins often show minimal to no signs prior to acute death. Survivors with chronic disease/infection are thought to have reduced longevity and fitness, as do other chronically infected bird species (Ings and Denk, 2022). Immune response to malaria varies depending on the malarial strain and host species. Usually, there is no overall immunity among all *Plasmodium* species (Paez et al., 2022). Previous exposure and antibody production will decrease the clinical signs and mortality (virulence) but will not inhibit the infection rate. In addition, infected birds may have a harder time managing secondary infections indicating some measure of immune compromise (Paez et al., 2022). The large number of

Plasmodium and vector species could lead to many different paths of malaria infection in many species, including endangered species (Paez et al., 2022).

Control of mosquitos is critical! This can be via pesticides, such as biopesticides. The biopesticide strategy is to place the bacterium *Bacillus thuringiensis* in standing water areas (Ragasruthi et al., 2024). This bacterium attacks and kills mosquito larvae which should control/reduce mosquito populations. Another strategy is to release infertile or genetically modified or sterilized male mosquitos to mate with female mosquitos which would lead to nonproductive reproduction.

Trichomonas gallinae is a small, flagellated protozoan which is generally localized to the oral-nasal cavity or anterior ends of the gastrointestinal or respiratory tract. It spread from wild Columbiformes (pigeon family) to various wild finch species – chaffinches (*Fringilla coelebs*) and green finches (*Carduelis chloris*) in Great Britain (Staley and Bonneand, 2015). In 2007, approximately half a million finches died from this disease. Since then, *Trichomonas* has spread to other species. It reproduces by simple binary fission and has no cyst stage, so it cannot survive for long outside the host. Transmission is directly between individuals (including mothers feeding nestlings), via contaminated water, food, or consumption of infected prey. Treatment is via antibiotic therapy, cleaning and disinfection of housing areas, and allowing these areas to dry out.

In summary, what do we know? Climate change and global warming are expanding the ranges of microbes, their vectors, and birds to new areas. Migratory birds, trade, and human movements are inadvertently spreading microbes to distant places. Habitat changes permit reassortment of species, genetic mutations in microbes, and increased virulence of pathogens. Habitat degradation and fragmentation will lead to greater congregations of birds, which will magnify the spread of infectious diseases/agents. All these facts are involved in the increased potential for exposure of pathogens to new hosts. These are what cause "emerging and reemerging diseases." Pathogens not previously known to cause epizootics or new agents are the emerging group. Previous pathogens that infect new and naive hosts are the reemerging diseases. These new emerging and reemerging diseases have already been observed. WNV spread across the world, and novel, more virulent strains have been found in birds and mammals (Fuller et al., 2012). In the Czech Republic, tick-borne encephalitis spread to higher altitudes as the range of the tick vector expanded its range to higher altitudes with increasing temperatures (Fuller et al., 2012). *Plasmodium* (the protozoan causing malaria) was found for the first time in the Galapagos Penguin (*Spheniscus mendiculus*) in the early 2000s from samples collected in 1996 (Levin et al., 2009). The prevalence was low (<10%), and the disease was mild. However, this population of penguins is endangered and has low genetic diversity (Levin et al., 2009). Subsequently, *Plasmodium* has spread to several different species in the Galapagos (Levin et al., 2013).

Some change in the host, microbe, and vector opens the possibility for infection of new hosts. New infection in naive hosts often causes intense epizootics with high initial mortality. But this tactic does not ultimately serve the microbe because if its host dies, the microbe can no longer reproduce and will also die out. Eventually, the microbe becomes less virulent so as not to kill its host, but it retains or increases its infectivity. If a new epizootic infects an endangered species, the resulting mortality may be too much for it to survive. Again, with various biotic and abiotic stressors, the new host may not be able to defend against the new pathogen and will succumb possibly to extinction. This is one of the biggest health issues facing birds in our changing environments.

The other major issue is the increasing contribution to the increase and spread of antibiotic-resistant microbes. All the factors above contribute to this. For example, high density of birds permits close association of different microbes that can transfer antibiotic resistance genes to each other. Then these new resistant microbes get transferred to the next location the birds fly to spreading it around. Antibiotic resistance makes it difficult to treat animals and people with infections of these bacteria. This is an incredibly difficult issue to tackle as *all* environments sampled, soil and water, have antibiotics or their residues in them. In a single year (2025), a search for antimicrobial resistance yielded over 500 peer-reviewed scientific papers!

So, what can "we" (the multidisciplinary group of avian scientists) do? In areas where we have captive birds, we can reduce mosquito prevalence by reducing standing water, clearing objects and vegetation that may contribute to small areas of water accumulation, and use ecofriendly pesticides; keep in contact with other facilities and researchers locally to share information on what diseases or agents have been found in other species; clean and disinfect housing and feeding areas of captive species which will help minimize direct close contact with any pathogen; continue researching new therapies and new antibiotics for treating infections; vaccinate when possible; and ideally, be vigilant and survey our local areas to assess what pathogens/parasites/vectors are already present.

In wild populations, well, that is harder. We certainly can do several of those environmental actions in cities; however, the larger the population of the city, the harder it may be. We can track bird movements and sample them for the presence of pathogens year after year (mark and recapture studies) to try and understand new and impending threats. We can try to "clean up" polluted areas/lakes. Perhaps the two most important factors are (i) to understand the life cycles (biology) and transmission modes of the infectious agents so we can design targeted therapies and preventions and (ii) to educate people (especially children) about birds, their uniqueness and diversity, and what changes we are already observing in bird populations and why. "We can only love what we know" (Aldous Huxley, 1894–1963), and we will only work to save what we love. Let's get others familiar with birds beyond pigeons, gulls, and parrots; enlighten them on how environmental change affects birds, how it can interact with humans; and show them how *they* can help. One little action every day goes a long way.

Literature Cited

Atkinson, C. T. (2023). Avian malaria and extinction of Hawaiian forest birds. In: *Wildlife Disease and Health in Conservation*, D. A. Jessup and R. W. Radcliffe (eds.). pp. 326–347. Johns Hopkins University Press.

Braga, E. M. and Vieira, L. M. (2025). Hidden effects of avian malaria under climate warming. *Trends in Ecology & Evolution* 41:15–17.

Caffrey, C., Smith, S. C. R., and Weston, T. J. (2005). West Nile virus devastates an American crow population. *Condor: Ornithological Applications* 107(1):128–132. https://doi.org/10.1093/condor/107.1.128.

Carlson, C. J., Bannon, E., Mendenhall, E., et al. (2023). Rapid range shifts in African Anopheles mosquitoes over the last century. *Biology Letters* 19(2):20220365. https://doi.org/10.1098/rsbl.2022.0365.

Couper, L. I., Nalukwago, D. U., Lyberger, K. P., et al. (2024). How much warming can mosquito vectors tolerate? *Global Changing Biology* 30(12):e17610. https://doi.org/10.1111/gcb.17610.

Cullen, J. A., Masto, N. M., Sullivan, J. D., et al. (2025). Spatiotemporal overlap of mallards with poultry farms is associated with greater risk of avian influenza wild bird spillover events. *Ecology & Evolution* 15(10):e72221. https://doi.org/10.1002/ece3.72221.

Daoust, P. and Prescott, J. F. (2007). Salmonellosis. In: *Infectious Diseases of Wild Birds*, N. J. Thomas, D. B. Hunter, and C. T. Atkinson (eds.), pp. 270–288. Blackwell Publishing.

Doneley, B. and Xie, S. (2025). *Avian Medicine and Surgery in Practice*, 3rd Ed. CRC Press.

El-Ghany, W. A. A. (2021). An updated comprehensive review on ornithobacteriosis: A worldwide emerging avian respiratory disease. *Open Veterinary Journal* 11(4):555–568. https://doi.org/10.5455/OVJ.2021.v11.i4.5.

European Food Safety Authority, European Centre for Disease Prevention and Control, European Union Reference Laboratory for Avian Influenza; Alexakis, L., Buczkowski, H., et al. (2024). Avian influenza overview June–September 2024. *EFSA Journal* 22(10):e9057.

Fernández-Bellon, H., Vergara-Alert, J., Almagro, V., et al. (2016). Vaccination against H5 avian influenza virus induces long-term humoral immune responses in flamingoes (*Phoenicopterus* spp.). *Vaccine* 34(27):3082–3086. https://doi.org/10.1016/j.vaccine.2016.04.078.

Fuller, T., Bensch, S., Müller, I., et al. (2012). The ecology of emerging infectious diseases in migratory birds: An assessment of the role of climate change and priorities for future research. *EcoHealth* 9(1):80–88. https://doi.org/10.1007/s10393-012-0750-1.

Gancz, A. Y., Barker, I. K., Lindsay, R., et al. (2004). West Nile virus outbreak in North American owls, Ontario. *Emerging Infectious Diseases* 10:2135–2142. https://doi.org/10.2903/j.efsa.2024.9057.

George, T. L., Harrigan, R. J., LaManna, J. A., et al. (2015). Persistent impacts of West Nile virus on North American bird populations. *Proceedings of National Academy of Sciences* 112(46):14290–14292. https://doi.org/10.1073/pnas.1507747112.

Giotis, E. S. and Skinner, M. A. (2019). Spotlight on avian pathology: Fowlpox virus. *Avian Pathology* 48(2):87–90. https://doi.org/10.1080/03079457.2018.1554893.

Guo, J., He, J., Liang, Z., et al. (2024). Birds as reservoirs: Unraveling the global spread of Gamma- and Deltacoronaviruses. *mBio* 15(10):e0232424. https://doi.org/10.1128/mbio.02324-24.

Hansen, W. R. and Gough, R. E. (2007). *Duck plague (Duck Virus Enteritis)*. In: *Infectious Diseases of Wild Birds*, N. J. Thomas, D. B. Hunter, and C. T. Atkinson (eds.), pp. 87–107. Blackwell Publishing.

Ings, K. and Denk, D. (2022). Avian malaria in penguins: Diagnostics and future direction in the context of climate change. *Animals* 12(5):600. https://doi.org/10.3390/ani12050600.

Jaeger, A., Gamble, A., Lagadec, E., et al. (2020). Impact of annual bacterial epizootics on albatross population on a remote Island. *EcoHealth* 17:194–202. https://doi.org/10.1007/s10393-020-01487-8.

Jaeger, A., Lebarbenchon, C., Bourret, V., et al. (2018). Avian cholera outbreaks threaten seabird species on Amsterdam Island. *PLoS One* 13(5):e0197291. https://doi.org/10.1371/journal.pone.0197291.

Jessup, D. A. (2023). Waterfowl diseases: A catalyst for wildlife health professions in North America. In: *Wildlife Disease and Health in Conservation*, D. A. Jessup and R. W. Radcliffe (eds.). pp. 293–308. Johns Hopkins University Press.

Kaleta, E. F. and Docherty, D. E. (2007). Avian herpesviruses. In: *Infectious Diseases of Wild Birds*, N. J. Thomas, D. B. Hunter, and C. T. Atkinson (eds.), pp. 63–86. Blackwell Publishing.

Kozlov, M. (2023). US will vaccinate birds against avian flu for first time – what researchers think. *Nature* 618(7964):220–221. https://doi.org/10.1038/d41586-023-01760-0.

Kuiken, T., Vanstreels, R. E. T., Banyard, A., et al. (2025). Emergence, spread, and impact of high-pathogenicity avian influenza H5 in wild birds and mammals of South America and Antarctica. *Conservation Biology* 40:e70052. https://doi.org/10.1111/cobi.70052.

LaDeau, S. L., Kilpatrick, A. M., and Marra, P. P. (2007). West Nile virus emergence and large-scale declines of North American bird populations. *Nature* 447(7145):710–713. https://doi.org/10.1038/nature05829.

Lamb, J. S., Tornos, J., Lejeune, M., et al. (2024). Rapid loss of maternal immunity and increase in environmentally mediated antibody generation in urban gulls. *Scientific Reports* 14(1):4357. https://doi.org/10.1038/s41598-024-54796-1.

Laratta, E., Masci, D., Procopio, A. C., et al. (2025). One health approach in the era of emerging viruses: The challenge of Usutu virus. *International Journal of Molecular Science* 26(17):8150. https://doi.org/10.3390/ijms26178150.

Leguia, M., Garcia-Glaessner, A., Muñoz-Saavedra, B., et al. (2023). Highly pathogenic avian influenza A (H5N1) in marine mammals and seabirds in Peru. *Nature Communications* 14(1):5489. https://doi.org/10.1038/s41467-023-41182-0.

Leighton, F. A. and Heckert, R. A. (2007). Newcastle disease and related avian paramyxoviruses. In: *Infectious Diseases of Wild Birds*, N. J. Thomas, D. B. Hunter, and C. T. Atkinson (eds.). pp. 3–16. Blackwell Publishing.

Levin, I. I., Outlaw, D. C., Vargas, F. H., et al. (2009). *Plasmodium* blood parasite found in endangered Galapagos penguin (*Spheniscus mendiculus*). *Biological Conservation* 142(12):3191–3195. https://doi.org/10.1016/j.biocon.2009.06.017.

Levin, I. I., Zwiers, P., Deem, S. L., et al. (2013). Multiple lineages of avian malaria parasites (*Plasmodium*) in the Galapagos Islands and evidence for arrival via migratory birds. *Conservation Biology* 27(6):1366–1377. https://doi.org/10.1111/cobi.12127.

Liu, J., Guo, S., Jin, Z., et al. (2023). Adjuvanted quaternized chitosan composite aluminum nanoparticles-based vaccine formulation promotes immune responses in chickens. *Vaccine* 41(18):2982–2989. https://doi.org/10.1016/j.vaccine.2023.03.067.

Malekian, M., Shagholian, J., and Hosseinpour, Z. (2021). Pathogen presence in wild birds inhabiting landfills in central Iran. *EcoHealth* 18:76–83. https://doi.org/10.1007/s10393-021-01516-0.

McLaughlin, A., Giacinti, J., Sarma, S. N., et al. (2025). Examining avian influenza virus exposure in seabirds of the northwest Atlantic in 2022 and 2023 via antibodies in eggs. *Conservation Physiology* 13(1):coaf010. https://doi.org/10.1093/conphys/coaf010.

McLean, R. G. and Ubico, S. R. (2007). Arboviruses in birds. In: *Infectious Diseases of Wild Birds*, N. J. Thomas, D. B. Hunter, and C. T. Atkinson (eds.), pp. 17–62. Blackwell Publishing.

McNamara, T. (2015). Updates on West Nile Virus. In: *Zoo and Wild Animal Medicine Current Therapy*, M. E. Fowler and R. E. Miller (eds.). vol. 8, pp. 710–713.

Nelson, A. N. and Ploss, A. (2024). Emerging mosquito-borne flaviviruses. *mBio* 15(12):e0294624. https://doi.org/10.1128/mbio.02946-24.

Paez, A. M., Chalkowski, K., Zohdy, S., et al. (2022). Management of avian malaria in populations of high conservation concern. *Parasite Vectors* 15(1):208. https://doi.org/10.1186/s13071-022-05327-2.

Pare, J. A. and Robert, N. (2007). Circovirus. In: *Infectious Diseases of Wild Birds*, N. J. Thomas, D. B. Hunter, and C. T. Atkinson (eds.). pp. 194–205. Blackwell Publishing.

Philippa, J. D. (2008). *Avian Influenza in Zoo and Wild Animal Medicine*, M. E. Fowler and R. E. Miller (eds.). vol. 6, pp. 79–87. Saunders Elsevier.

Pohlmann, A., King, J., Fusaro, A., et al. (2022). Has epizootic become enzootic? Evidence for a fundamental change in the infection dynamics of highly pathogenic avian influenza in Europe, 2021. *mBio* 13(4):e0060922. https://doi.org/10.1128/mbio.00609-22.

Puryear, W. B. and Runstadler, J. A. (2024). High-pathogenicity avian influenza in wildlife: A changing disease dynamic that is expanding in wild birds and having an increasing impact on a growing number of mammals. *Journal of American Veterinary Medicine Association* 262(5):601–609. https://doi.org/1.02460/javma.24.01.0053.

Qiu, Y., Lv, C., Chen, J., et al. (2025). The global distribution and diversity of wild-bird-associated pathogens: An integrated data analysis and modeling study. *Medicine* 6(4):100553. https://doi.org/10.1016/j.medj.2024.11.006.

Ragasruthi, M., Balakrishnan, N., Murugan, M., et al. (2024). *Bacillus thuringiensis* (Bt)-based biopesticide: Navigating success, challenges, and future horizons in sustainable pest control. *Science Total Environment* 954:176594. https://doi.org/10.1016/j.scitotenv.2024.176594.

Ramey, A. M. (2023). Avian influenza in wild birds. In: *Wildlife Disease and Health in Conservation*, D. A. Jessup and R. W. Radcliffe (eds.). pp. 309–325. Johns Hopkins University Press.

Ramey, A. M., Reeves, A. B., Drexler, J. Z., et al. (2020). Influenza A viruses remain infectious for more than seven months in Northern Wetlands of North America. *Proceedings of the Royal Society B* 287:20201680.

Rayment, K. M., Franzen-Klein, D., Kurimo-Beechuk, E., et al. (2025). Exposure and survival of wild raptors during the 2022–2023 highly pathogenic influenza A virus outbreak. *Scientific Reports* 15(1):6574. https://doi.org/10.1038/s41598-025-90806-6.

Rijks, J. M., Kik, M. L., Slaterus, R., et al. (2016). Widespread Usutu virus outbreak in birds in the Netherlands, 2016. *European Surveillance* 21(45):30391. https://doi.org/10.2807/1560-7917.ES.2016.21.45.30391.

Saarman, N., Graybeal, K., Seeley, T., et al. (2025). Range expansion of *Culex quinquefasciatus* and *Culex pipiens* hybrids across mid-latitudes of North America. *One Health* 21:101205. https://doi.org/10.1016/j.onehlt.2025.101205.

Samuel, M. D., Botzler, R. G., and Wobeser, G. A. (2007). Avian cholera. In: *Infectious Diseases of Wild Birds*, N. H. Thomas, D. B. Hunter, and C. T. Atkinson (eds.). pp. 239–269. Blackwell Publishing.

Staley, M. and Bonneaud, C. (2015). Immune responses of wild birds to emerging infectious diseases. *Parasite Immunology* 37(5):242–254. https://doi.org/10.1111/pim.12191.

Stettler, M., Hoby, S., Wenker, C., et al. (2025). RNA replicon vaccination confers long-lasting protection against H5N1 avian influenza in 23 zoo bird species. *Nature Communications* 16:9245. https://doi.org/10.1038/s41467-025-64301-5.

Stokes, H. S., Berg, M. L., and Bennett, A. T. D. (2021). A review of chlamydial infections in wild birds. *Pathogens* 10(8):948. https://doi.org/10.3390/pathogens10080948.

Taylor, L. U., Ronconi, R. A., Spina, H. A., et al. (2023). Limited outbreak of highly pathogenic influenza A (H5N1) in herring gull colony, Canada, 2022. *Emerging Infectious Disease* 29(10):2150–2154. https://doi.org/10.3201/eid2910.230536.

Theodosopoulos, A. N., Andreasson, F., Jönsson, J., et al. (2025). Climate-driven increase in transmission of a wildlife Malaria Parasite over the last quarter century. *Global Change Biology* 31(10):370550. https://doi.org/10.1111/gcb.70550.

Tolf, C., Latorre-Margalef, N., Wille, M., et al. (2013). Individual variation in influenza A virus infection histories and long-term immune responses in Mallards. *PLoS One* 8(4):e61201. https://doi.org/10.1371/journal.pone.0061201.

Tomás, G., Marandino, A., Panzera, Y., et al. (2024). Highly pathogenic avian influenza H5N1 virus infections in pinnipeds and seabirds in Uruguay: Implications for bird-mammal transmission in South America. *Virus Evolution* 10(1):veae031. https://doi.org/10.1093/ve/veae031.

Ul-Rahman, A., Ishaq, H. M., Raza, M. A., et al. (2022). Zoonotic potential of Newcastle disease virus: old and novel perspectives related to public health. *Reviews in Medical Virology* 32:e2246. https://doi.org/10.1002/rmv.2246.

Vestal-Laborde, A. A., Christofferson, R. C., Ringelman, K. M., et al. (2025). A review of coronaviruses in wild birds and opportunities for future research on migratory waterfowl. *Birds* 6(4):52. https://doi.org/10.3390/birds6040052.

Yadav, J. P., Tomar, P., Singh, Y., et al. (2022). Insights on *Mycoplasma gallisepticum* and *Mycoplasma synoviae* infection in poultry: A systematic review. *Animal Biotechnology* 33(7):1711–1720. https://doi.org/10.1080/10495398.2021.1908316.

11

Stress and Welfare

What Is Stress?

Stress in life is ubiquitous. Recall that homeostasis is the narrow range of conditions in which a cell or organism functions normally. *Stress* is defined as a temporary, relatively short-lived, alteration in homeostasis. At the end of the stressful event, the body returns to normal homeostasis. If the stressful situation is not resolved, then the animal is said to be in *distress.* Stress is often unpleasant. But *distress*, or a negative stress response, involves negative effects and physiological reactivity. It can generate physical, behavioral, and/or psychological maladaptation and pose serious health risks for individuals. The term "acute" refers to a short time, but this time period can vary (minutes, hours, days, etc.) depending on the stimulus (or cause) of the stress. "Chronic" refers to a protracted period of time significantly longer than the "acute" time period. Stress can be persistent, triggered by one continuous stimulus which then disappears, or stress can be intermittent when the stimulus comes and goes.

Animals experiencing stress can decrease their stress response by habituating or acclimating to the triggering stimulus. *Habituation* is the diminishing of a physiological or emotional response to a frequently repeated stimulus. Some have referred to this as "stress inoculation." The animal will learn to predict its occurrence and control their response to it (Whitham and Miller, 2025). *Coping* with stress (especially if it is chronic and/or recurring) is another method to mitigate its effects. Coping behavior is the use of behavioral and/or cognitive strategies (compensatory mechanisms) to manage a situation or emotions (Badas et al., 2025). It can vary and, in the extreme, may become stereotypical. *Stereotypical behaviors* are those that are repeated over and over and are the same every time. Typical repetitive behaviors that have been described in managed care include pacing, excessive feather picking, and head pressing. These are usually interpreted as negative or indicative of poor welfare. Some repetitive behaviors, for example, head pressing or feather picking are obviously destructive to the animal. However, I assert that not all stereotypical behaviors are representative of negative welfare. I avoid the term "stereotypical" because of the negative connotation attributed to it.

Resilience to stress is a recent approach (in the avian literature) to deal with stress. Resilience implies the animal can be affected minimally by a disturbance and/or can quickly return to normal or to the state before the disturbance occurred (Whitham and

Miller, 2025). It can include behavioral, physiological, or cognitive changes. Some recommended strategies to encourage development of resilience in birds in zoos include enriching the physical, cognitive, and social environment.

Stress and Health

Stress is an advantageous response that evolved for self-preservation. Epinephrine and norepinephrine stimulated by fear and/or anxiety trigger increased adrenal activity and release of ACTH, cortisol/corticosterone, and aldosterone and affect thyroid hormone secretion (Figure 11.1). Consider the fight or flight response which arises when an animal is faced with an acute *life or death* decision. It involves a series of hormonal and neurochemical changes that prepare the animal to fight or flee, quickly! Epinephrine and/or norepinephrine are secreted resulting in an increased heart rate and increased blood flow,

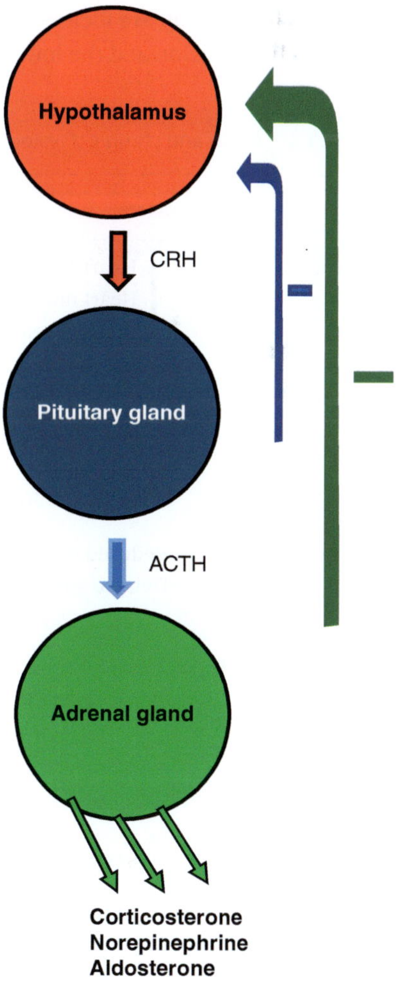

Figure 11.1 HPA axis: the hypothalamic-pituitary axis controls hormone secretion in the body. A stressful stimulus is sensed, and the hypothalamus in the brain sends corticotropin-releasing hormone (CRH) to the pituitary gland at the base of the brain. The pituitary gland secretes adrenocorticotropic hormone (ACTH) to act on the adrenal gland to produce a glucocorticoid (cortisol or corticosterone), aldosterone, and/or norepinephrine. The "–" arrows represent negative feedback loops to the brain to decrease their signal.

especially to muscles, heart, and brain. This results in increased glucose availability for utilization by muscles (to run). When the fear from a predator dissipates, the hormonal feedback decreases resulting in decreased secretion of epinephrine and other hormones.

It is easy to see how the acute stress response facilitates survival. Nowadays in humans and animals, however, the stress response is stimulated by non-life-threatening events and is often chronic and/or recurrent in nature. The stress response follows the same path, though, regardless of how life-threatening the stimulus is. The stress response in animals involves neurologic, endocrine, physiologic, and immunologic components. These systems share interrelated signaling via neurotransmitters, hormones, and cytokines. Table 11.1 summarizes the acute and chronic effects of stress on the major organ systems.

Perhaps one of the most important and investigated consequences of stress on health is its effects on the immune system. Recall that the adrenal glands help with glucose metabolism and energy by producing glucocorticoids (corticosterone in birds), which is a good thing for the *fight or flight* response. However, continuous release of glucocorticoids and other changes experienced in chronic stress can have long-term consequences that can negatively impact the health and well-being of animals (Table 11.1). During acute fight or flight, all the resources in the body are focused on the muscles and parts of the body that are needed to run quickly. Digestion and the immune system are examples of systems that are not needed

Table 11.1 Acute and chronic physiological and systemic consequences of stress.

System	Acute	Chronic
Cardiovascular	↑ Heart rate Heart muscle contraction Blood pressure	Sympathetic activation Endothelial dysfunction Inflammation Atherosclerosis Vascular disease
Respiratory	Bronchial hyperresponsiveness Inflammation Shortness of breath	↑ Susceptibility to infection Exacerbate asthma COPD
Gastrointestinal	Reduced motility Delayed gastric emptying	Decreased nutrient absorption ↑ Susceptibility to infection Altered gut microbiota
Musculoskeletal	Tension headaches Temporomandibular joint aches	Muscle wasting Decreased bone density Prolonged healing time
Immune	Reduction in pro-inflammatory signals Reduced activity of immune cells ↑ Susceptibility to infection	Systemic inflammation Delayed wound healing Autoimmune diseases Inflammatory disorders
Reproductive	Impairs ovarian function Impairs testosterone production	Infertility

Source: Adapted from Chu et al. (2024).

during this response and are therefore not serviced or inhibited. When stress persists for a long time, physiologic and immunologic dysfunctions accumulate, and chronic immunosuppression may result, putting the animal at greater risk of infection and illness.

Assessing and/or Quantifying Stress

In the recent few decades, research into defining and identifying stress in birds has burgeoned due to questions regarding animal welfare on poultry farms and zoos. Measuring stress in an animal, however, can be difficult as stress is a subjective human concept. While it seems logical that animals *can* get stressed, it can be hard to demonstrate it using objective data. To identify stress in an animal, changes in cortisol/corticosterone levels in the body are commonly evaluated. In birds, corticosterone is the main glucocorticoid released from the adrenal gland. In response to stress, glucocorticoids will increase in the bloodstream within 30 minutes and can remain elevated for hours after the stressor ceases.

Increases in corticosterone to presumably acutely stressful situations have been documented in birds in managed care settings and in free-ranging birds. Wild Clark's nuthatches (*Nucifraga columbiana*) were captured and brought into captivity. They were provided with enrichment, which was then removed (the stressor). When the enrichment items were removed after 10 days, the birds had increased corticosterone (assayed using feathers; Fairhurst et al., 2011). Red jungle fowl (*Gallus gallus*) had a stronger behavioral reaction and higher corticosterone response to restraint stress than did domestic chickens (Ericsson et al., 2014).

Extensive or recurrent stress can lead to immune modulation or a decrease. The most common measure of immunologic impairment in birds is the heterophil : lymphocyte ratio (H : L ratio). Normally in avian blood, lymphocytes outnumber heterophils. Stress affects the WBC distribution resulting in increased heterophils and increased H : L ratio. Numerous studies have documented stress-induced increases in H : L ratio in both wild and captive birds. Mexican house finches (*Haemorhous mexicanus*) who were infected with both *Mycoplasma* and *Haemosporidia* had a greater H : L ratio than did birds infected with only one of these agents (Reinoso-Pérez et al., 2025). In addition, the greater the concentration of infectious agent, the greater the H : L ratio. Evaluation of multiple wild avian species in and around Brasilia, Brazil, documented increased H : L ratio associated with intensity of urbanization (closer to the large city) and the ratio was inversely related to body condition (Santos et al., 2025). These are only a few of the studies documenting increased H : L ratio and stress.

Chronic stress and increased corticosterone have been associated with increased susceptibility to and prevalence of disease. Applegate (1971) first documented this in wild-caught house sparrows (*Passer domesticus*) experimentally treated with corticosterone. They had a higher *Plasmodium* parasitemia (high levels of parasites in the bloodstream) and a greater number of RBC infected than did control birds. Experimentally induced increase in corticosterone in the Hawaiian Amakihi (*Chlorodrepanis virens*) resulted in decreased hematocrit and increased *Plasmodium* spp. parasitemia (Names et al., 2021). Interestingly, populations of this bird at lower elevations appear to have increased resilience in their ability to recover from malaria (*Plasmodium* infection) than do the birds from the higher elevation population.

Increased susceptibility to other pathogens is also evident. Zylberberg et al. (2013) surveyed seven species of Galapagos finches in various habitats in relation to avipox (avian pox virus) infection. They found a positive association between the degree of immune suppression and prevalence and susceptibility to poxvirus infection. Captive zebra finches (*Taeniopygia castanotis*) given corticosterone and then challenged with West Nile Virus had greater viremias (viral levels in blood) than did control birds not given corticosterone (Gervasi et al., 2017). The authors termed them "superspreader hosts." House finches infected with *Mycoplasma gallisepticum* had increased infection load if they had greater corticosterone levels (Dhondt and Dobson, 2017). In addition, zebra finches (*T. guttata*) experimentally implanted with corticosterone were more likely to be bitten and fed upon by mosquitos, suggesting the effects of increased stress extend to vectors as well.

Stress can also be assayed by changes in body and cellular physiology. When separated from its group of conspecifics and housed alone in a new cage, pigeon (*Columba livia*) body temperature increased and then returned to normal after two hours, suggesting this move was an acute stressor (Bittencourt et al., 2015). Song sparrow (*Melospiza melodia*) nestlings treated with corticosterone showed sex specific responses to stressors. Corticosterone-treated male nestlings gained more weight (were heavier, larger) than controls, while female nestlings gained less weight (Schmidt et al., 2012). Female nestlings had greater basal metabolic rates as adults if treated with corticosterone, while males did not. These differences, they suggested, likely give males an advantage especially in poorer quality habitats. Jimenez and Williams (2014) took a different approach to investigate physiological effects due to extreme heat stress. They exposed house sparrows to 43 °C (109 °F) for 24 hours, exposed some to 43 °C, and then returned them to room temperature, and birds only at room temperature served as controls. The skin was sampled, and the metabolism of dermal fibroblasts was measured. Exposure to the increased temperature resulted in an increased rate of glycolysis and oxygen consumption in fibroblasts relative to those from birds held at room temperature. However, when they tested the birds that returned to room temperature after 24 hours, they saw that the metabolic changes returned to normal (same as controls). This, they suggested, indicates that some changes are reversible, enabling adaptation or resilience to heating (high temperature) events. Other physiologic changes, such as surface body temperature, are related to stressors. Increased ambient temperature led to increased body temperature in the eye region of little auks (*Alle alle;* Grunst et al., 2026). This increase in temperature is consistent with increased heat dissipation in the animals. Some studies have documented decreased vocal learning in birds exposed to various stressors when young and when adult. Nestling zebra finches (*Taeniopygia castanotis)* exposed to a nutritional stress showed decreased neuronal response and memory to songs heard later when they were adults (Bell et al., 2018). Similarly, male budgerigars (*Melopsittacus undulatus*) exposed to variable stressors as adults showed lower vocal plasticity than unstressed males (Wright et al., 2026).

Usually, a combination of parameters will provide the best picture of an animal's stress level. In addition to increasing corticosterone, physiologic, and immunologic changes, changes in behaviors and vocalizations are useful indices to assess stress in relation to environmental and/or social conditions. Wild hooded crows (*Corvus cornix*), common mynas (*Acridotheres tristis*), and cattle egrets (*Bubulcus ibis*) had modified cognitive and exploratory behaviors after seven days in captivity (Hassaneen et al., 2025). The researchers used videography and deep learning (machine learning) to analyze subtle behaviors that may be more reliable cues for stress.

We know, in managed care, if animals are stressed, it is not likely to be due to illness or poor nutrition. What might be triggering their stress? Interactions with other animals, facility, or environmental issues, external conditions (like weather events and visitors) are all possibilities. Close observation of the animal in question is needed. The people who usually detect early signs of stress are the zookeepers who can pick up on subtle behavioral changes in the animals. This animal could then receive a health assessment by the veterinarian. If the health exam is normal, other factors would need to be considered. How this is done will likely vary by species and facility. Continual observation and comparison of behaviors over time, vocalizations, willingness to respond to zookeepers, etc. should help clarify if the stress has been resolved or is continuing.

Treating or Managing Stress

Depending on the stimulus for stress in managed care, the animals' social groupings/environment may need to be changed, or the animal may need to be removed from public view for further evaluation. The health status of the other animals may need to be assessed as well. If all else fails and the animal is truly stressed, then modern medicine may provide medication that would help alleviate stress or anxiety if present. The main point is that IF a cause of stress is found, it can usually be managed and/or eliminated in managed care/zoo situations.

In rehabilitation, I would assert that most animals are stressed, especially at initial entry into rehabilitation. They clearly are out of their normal environment, in a smaller enclosure than they are accustomed to, close to other animals (people) who may be very foreign to them and are separated from their social groups. Studies assessing stress levels during rehabilitation are rare. But we can approximate what may be happening by evaluating the initial stress levels of wild birds brought into captivity. Three Antarctic penguin species showed increased corticosterone levels in feces within one hour of capture, as did hooded crows (*Corvus cornix*), common mynas (*Acridotheres tristis*), and cattle egrets (*Bubulcus ibis*) (Hassaneen et al., 2025; Pinto et al., 2025). In the first 10 days, chukar birds (*Alectoris chukar*) lost weight, had a decrease in hematocrit, and corticosterone baseline and stress-induced levels (by handling) significantly decreased (Dickens et al., 2009). By day 10, the values had normalized. The inability to mount a corticosterone increase (as well as other tests they did) resulted from alterations to the HPA axis, which is more likely to be seen in chronic stress situations.

Free-ranging Populations

Free-ranging animals likely are experiencing levels of anthropogenically induced stress (acute and chronic) that are variable and recurrent. For these animals, the easiest way to assess if they are affected by an external stimulus is to observe their behavior and movements. Changes in behaviors and movement patterns due to some external stimulus may not necessarily be "stressful." They may just be changes in behavior. However, if these behavioral changes are recurrent, cause animals that were foraging to move into areas without appropriate prey, and result in increased mortality or decreased reproductive success, then we could define these altered movement patterns and behaviors as likely stressful and/or distressful.

Another useful method to assess stress in free-ranging animals without capturing them is monitoring of sounds and vocalizations. In areas where we know or have reasonable expectations of potential interference from the presence of, and noise from, people, cars, etc., we can eavesdrop or listen to bird vocalizations. Microphones can be deployed and can record sounds and vocalizations before, during, and after a stimulus. Any vocalization changes, coupled with behavioral observations, can provide good information on the effects of the increased urban noise as stressful stimuli. This topic was discussed in more detail in Chapter 8.

Additional less- and noninvasive methods of collecting physiological information without capturing animals would also be very useful. Unoccupied aerial systems, or drones, could be useful in some situations. Collection and analysis of feces or feathers that drop off/from the birds are not invasive. While these samples are interesting, their potential utility can only be fully understood if we understand what "normal" baselines are for these animals. However, we often do not know these for wild species. Therefore, interpretation of these data may be difficult. Consistent behavioral observations combined with these methodologies over time are the best bet for free-ranging populations. In Chapters 8 and 9, we discussed anthropogenic stressors on birds and their responses to those stressors. These data are critical if we are to understand how to mitigate stress. We may discover that some aspects of urbanization (for example) we had not previously considered as stressful are actually stressful. Thus, we need to keep studying birds in all situations and their response to all stressors.

There is not always a definitive way to *prove* that anthropogenic effects impose stress on wild birds. We can glean data from experimental animals (rodents and fish) exposed to contaminants or toxins and use observational and correlative data to build the case that anthropogenic activities do stress and/or injure birds. Most diagnostic interventions assess health impacts on individual animals; however, the success of these interventions is most often defined at the population level, which may take years to be fully realized. In populations where capture/recapture projects or long-term repetitive monitoring are possible, we could establish stress "profiles" for individual animals. However, from the viewpoint of management of populations and conservation efforts, the unit remains the population. Ultimately, successful management of stress on free-ranging populations will need to be investigated in concert with people from other disciplines, such as population conservationists, oceanographers, chemists, and microbiologists. Until then, every bit of data collected on different species, data from tissues evaluated, locations, etc. provides another piece of the puzzle we can use to optimize sampling, diagnostics, and problem-solving stressful situations in the wild. Decreasing pollution emissions, cleaning up the environment when we can, continuing to lobby and voice concerns for the environment are important ways to help free-ranging populations of animals live in a less stressful and healthier environment.

Does Increased Stress Equal Decreased Welfare?

Why do we want/need to measure and document stress in individual animals (i.e., in managed care or rehabilitation)? One reason is to contribute to the health assessment of the animals under care. Normal physical exams and blood chemistry parameters may not always tell the entire story of how an animal is doing. Methods to evaluate stress-induced health changes (in combination with blood diagnostics) include behavioral and vocalization assessments. There may be a low level (or mild) stressor that causes the animal to alter their behavior. This may suggest some sort of stress.

Another reason may be to combat the animal activists who claim that captive animals are *distressed,* have poor welfare, and need to be released. Activists are a reality of life for zoos. We can see if the animals are showing behaviors or have physiologic parameters consistent with a stress response and use this information to amass objective data. Acute and chronic stress are different; however, often animal activists fail to appreciate this difference. Does acute stress present a welfare issue? Does chronic stress? And what exactly is animal welfare?

Avian Welfare

Welfare can be defined as a balance between positive (reward, satisfaction) and negative (stress) experiences and affective states. The balance may range from positive (good welfare) to negative (poor welfare; Spruijt et al., 2001). Historically, pre-1970, the welfare of animals in zoos and aquaria had focused on the basic needs/resources that humans provide for animals to survive. Is the environment appropriate? Does the animal have sufficient food and water? Is medical care adequate and timely? In 1966, the US government ratified the Animal Welfare Act (AWA). The publication resulting from this act specifically defines minimum standards for these "resource based" measures for various warm-blooded species, but only recently incorporated oversight of birds in 2023. These AWA standards are logical, reasonable, and achievable, and were developed by the opinions of experts in the field. They do not take into consideration the animal itself, just the resources the animal needs to survive in captivity.

A newer, holistic approach has been developed, which incorporates not only the resources needed for the animals (including medical diagnostics) but also the animal's perspective (the Five Freedom's model; Littlewood et al., 2023; Mellor, 2016). How does the animal respond to its environment? Does the animal interact with the zookeepers? With conspecifics (social interactions)? What is their affective state? And how do these all interact with the animal's physiology?

The *affective state* of an animal is their mood, emotional state, state of mind, disposition, and temperament. While these are clearly human terms, anyone who has spent time with animals knows that they have "moods," or times when they are more willing to engage with you than other times. Animals have times when they are hyperactive and other times when they are calmer. Clegg et al. (2019) demonstrated that bottlenose dolphins in managed care were willing to participate in positive reinforcement training sessions more often when they were in better health status than when in poorer health status. This suggests that willingness to participate is an example behavior that can indicate affective and welfare state and can be an early signal of a change in health status. Košťál et al. (2020) described several test designs in birds to investigate if/how cognition affects emotional responses. This type of approach opens the door to new ways to assess welfare (quality of life) in birds and all animals in managed care.

In the United States, the AWA oversees and ensures facilities provide resources to promote good health and are under appropriate veterinary management. Adherence to the AWA directives effectively removes health status from the welfare discussion. While this discussion is not meant to detail both sides of the activist's argument that captive animals have poor welfare, I believe it is safe to say that judgments/complaints of activists are largely made without considering objective data on the animals' welfare and are made through a human-only lens.

Let's look at assessing welfare in zoo/managed care animals. One way to assess the health and welfare of animals in managed care is to evaluate their stress level in addition to traditional health parameters. We already discussed that, in fact, we can demonstrate acute stress responses in certain situations in a managed care setting. Does this suggest that these animals are in a poor welfare state? Or that they have a poor quality of life? Perhaps if we evaluate stress levels at other times (not during expected stressful events like transport, for example), we could see data indicating little and/or no stress, thus balancing out the short periods of acute stress. Then taken together, all these data points could reveal a different overall picture.

The answer to the question of "Does stress equal poor welfare?" is "not necessarily." The type of stress is important – is it acute or chronic? Is the stressor a routine activity (such as a physical examination) or is it a surgical procedure? Acute stress is, by definition, short-lived. While that moment of stress may be perceived as "negative" to the animal, when the stressor is gone, then the negativity is also gone. Chronic stress is a different story. In chronic stress, the type of stressor is important. The magnitude of the "stress" is also important. Does the chronic stressor impact the animal's physiology acutely or put the animal at risk of physical injury or illness? Importantly, since chronic stress can lead to long-term health sequelae, can veterinarians treat, prevent, and/or mitigate those expected issues? If veterinarians can, then the magnitude and duration of those negative health sequelae can be minimized and/or negated. So, then how stressful is it really?

Clearly, assessment of overall welfare status requires a continuous analysis over the lifetime of the animal. In many avian species that can be easily 20+ years. Despite an occasional acute stressor, the general welfare may be very positive and stress free. Health assessments by zookeepers are one method to evaluate health of individuals (Whitham and Wielebnowski, 2009). Several "tools" have been promoted for use to monitor birds over time (Mels et al., 2023; Ward et al., 2018; Justice et al., 2017; Main et al., 2012; Butterworth et al., 2009). These are basically matrices which allow grading (e.g., using a scale of 1–5) of behaviors, physiologic data, etc. over time. The summation of these grades yields a composite score at each assessment date. Evaluation of the composite scores over time can reveal decreasing or increasing welfare and/or indicate possibly seasonal, individual, or age-related changes. Each individual animal is compared to itself, not to other animals. These tools are based heavily on behavioral assessments and provide a strong argument to include ethograms/behavioral assessments at regular intervals such as we do for veterinary assessments (such as blood work and cytology; Wolfensohn et al., 2018).

Are there any facility changes or activities that we can do with or for our animals in managed care that could help enhance their welfare? Environmental enrichment (EE) is a big focus in the field of animal welfare. How can the environment be enriched/improved to stimulate increased natural behaviors and enhance welfare? Toys, manipulata, three-dimensional (3-D) variation in the enclosure itself, etc. are examples of EE approaches. Placing food items in complex 3-D containers which encourage the animals to figure out how to get at the food (foraging) is also common. Music, olfaction, human interaction, and random and variable enrichment EE items or schedules are other approaches (Lubke et al., 2025). Finally, cognitive enrichment attempts to stimulate cognition and problem-solving processes in animals (Lubke et al., 2025; Kaplan, 2024). We know birds, especially parrots and corvids, are highly intelligent! So, engaging this part of their life is desirable and seen as encouraging positive welfare.

What do the data show? In zoo or other managed care facilities, enrichment is a priority. Habitat enrichment by the addition of physical structures or mazes in which food can be hidden or by modifying the substrate in which the animals forage can lead to increased time foraging and interacting with conspecifics (Claydon et al., 2024; Contardo et al., 2026). Zoo visitors approaching cages/habitats or children's playgrounds near bird cages can create visual enrichment for some species (Collins and Marples, 2015). Auditory and olfactory stimuli work well to stimulate the interest of captive birds especially for psittacines (Robbins and Margulis, 2016; Slater and Hauber, 2017; Lubke et al., 2025). Interaction with zookeepers/handlers is a source of enrichment as is positive reinforcement training for common medical behaviors (Mattison, 2012; Fernandez et al., 2019).

Data from poultry farms indicate that enriched environments (by whatever manner) in general promote increased activity in broilers (Meyer et al., 2020; Riber et al., 2018). Feather pecking and feather damage decreased with enrichment and increased in conventional cage systems and with age (van Staaveren et al., 2021; Colton and Fraley, 2014). EE and/or more complex environments resulted in decreased stress (decreased H : L ratio and startle response), did not alter immune function, prevented an increase of comb temperature, and promoted resilience as any effects returned to normal/baseline more rapidly than in chickens without EE (Ross et al., 2020; Campderrich et al., 2019). The data also show that there is a lot of variability in responses to EE dependent on age, chicken variety, and housing system. However, overall EE and novelty have a positive effect on birds.

Summary

Data on physiologic and immunologic changes from stress are variable depending on species life history, sex, and age; however, data do indicate acute stress responses to handling/restraint, heat, social changes, and pollution (see Chapter 8). These data are important but not always sufficient to determine overall welfare or chronic stress. Welfare (and stressors) perhaps should be better viewed over a longer time scale (months, years, lifetime). Newer welfare approaches assess changes in various factors (resource and animal based) over time. The data over time are a more realistic indication of overall welfare rather than a single stressful event.

The welfare of birds (and other animals) in managed care settings is topical. This section presents a high-level overview. There is still a lot to do in this arena as we face lots of change in the environment. How will those changes impact stress and welfare of birds in zoos/managed care settings? How will those changes impact wild bird populations? What role, if any, will zoos play in the future?

Post-script: Poultry Stress and Welfare in Brief

The poultry industry – chickens raised for meat (broilers) or eggs (layers) – has a long history and evolution to get where they are today. From egg laying to processing and distribution to waste management, the business of poultry for consumption is a thoroughly thought-out and efficient business operation! (I was impressed when I read about it!) However, when viewed from the "outside," things can look very different.

Housing types for these chickens include conventional (original), free-ranging, cage-free, pasture raised, and organically raised. Conventional systems have lots of birds that live in cages, have access to food and water, and held under defined lighting (14 : 10 light : dark hours) and temperature regimens (Figure 11.2a). This system is the type that stirs the most welfare arguments. Cage-free birds do not live in cages, but rather live in large aviaries with 1 square foot/bird (on average). Free-range birds do not live in cages (cage-free) and have access to go outdoors (Figure 11.2b). Pasture-raised birds are outdoors most to all of the time. Organically raised chickens are housed free-range, and their diet is all organically produced.

Data show that 1–1.5 square feet/bird is optimal size for growth and health (Zabir et al., 2021). The main "stressor" in conventional chicken production seems to be heat stress (if the temperature rises in the facility). Heat stress can be managed by adequate air flow/ventilation

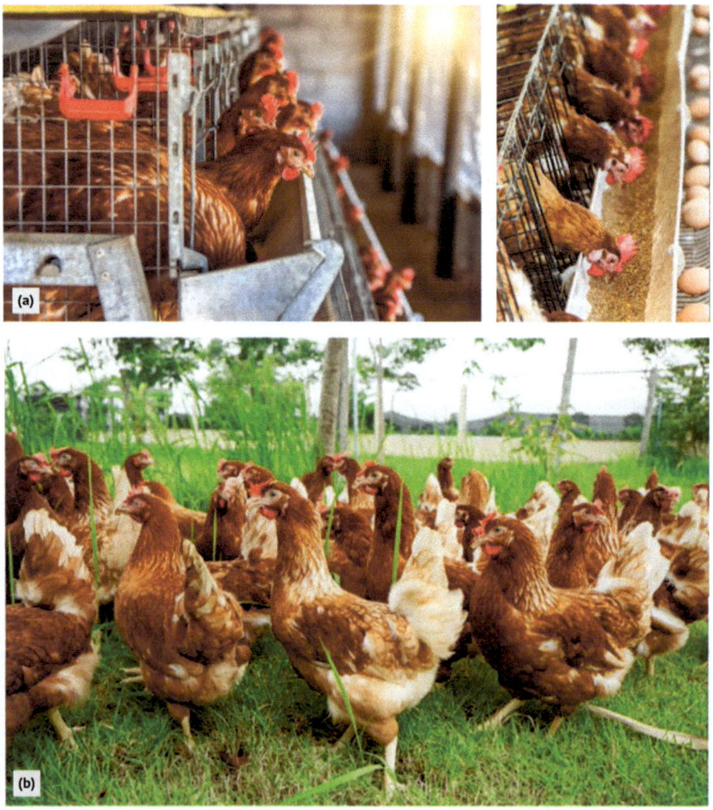

Figure 11.2 Housing systems of egg-laying hens in (a) conventional housing conditions and (b) free-ranging conditions.

and cooling systems. In addition, the poultry industry is trying to select and breed more "heat tolerant" chickens, and they are working on ways to condition young chicks to tolerate increasing heat (Goel et al., 2023). Those last two are intense mitigation strategies and raise ethical considerations for some. These are but a few of the studies on stress in poultry.

Another consideration is keeping the birds healthy and free from disease. This is a welfare issue. Evaluating large flocks or aviaries of birds can be challenging. Several approaches have been put forward for health assessments of flocks. All involve evaluation of numerous parameters that cover both resource and animal-based approaches, rank the responses, then sum them up to yield a single overall "score." This process then would be repeated at regular intervals. The "animal welfare assessment grid," "Welfare Quality," and "AssureWel" approaches are a few examples used in poultry (similar to the matrix presented in Chapter 6; Mels et al., 2023; Ward et al., 2018; Justice et al., 2017; Main et al., 2012; Butterworth et al., 2009). Assessing flock health as a unit can be done by walking a planned route in the aviary (like a transect) and recording numbers of birds seen with illness, etc. (Mels et al., 2023).

Birds raised in large densities, such as poultry for food, always carry the risk of rapid spread of infectious disease should any new agent get introduced into the facility. There is an extensive chicken vaccination protocol for each type of housing, use, and age (recall Chapter 6). Chickens roaming outside in an enclosed environment are more likely to encounter a pathogenic agent because nature is not controlled. Then they can bring it back to the group and the disease can spread. When this occurs, often the entire flock needs to be culled (euthanized) to avoid any spread to other birds, animals, and/or humans.

Euthanasia (humane killing) is also a welfare concern. The goal of euthanizing is to get the animal to an unconscious state as quickly as possible, so they do not feel anything or stress (AVMA, 2020). Then while in this state the animal dies. While witnessing or performing euthanasia, it is hard to avoid thinking that the animal is in distress. I think this is a typical response for a human. There may be a very short (hopefully) period of time where the animal does feel stressed or potentially distressed. I am not sure it is possible to euthanize many animals simultaneously and safely without stress. However, it is clear from the literature that euthanasia methodology is an important and heavily researched issue in the poultry world. More details on euthanasia methods are presented in Box 11.1.

Box 11.1 Euthanasia

Euthanasia refers to ending the life of an animal in a way that minimizes or eliminates pain and/or distress (AVMA, 2020). It involves humane techniques that induce the most rapid, painless, and distress-free death possible. The American Veterinary Medical Association created a guiding document with practices recommended (and prohibited) for use in various vertebrate species. This document states that euthanasia should be performed by a veterinarian or overseen by the veterinarian. The veterinarian should assess the discomfort or stress potentially induced by physical setting, handling, social setting, pheromones or odors from other animals, including those previously euthanized, and the presence of humans. Personnel performing euthanasia should be trained and skilled in euthanasia techniques. Other factors such as infectious disease concerns,

(Continued)

Box 11.1 (Continued)

conservation status, regulatory oversight, equipment used, and disposal of carcasses should be considered.

Euthanasia of individual poultry (chickens, turkeys, quail, pheasants, ducks, geese) includes gas (CO_2, CO, N, Ar) inhalation, overdose of injectable anesthetics (e.g., barbiturates or their derivatives), and various physical methods that produce rapid and complete loss of consciousness and death. Depending on the bird's size, these may include cervical dislocation, decapitation, blunt force trauma, gunshot, and captive bolt (AVMA, 2020). Other methods include anesthetization plus exsanguination or potassium chloride administration. For embryonated eggs and hatchlings ≤72 hours old, exposure to carbon dioxide for 20 minutes, or maceration. If the eggs are <80% incubated, then cooling (4 hours at 40 °F), freezing, or maceration are acceptable. Maceration is fragmentation and death by a device with rotating blades or projections. Sometimes a secondary method of euthanasia may be required to ensure death for maceration and other methods.

Due to infectious and zoonotic diseases in the past few decades, there has been an urgent need to cull thousands of birds rapidly to mitigate further spread. Currently, using carbon dioxide in a closed container is the method used for many animals at a time (Kingston et al., 2005). This unfortunate circumstance has led to research on the best way to euthanize poultry with the least disruption of the farm and personnel. Infected/contaminated birds should be euthanized separate from uncontaminated individuals who need to be euthanized to minimize infectious spread. In these types of situations, gas inhalation is the main method used. Gas is injected into a closed container or enclosure which contains numerous individuals. The gases (mentioned above) cause stunning and death by hypoxia. In 2024, the European Food Safety Panel on Animal Health and Welfare described the use of portable containers, separate from areas on the farm, in which to euthanize infected animals. This method includes use of high expansion foam as a vehicle to deliver nitrogen, which is sprayed into a closed container over the chickens.

Within the foam, there is gas (e.g., CO_2 and N) which the poultry will inhale as the foam settles down onto them. Stunning and death occur rapidly due to hypoxia with minimum stress. The use of separate and mobile enclosures has been used in emergency situations such as mass euthanasia due to influenza virus. These enclosures separate the infected carcasses and waste. Efforts are being made to utilize as much of the uncontaminated carcass as possible for animal feed or human consumption to minimize waste and monetary loss. The panel determined that the level of welfare of the animals until death was the same or better than current methods, is valid for layers and broilers, and to only be used on animals not intended for food. Euthanasia of animals for human consumption (slaughter) involves pre-stunning transport to the location where slaughter will occur, stunning, and then bleeding (EFSA, 2019).

There are numerous publications evaluating all aspects of housing and care and their welfare impact on chickens. It is in the best interest of the poultry industry to mitigate/decrease stress in broilers and egg-laying chickens, as their growth rate slows, breast muscle size or number of eggs laid decreases also. This affects the bottom line for the poultry company. In general, the industry has modified its standards to optimize welfare, including larger and/or more complex caging, no more beak trimming unless medically necessary, improvements in ventilation and temperature controls, and commitment of industry personnel to optimize welfare.

How do we weigh the presumed welfare issues of chickens raised in these ways? The animals are born into the "system." They are not brought in from outside in the field. The system they are born into is all they know. They don't know what other living arrangements there are. Both chickens for meat and eggs have been genetically modified and/or selectively bred to maximize the amount of meat and number of eggs, respectively. In this process, some disease issues may be observed in relatively low prevalence. These include metabolic type diseases, bone issues, etc., as the chicken has been bred to allocate minerals and resources to meat or egg production sometimes at the expense of the rest of its body. Many of these health issues can be resolved with nutritional adjustments. All diseases are managed by veterinary care, food supplementation, or the animals are culled.

How DO we (or should we) weigh the presumed welfare of the chickens raised for food? Considering the nutritional value chicken meat and eggs provide at a more economical price than other meats? In light of increasing human poverty, inability to purchase food, and food shortages in the world? In light of the concept that good nutrition in humans helps mitigate the prevalence and/or severity of human diseases? Could the chickens in these facilities even survive if set free in the environment? Would mitigating measures (such as providing free food to people in need in the United States and the world) performed by the companies that raise the chickens make a difference?

The welfare debate regarding poultry production is not an easy issue. The industry has advanced and responded to consumer concerns regarding housing and welfare. For example, antibiotics fed to enhance chicken growth rate have been discontinued in the United States in part due to public opinion and customer pressure. This change resulted in a slight change in feed efficiency and a marginal increase in costs to raise the chickens (Korver, 2023). Other products, such as probiotics and other natural additives, are being investigated as alternatives. Similarly, legislative and consumer-driven pressure is now focused on restricting (slowing) the growth rate of broilers. There is an increasing call for "reduced growth rate" chicken meat, which is apparently deemed as more humane or an improvement (Korver, 2023). However, slower growth rate of genetically fast-growing birds may present other physiologic problems. And slower-growing flocks would produce more waste and a larger carbon footprint. Again, not an easy issue.

Literature Cited

Applegate, J. E. (1971). Spring relapse of *Plasmodium relictum* infections in an experimental field population of English sparrows (*Passer domesticus*). *Journal of Wildlife Diseases* 7(1):37–42. https://doi.org/10.7589/0090-3558-7.1.37.

AVMA (2020). AVMA euthanasia guidelines for the euthanasia of animals. *American Veterinary Medical Association.*

Badas, E. P., Romero-Haro, A., and Morales, J. (2025). What doesn't kill you makes you (and your descendants stronger: A perspective on early-life exposure to human-induced challenges as a trigger of compensatory mechanisms. *Journal of Avian Biology* e03418. https://doi.org/10.1002/jav.03418.

Bell, B. A., Phan, M. L., Meillère, A., et al. (2018). Influence of early-life nutritional stress on songbird memory formation. *Proceedings of the Royal Society B: Biological Sciences* 285(1887):20181270. https://doi.org/10.1098/rspb.2018.1270.

Bittencourt, Mde. A., Melleu, F. F., and Marino-Neto, J. (2015). Stress-induced core temperature changes in pigeons (*Columba livia*). *Physiology & Behavior* 139:449–458. https://doi.org/10.1016/j.physbeh.2014.11.067.

Butterworth, A., Arnould, C., and van Niekerk, T. (2009). *Assessment Protocol for Poultry*. Lelystadt, Netherlands: Welfare Quality® Consortium.

Campderrich, I., Nazar, F. N., Wichman, A., et al. (2019). Environmental complexity: A buffer against stress in the domestic chick. *PLoS One* 14(1):e0210270. https://doi.org/10.1371/journal.pone.0210270.

Chu, B., Marwaha, K., Sanvictores, T., et al. (2024). Physiology, Stress Reaction. [Updated 2024 May 7]. In: StatPearls [Internet]. Treasure Island (FL): StatPearls Publishing; 2026 Jan. Available from: https://www.ncbi.nlm.nih.gov/books/NBK541120/ /.

Claydon, M., Brereton, J., and Rose, P. (2024). Never be mute about bird welfare: Swanning around with environmental enrichment. *Zoo Biology* 43(1):83–91. https://doi.org/10.1002/zoo.21808.

Clegg, I. L. K., Rodel, H. G., Mercera, B., et al. (2019). Dolphins' willingness to participate (WtP) in positive reinforcement training as a potential welfare indicator, where WtP predicts early changes in health status. *Frontiers in Psychology*, 10:2112. https://doi.org/10.3389/fpsyg.2019.02112.

Collins, C. K. and Marples, N. M. (2015). Zoo playgrounds: A source of enrichment or stress for a group of nearby cockatoos? A case study. *Journal of Applied Animal Welfare Science* 18(4):375–387. https://doi.org/10.1080/10888705.2015.1034278.

Colton, S. and Fraley, G. S. (2014). The effects of environmental enrichment devices on feather picking in commercially housed Pekin ducks. *Poultry Science* 93(9):2143–2150. https://doi.org/10.3382/ps.2014-03885.

Contardo, J., Labra, A., and Cubillos, G. (2026). Environmental enrichment increases foraging duration in Chilean flamingos under human care. *Journal of Applied Animal Welfare Science* 29(1):144–159. https://doi.org/10.1080/10888705.2025.2524415.

Dhondt, A. A. and Dobson, A. P. (2017). Stress hormones bring birds, pathogens and mosquitoes together. *Trends in Parasitology* 33(5):339–341. https://doi.org/10.1016/j.pt.2017.01.001.

Dickens, M. J., Earle, K. A., and Romero, L. M. (2009). Initial transference of wild birds to captivity alters stress physiology. *General and Comparative Endocrinology* 160(1):76–83. https://doi.org/10.1016/j.ygcen.2008.10.023.

EFSA AHAW Panel (EFSA Panel on Animal Health and Welfare), Nielsen, S. S., Alvarez, J., et al. (2024). The use of high expansion foam for stunning and killing pigs and poultry. *EFSA Journal* 22(7):e8855. https://doi.org/10.2903/j.efsa.2024.8855.

EFSA Panel (2019). Slaughter of animals: Poultry. https://doi.org/10.2903/j.efsa.2019.5849.

Ericsson, M., Fallahsharoudi, A., Bergquist, J., et al. (2014). Domestication effects on behavioral and hormonal responses to acute stress in chickens. *Physiology & Behavior* 133:161–169. https://doi.org/10.1016/j.physbeh.2014.05.024.

Fairhurst, G. D., Frey, M. D., Reichert, J. F., et al. (2011). Does environmental enrichment reduce stress? An integrated measure of corticosterone from feathers provides a novel perspective. *PLoS One* 6(3):e17663. https://doi.org/10.1371/journal.pone.0017663.

Fernandez, E. J., Kinley, R. C., and Timberlake, W. (2019). Training penguins to interact with enrichment devices for lasting effects. *Zoo Biology* 38(6):481–489. https://doi.org/10.1002/zoo.21510.

Gervasi, S. S., Burgan, S. C., Hofmeister, E., et al. (2017). Stress hormones predict a host superspreader phenotype in the West Nile virus system. *Proceedings of the Biological Sciences* 284(1859):20171090. https://doi.org/10.1098/rspb.2017.1090.

Goel, A., Ncho, C. M., Gupta, V., et al. (2023). Embryonic modulation through thermal manipulation and in ovo feeding to develop heat tolerance in chickens. *Animal Nutrition* 13:150–159. https://doi.org/10.1016/j.aninu.2023.01.005.

Grunst, M. L., Grunst, A. S., Grémillet, D., et al. (2026). Arctic seabirds exposed to acute stress display state- and environment-dependent patterns of surface temperature change, independent of mercury contamination. *Comparative Biochemistry Physiology Pt A, Molecular & Integrative Physiology* 311:111948. https://doi.org/10.1016/j.cbpa.2025.111948.

Hassaneen, R. K., Mobarak, Y. M., El-Baz, L. M. F., et al. (2025). Short- and long-term captivity impacts on bird memory, corticosterone level, and oxidative stress genes: Perspectives on deep learning analysis. *Physiology & Behavior* 301:115064. https://doi.org/10.1016/j.physbeh.2025.115064.

Jimenez, A. G. and Williams, J. B. (2014). Rapid changes in cell physiology as a result of acute thermal stress house sparrows, *Passer domesticus. Journal Thermal Biology* 46:31–39. https://doi.org/10.1016/j.jtherbio.2014.10.001.

Justice, W. S. M., O'Brien, M. F., Szyszka, O., et al. (2017). Adaptation of the animal welfare assessment grid (AWAG) for monitoring animal welfare in zoological collections. *Veterinary Record* 181(6):143. https://doi.org/10.1136/vr.104309.

Kaplan, G. (2024). The evolution of social play in songbirds, parrots and cockatoos – emotional or highly complex cognitive behaviour or both? *Neuroscience & Biobehavioral Reviews* 161:105621. https://doi.org/10.1016/j.neubiorev.2024.105621.

Kingston, S. K., Dussault, C. A., Zaidlicz, R. S., et al. (2005). Evaluation of two methods for mass euthanasia of poultry in disease outbreaks. *Journal of the American Veterinary Medical Association* 227(5):730–738. https://doi.org/10.2460/javma.2005.227.730.

Korver, D. R. (2023). Review: Current challenges in poultry nutrition, health and welfare. *Animal* 17:100755. https://doi.org/10.1016/j.animal.2023.100755.

Košťál, Ľ., Skalná, Z., and Pichová, K. (2020). Use of cognitive bias as a welfare tool in poultry. *Journal of Animal Science* 98(Supplement 1):S63–S79. https://doi.org/10.1093/jas/skaa039.

Littlewood, K. E., Heslop, M. V., and Cobb, M. L. (2023). The agency domain and behavioral interactions: Assessing positive animal welfare using the Five Domains model. *Frontiers in Veterinary Science* 10:1284869. https://doi.org/10.3389/fvets.2023.1284869.

Lubke, N., Held, S. D. E., Massaro, M., et al. (2025). Dance behaviour in cockatoos: Implications for cognitive processes and welfare. *PLoS One* 20(8):e0328487. https://doi.org/10.1371/journal.pone.0328487.

Main, D. C. J., Mullan, S., Atkinson, C., et al. (2012). Welfare outcomes assessment in laying hen farm assurance schemes. *Animal Welfare* 2(3):389–396. https://doi.org/10.7120/09627286.21.3.389.

Mattison, S. (2012). Training birds and small mammals for medical behaviors. *Veterinary Clinics North America Exotic Animal Practice* 15(3):487–499. https://doi.org/10.1016/j.cvex.2012.06.012.

Mellor, D. J. (2016). Updating animal welfare thinking: Moving beyond the "Five Freedoms" towards "A life worth living". *Animals (Basel)* 6:21. https://doi.org/10.3390/ani6030021.

Mels, C., Niebuhr, K., Futschik, A., et al. (2023). Development and evaluation of an animal health and welfare monitoring system for veterinary supervision of pullet farms. *Preventative Veterinary Medicine* 217:105929. https://doi.org/10.1016/j.prevetmed.2023.105929.

Meyer, M. M., Johnson, A. K., and Bobeck, E. A. (2020). A novel environmental enrichment device increased physical activity and walking distance in broilers. *Poultry Science* 99(1): 48–60. https://doi.org/10.3382/ps/pez581.

Names, G. R., Schultz, E. M., Krause, J. S., et al. (2021). Stress in paradise: Effects of elevated corticosterone on immunity and avian malaria resilience in a Hawaiian passerine. *Journal of Experimental Biology* 224(20):jeb242951. https://doi.org/10.1242/jeb.242951.

Pinto, J. A. M., Souza-Kasprzyk, J., Guilherme Padilha, J. A., et al. (2025). Comparative corticosterone responses to capture stress in sympatric Antarctic penguins. *General and Comparative Endocrinology* 374:114836. https://doi.org/10.1016/j.ygcen.2025.114836.

Reinoso-Pérez, M. T., Dhondt, K. V., Yánez Abad, A. A., et al. (2025). Pathogen-induced stress in wild house finches (*Haemorhous mexicanus*): Leukocyte dynamics as health indicators. *Journal of Wildlife Diseases* 61(2):334–347. https://doi.org/10.7589/JWD-D-24-00164.

Riber, A. B., van de Weerd, H. A., de Jong, I. C., et al. (2018). Review of environmental enrichment for broiler chickens. *Poultry Science* 97(2):378–396. https://doi.org/10.3382/ps/pex344.

Robbins, L. and Margulis, S. W. (2016). Music for the birds: effects of auditory enrichment on captive bird species. *Zoo Biology* 35(1):29–34. https://doi.org/10.1002/zoo.21260.

Ross, M., Rausch, Q., Vandenberg, B., et al. (2020). Hens with benefits: Can environmental enrichment make chickens more resilient to stress? *Physiology & Behavior* 226:113077. https://doi.org/10.1016/j.physbeh.2020.113077.

Santos, E. G., Herter, J. V., Wiederhecker, H. C., et al. (2025). Health stress in birds increase with Urbanization in a large tropical city. *Ecohealth* 22(2):233–243. https://doi.org/10.1007/s10393-025-01708-y.

Schmidt, K. L., Macdougall-Shackleton, E. A., and Macdougall-Shackleton, S. A. (2012). Developmental stress has sex-specific effects on nestling growth and adult metabolic rates but no effect on adult body size or body composition in song sparrows. *Journal of Experimental Biology* 215(Pt 18):3207–3217. https://doi.org/10.1242/jeb.068965.

Slater, M. N. and Hauber, M. E. (2017). Olfactory enrichment and scent cue associative learning in captive birds of prey. *Zoo Biology* 36(2):120–126. https://doi.org/10.1002/zoo.21353.

Spruijt, B. M., van den Bos, R., and Pijlman, F. T. A. (2001). A concept of welfare based on reward evaluating mechanisms in the brain: Anticipatory behavior as an indicator for the state of reward systems. *Applied Animal Behavior Science* 72:145–171. https://doi.org/10.1016/S0168-1591(00)00204-5.

van Staaveren, N., Ellis, J., Baes, C. F., et al. (2021). A meta-analysis on the effect of environmental enrichment on feather pecking and feather damage in laying hens. *Poultry Science* 100(2):397–411. https://doi.org/10.1016/j.psj.2020.11.006.

Ward, S. J., Sherwen, S., and Clark, F. E. (2018). Advances in applied zoo animal welfare science. *Journal of Applied Animal Welfare Science* 21(Supplement 1):23–33. https://doi.org/10.1080/10888705.2018.1513842.

Whitham, J. C. and Miller, L. J. (2025). Why measuring and building resilience is applicable to Zoo and Aquarium animal welfare. *Journal of Zoological and Botanical Gardens* 6:48. https://doi.org/10.3390/jzbg6030048.

Whitham, J. C. and Wielebnowski, N. (2009). Animal-based welfare monitoring: Using keeper ratings as an assessment tool. *Zoo Biology* 28(6):545–560. https://doi.org/10.1002/zoo.20281.

Wolfensohn, S., Shotton, J., Bowley H., et al. (2018). Assessment of welfare in zoo animals: Towards optimum quality of life. *Animals* 8:110.

Wright, T, F., Araya-Salas, M., Villalba, A., et al. (2026). Chronic stress raises baseline circulating corticosterone and reduces vocal plasticity in male budgerigars, an avian model for adult vocal learning. *Hormones & Behavior* 178:105884. https://doi.org/10.1016/j.yhbeh.2026.105884.

Zabir, M., Miah, M. A., Alam, M., et al. (2021). Impacts of stocking density rates on welfare, growth, and hemato-biochemical profile in broiler chickens. *Journal of Advanced Veterinary and Animal Research* 8(4):642–649. https://doi.org/10.5455/javar.2021.h556.

Zylberberg, M., Lee, K. A., Klasing, K. C., et al. (2013). Variation with land use of immune function and prevalence of avian pox in Galapagos finches. *Conservation Biology* 27(1): 103–112. https://doi.org/10.1111/j.1523-1739.2012.01944.x.

12

Environmental Change and the Future of Avian Health and Welfare

There are several recurrent themes in this text. These are the susceptibility of birds to airborne/respiratory insults, the energetically expensive lifestyle of birds, increasing ranges of birds and pathogens (and all other species) due to climate warming, and increasing anthropogenic impact (urbanization, organic contaminants, etc.) on birds. All of these are on a collision course that will magnify the avian losses we are already experiencing. We already know that these events not only affect birds but also affect humans and other animals (and plants) – zoonoses, viruses mutating and gaining the ability to infect new species, and bacteria becoming resistant to antimicrobial medications at an accelerating pace! Humans have created an environment polluted with metals, organic contaminants, plastics, and discarded pharmaceutical agents. Our activities on land have led to decreased biodiversity (of all species), modification of soil nutrients and conditions, decreased suitable areas for bird aggregation and foraging, and increasing (and increasingly toxic) air pollution from construction, transportation (cars, etc.). Human-derived waste (personal, agricultural, and commercial) has led to eutrophication of lakes, estuaries, and bays, which has led to increased algal blooms that may release toxins into the water and air. Ozone and carbon dioxide emissions into the atmosphere contribute to a rapidly magnifying cycle of global warming, increased air, and water surface temperatures. These changes have led to shifts in food webs, movement, or elimination of some aquatic species that are prey for aquatic birds and melting of ice sheets in the polar regions. Together with overfishing by humans, the result of decreasing ice is loss of habitat and foraging areas for seabirds (and other marine animals), resulting in an increase in severely threatened species and avian extinctions (see Box 12.1).

Box 12.1 Avian extinctions

Currently, there are approximately 11,000 extant species of birds. An additional 216 species of birds have already gone extinct since the 1500s, mostly due to hunting and/or out competition from invasive species. These included mostly the large, flightless species and island species. More recent extinctions have been due to anthropogenic and environmental impacts (such as pollutants and environment destruction). Of the

11,000 extant species, approximately 16% (1700 species) are critically endangered and/or at risk of extinction.

There are several "well-known" extinct species of birds. These include the great Auk, passenger pigeon, Carolina parakeets, large-bodied moas, and elephant birds. However, there are extinct species from each of the avian orders (listed below). Orders with an asterisk have experienced recent (20th–21st) century extinctions.

Passeriformes (perching birds) – 86 species*
Gruiformes (rails, cranes) – 35 species*
Psittaciformes (parrots, parakeets) – 20 species*
Columbiformes (pigeons, doves, dodo) – 19 species*
Anseriformes (ducks, geese, swan) – 11 species*
Charadriiformes (shore birds – sandpipers, auks, curlews, etc.) – 10 species*
Strigiformes (owls) – 8 species*
Pelecaniformes (pelicans, ibis, herons) – 7 species
Procellariformes (petrels, albatross) – 6 species*
Apodiformes (swifts, hummingbirds) – 5 species*
Caprimulgiformes (nightjars, poorwills) – 3 species*
Galliformes (quail, bustards) – 3 species
Podicipediformes (grebes) – 3 species*
Piciformes (woodpeckers) – 3 species*
Caraciformes (kingfishers) – 2 species*
Cuculiformes (cuckoos) – 2 species
Falconiiformes (falcons, kestrels) – 2 species
Suliformes (boobies, gannets) – 2 species
Aegotheliformes (owlets) – 1 species*
Apterygiformes (ratites, tinamous) – 1 species
Cathartiformes (vultures) – 1 species
Sphenisciformes (penguins) – 1 species

This all sounds very negative! After all, our human societies have become incredibly advanced in various technologies, medicine, and food production (among others). Do the positives of our advanced civilization outweigh the negatives created by, or by-products of, the actions of advanced civilizations?

There are some positive things humans have done other than discover and create medications, technologies, etc. The poultry industry is/has cleaned up its act by modifying the ways chickens are housed and managed, adopting humane techniques for handling and euthanasia, and recycling their waste as fertilizer for other uses. Humans have started to gather and work collectively to find ways to mitigate pollution, study birds, their ecology and life histories, and look for ways to preserve, conserve, rescue and/or rehabilitate birds and critical habitats. Let's look at these in more detail.

Breeding Endangered Avian Species in Captivity (*Ex situ* Breeding)

Breeding in captivity for release to replenish natural population numbers or to preserve a species is a great opportunity to learn about the birds' habits and intricacies of their lives that can increase the success of release projects and simply learn about their biology. The shear nature of the great variety of avian species on earth begs for information about their biology and behavior. Why are there so many varieties and lifestyles? What is unique about each of these varieties?

Breeding in captivity began in earnest in the late 1800s and early 1900s largely to replenish bird species for hunting (pheasants, geese, grouse, etc.). Breeding in captivity for conservation became popular in the 1960s after Rachel Carson published the book *Silent Spring* in 1962, and with the passage of the Endangered Species Act in 1966 (D'Elia, 2010). There have been notable successes in *ex situ* breeding, release, and repopulation of various endangered species. In the late 1980s, the California condor (*Gymnogyps californianus*) was bred in captivity and individuals were released to reconstitute that decimated population (Figure 12.1; see Chapter 9). The Peregrine falcon (*Falco peregrines*) population was severely declining, and by the year 2000, the Peregrine Fund organization had raised and released more than 7000 birds into the wild (D'Elia, 2010)! The Griffon vulture (*Gypsfulvus*) was successfully reintroduced in Bulgaria between 2010 and 2020 after captive breeding efforts (Stoyanov et al., 2023). It is now generally accepted that one of a zoo's main functions is captive (*ex situ*) breeding of endangered species including support and information sharing with other zoos and avian organizations (D'Elia, 2010). The consensus though is

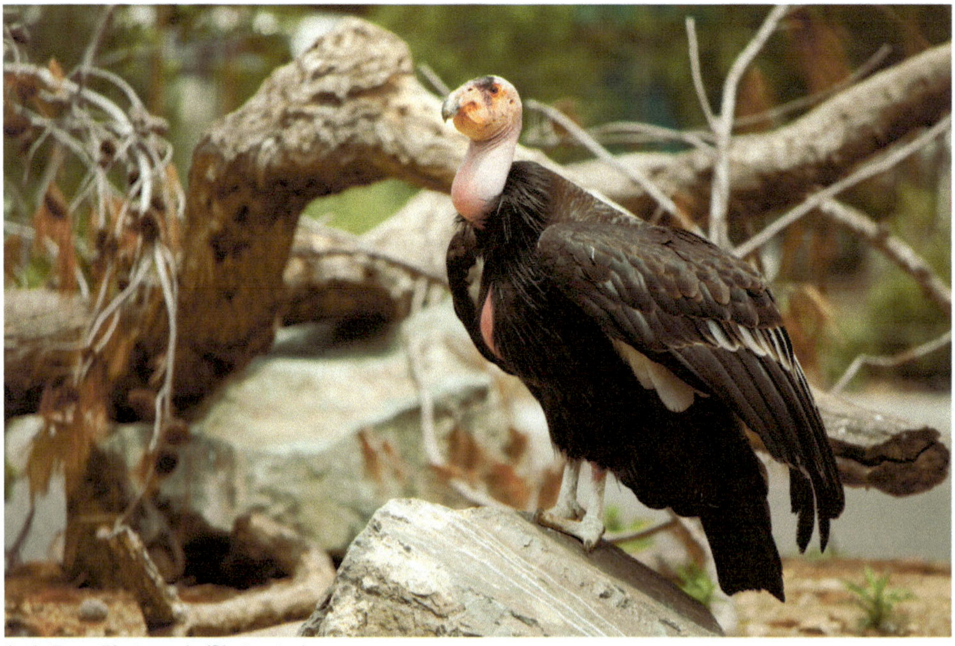

Andy Dean Photography/Shutterstock

Figure 12.1 California condor.

that if we do not try to mitigate the ongoing threats to these birds *in their habitats* as well, the effort is futile. They will most likely just perish again.

There is some controversy about the impacts of captive breeding selecting traits independent of natural selection. Decisions on which species to select for captive breeding are also a concern. How do we choose among the numerous species at risk? Do we select species that are similar or related to those for whom we have captive breeding information? Should we aim to breed the widest variety of species? A survey of zoos around the world suggests that species with the greatest "evolutionary distinctness" are more likely to be resident in zoos (Biega et al., 2019). The authors suggest that the more distinct species have fewer close relatives; therefore, their extinction would result in an overall greater loss of avian diversity. A survey of captive breeding in British zoos found that between 1988 and 1997, the number of birds in captive *ex situ* breeding programs increased in each IUCN category, the majority of whom were threatened species (Whitfort and Young, 2004). Zoos that have congeners (members of the same genus) of an endangered species would have valuable information on how to rear that endangered bird, permitting a greater chance of success (Che-Castaldo et al., 2018). Should only those endangered or threatened species be prioritized for breeding? Should only species that are planned to be released be bred in captivity? Or should we breed in captivity to maintain a species that we cannot/should not release back to the wild (e.g., the Guam kingfisher; Ramont et al., 2025)?

Zoos and aquaria contribute far more than simply captive breeding opportunities. Many zoos can transfer individuals to other zoos with the same species to increase genetic diversity of the breeding group. Conservation and basic biology education are primary activities of zoos (see Box 12.2). *In-situ* conservation and field research projects sponsored by zoos are integral for the conservation of migratory and nonmigratory birds (Che-Castaldo et al., 2018; Hutchins et al., 2017).

Box 12.2 Zoos – Challenges and opportunities

Zoos (and aquaria) are the main institutions that can hold, breed, and exhibit non-domestic animals. They are attractions that reach people of all ages and offer amazing opportunities to educate the public about animals around the world. They assume a prominent role in conservation management for a variety of species – many of which would be extinct if not for zoos. Zoos around the world are members of zoological organizations such as the American Zoological Association and the European Association of Zoos and Aquaria. These associations provide a network of support and emphasize the importance of animal welfare, population management, and research.

Zoos and aquaria face an ongoing dilemma. We know that the most charismatic, attractive, and unique species drive (in part) attendance. This leaves fewer resources (housing space and money) for other, perhaps less attractive but diminishing species. Will people flock to the zoo to see a rare, endangered species of rat? Probably not a huge draw! There is a precarious balance in how resources are allocated between exhibited species and those that need to be bred for conservation. Successful breeding requires an appropriate environment and food for each species. If the animals are destined for release to the environment, then those factors need to be assessed in

(Continued)

Box 12.2 (Continued)

the expected location of release. This is a potentially daunting task which requires time, people, and other resources. Zoos rely on donations, grants, and other methods to raise money. How do they balance how to distribute those resources while working to increase/maintain zoo visitors?

Research in the wild focusing on breeding and foraging behaviors (among others) is critical to the eventual success of breeding in captivity. The Raggiana Bird-of-Paradise (*Paradisaea raggiana*) is a lekking (lek using) species. Leks are congregations of males that perform courtship displays so that a female has a forum to choose her mate. Initially, reproductive success in the zoo was very poor in this species. Once they instituted a lek system so the males could display, females chose their mates, and nesting soared (Theule and Rimlinger, 2023). The eggs were collected, incubated, and the chicks hand reared. The change to allow natural breeding behavior was the key to their success! One of the Hawaiian honeycreepers, the 'Akikiki (*Oreomystis bairdi*), that was decimated by malaria has been in captivity to save what is left of this population/species. Reproductive success in captive breeding of this species was low until the husbandry and breeding scheme was changed to better reflect their practices in the wild. They are a territorial species, so the density of the breeding pairs was decreased (pairs had more space) and the insect prey were mixed with leaves, soil, detritus, etc. to simulate their natural foraging style (Flanagan et al., 2024). These changes, derived from observations in the wild, were critical to improving nesting success.

Not all species are easy to house or breed in captivity. Artificial reproductive practices, such as sperm collection, artificial insemination, and using germ cells to create embryos, can also be used. The Houbara bustard (*Chlamydotis undulata*) lives in North Africa and the Middle East, has been in decline due to hunting, and is now an IUCN vulnerable species. Breeding in captivity was difficult and largely unsuccessful. Germ cells obtained from one of these birds were injected into a chicken embryo, creating a chimera (a mixture of bustard and chicken; Wernery et al., 2010). One egg successfully hatched and genotyping revealed it to be 100% Houbara bustard! So modern reproductive and genetic techniques have great potential for species breeding and conservation. As of 2023, there are less than 30,000 Houbara bustards in the wild and it remains classified as a vulnerable species.

Let's look at some examples of successful captive *ex situ* breeding in more detail. Endangered African penguins (*Spheniscus demersus*) have been breeding in captivity for a long time (Figure 12.2). The South African population was designated as endangered due to a global population decrease of >70% between 2001 and 2013 (Sherley et al., 2014). The estimated population size in 2023 was 10,000 pairs. This decrease was due to the decrease in their prey species, sardines and anchovies, and competition with fisheries. In 2006–2007, 1282 chicks were abandoned by their parents and were taken into rehabilitation for captive rearing (Sherley et al., 2014). Zoo personnel began incubating and hand rearing abandoned eggs and chicks. Many of the chicks had various diseases, including malaria and bacterial infections, which were treated. Overall, 82% of these chicks were successfully raised and were released back into their habitat in South Africa. Their survival rates (32% for juveniles, 76% of adults) were similar to those of penguins that were reared in the wild and to those that were rehabilitated because of oil spills. In 2012–2016, after the adoption of an enhanced

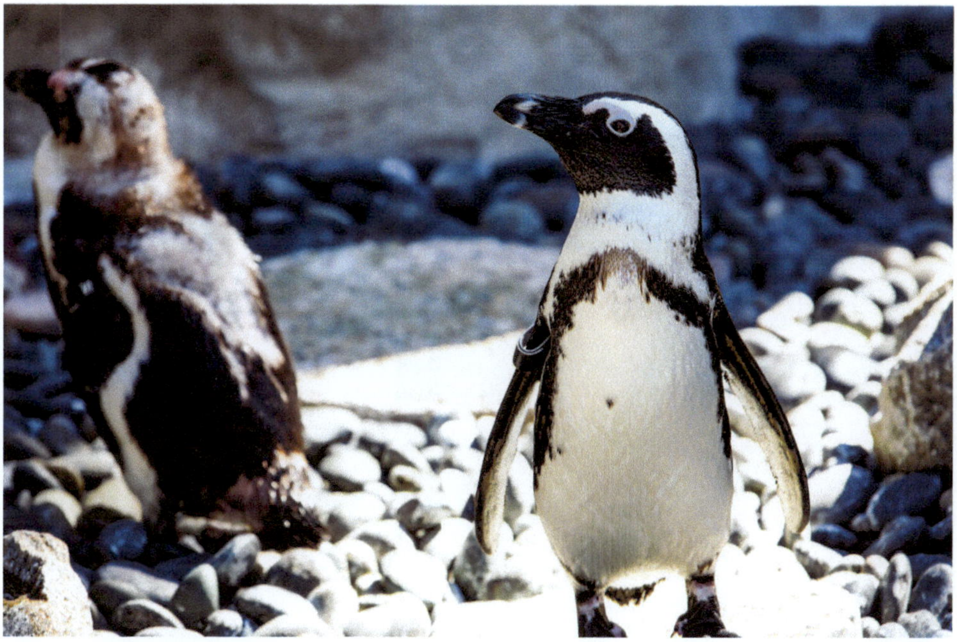

Jianwei Zhu/Adobe Stock Photos

Figure 12.2 African penguin (*Spheniscus demersus*) (Wiley #147195359).

rearing process, 77% of more than 2800 chicks and almost 700 eggs were raised and released, all with flipper tags so they can be tracked for follow-up (Klusener et al., 2018). Five years later, 12 of the released birds were breeding in the wild. That may not seem like many birds, but it is a start. Penguins are common residents in zoos, so we have a good handle on their husbandry and disease management. We know that malaria in captive penguin colonies is more prevalent than in wild penguins, and we can enhance monitoring of captive animals to be able to mitigate disease and mortality. We just cannot control the environment they return them to, especially the species that live at the farthest latitudes.

Flamingos (family Phoenicopteridae) are one of the most iconic avian species (Figure 12.3). Their pink-white coloration, long neck, and downward curved beaks are highly recognizable. There are six extant flamingo species of varying conservation statuses. The Greater and American flamingo species are considered of least concern (by IUCN). The Chilean, Lesser, and Puna (aka James's) species are considered near threatened. The Andean flamingo is classified as vulnerable. Threats to flamingos in the wild include increased industrialization, associated pollution and heavy metal waste, habitat encroachment, increasing temperature, and, in the Andes, mining operations. Their natural habitat includes hypersaline, high alkaline lakes where they forage. Small precipitation or temperature changes can cause large changes in this extreme environment and result in decreased reproductive success of flamingos (Mooney et al., 2023).

Flamingos are and have been common residents of zoos (and the like) and have been bred in captivity for a long time. While breeding has been relatively successful, there are still hurdles that need to be overcome. For example, often new adults need to be brought in from the wild to help replenish stocks (Mooney et al., 2023). Flamingos are obligate colonial breeders and

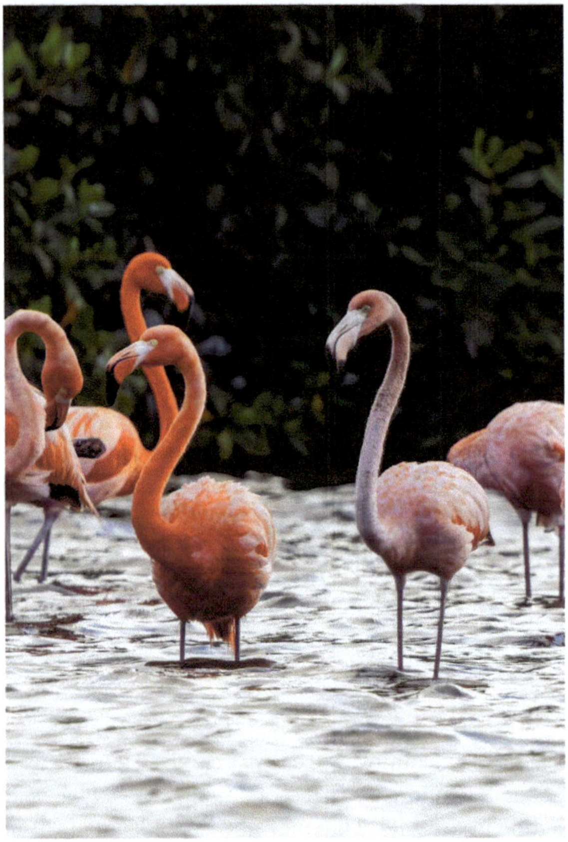

Figure 12.3 American Flamingos in the wild in Trinidad. *Source:* With permission of Jed Steiner.

live in large, dense flocks. Data amassed from over 500 zoos across the world indicate a minimum flock size of 40 birds to encourage reproduction. Flocks of up to 100 birds give a greater likelihood of reproduction and chick production (Mooney et al., 2023). A single egg is laid, and both parents share incubation duties. After 27–31 days, a precocial chick (with downy feathers) hatches. Parents feed it crop milk even after the chick learns to forage on its own at about six weeks or so. Chicks fledge between 9 and 13 weeks of age. During the nestling and fledgling period, chicks congregate in groups called creches. In these groups, they begin forming social bonds and learn foraging and social behaviors from each other. The creches are accompanied by some adult caretakers (Mooney et al., 2023).

By 6–10 months, the young flamingo will grow regular feathers, and their bill will develop the characteristic downturned shape. Reproductive maturity is not reached until 3–6 years of age! Reproducing pairs lay a single egg in a year. Some flamingos migrate while others do not. Life expectancy is long, 20–40 years in the wild, up to 50 or more in captivity. Interestingly, resident flamingos appear to have longer lifespans (by approximately 6–7 years) than migratory birds (Cayuela et al., 2025). In addition, their peak reproductive success occurs by the midpoint of their life and it decreases with age, consistent with senescence.

What we have learned from *ex situ* breeding over the years is that in addition to large flock sizes, an even flock sex ratio, long-term pair bonding, and the introduction of new birds lead to increased reproductive success (Mooney et al., 2023). These data are largely from American and greater flamingos; however, they are regularly applied to breeding of the other threatened flamingo species. Given their unique habitat, long lifespan, and long time to become reproductively active, it is easy to see how it may be difficult for these birds to adapt to the rapid environmental changes we are experiencing.

Questions always arise regarding the welfare of animals in zoos. We discussed welfare in the last chapter and the methods available to assess individual and group welfare. Qualitative behavioral assessment is the basis for welfare tools/assessments. While behavior (frequency and types) in captivity may differ from that in the wild, information on behavior in the wild allows facility and husbandry characteristics to be designed as close as possible to natural conditions (Rose and Riley, 2019). Then each individual's behavior/activity should be regularly evaluated in the zoo environment. Welfare comparisons zoo to zoo are not a good measure of actual welfare because all facilities are different, especially personnel/zookeepers. However, they do serve to identify if particular practices or aspects of husbandry may be improved or changed to improve welfare.

Public perception drives the claims of poor welfare. There is a growing literature base on zoo visitors' perceptions of zoo animal welfare, which are mostly positive. Zoos (aquaria, etc.) are held to the USDA standards of care, and most importantly, the animals are under veterinary oversight and veterinary technician/zookeeper care, all of whom are there *to ensure* the best welfare as possible. The main criticism is that the animals are not in the wild and likely not in their native location. Is that difference a welfare concern? Is it enough of a welfare concern to override the likelihood of starvation, stress, (both negative welfare states), and extinction of the animal in its imperiled habitat?

Research on Wild Populations and Habitats

Research on wild populations and in native habitats is critical. In addition to observing behaviors, we need to understand the presence/prevalence of any infectious, zoonotic, and other diseases or parasites. Knowing this we can predict and/or anticipate how the range expansion of influenza virus, for example, may affect the population. If birds cannot be captured and sampled, the collection of feces or feathers dropped on the ground can provide information, and new storage methods allow preservation of information (such as DNA and metals) from these samples for long periods of time (Zhang et al., 2026). If the existing population has no previous exposure to influenza virus (in this example), and we predict a potential outbreak, perhaps we can translocate or capture some birds to bring into captivity as a "reserve" population. Newer genetics and isotope methodology can extract information on migration routes, potential exposure to pathogens, etc. from a single feather. This can help target areas for screening or hotspots (Fuller et al., 2012). Mark and recapture information are optimal and provide temporal patterns of exposure to pathogens and continual assessment of welfare. Unfortunately, these data may be difficult or expensive to obtain. If we can capture individuals, we can also collect physiologic data, which can give us information on the individual's health status. Repeated sampling can tell us if and how the health changes. This is the basis of conservation physiology.

Similar to pathogen information, we should research the contaminants in the area and their sources. There are data already on the interactive effects of heavy metals and the likelihood of infection with infectious agents, such as *Haemosporidia* infection in passerines

(Werner et al., 2026). Depending on what we find, we can predict or anticipate possible immune suppression, eggshell thinning, etc. and create a plan to intercede if the risk of extinction is that extreme. Collaboration with other scientists is needed to work on ways to mitigate or remove pollutants, model environmental changes, so we can improve predictions and plan for future changes including data sharing and coordinated planning. Inclusion of community leaders and environmentalists relevant to habitats of interest is important to better understand if there are any societal/ethnic aspects of the species/habitat that should be taken into account (Jennings et al., 2025).

Education of the public in zoos or via ecotourism is important. Zoos and aquaria used to be the main way people were exposed to animals from other locations and parts of the world. Now we have video and social media exposure. But the vast majority of people still get a greater emotional connection from seeing the animals in person. Exposing people to the birds, their habitat, the factors impinging on their habitat, how those factors are affecting the bird's welfare and survival – these are topics to research and teach the public about. What is the biodiversity of the imperiled habitat? What does biodiversity mean in relation to ecology and evolution? What is the impact of birds on the environment and plants? What bird species may serve as good sentinels of what is happening in the environment? Which can we study *before* a major outbreak occurs?

How will we know how some birds/species modify their behavior or activities to cope with the environmental change? Do birds move nesting locations to shadier areas to deal with the increased heat? How does the heat affect where and what the birds prey on? Is the new prey nutritious enough? Do they have to forage for a longer amount of time to get the same nutritive gain? Does increased foraging time lead to an increased predation risk? Do the birds reduce their clutch size? Or do only some nestlings get fed and survive? There are many potential avenues for adaptation or resilience to a changing environment. All habitats are not equally permissive to behavioral changes. Melting sea ice modifying foraging opportunities may entail longer movements/flight in seabirds to find appropriate prey, while in a forest, the extra movement may be only a few feet or so, entailing a much lower cost to the bird. Data show that birds can decrease their metabolic rate in response to heat stress (Voges et al., 2024). In doing so, they generate less body heat and avoid losing as much water, thus avoiding dehydration. However, different species vary in their ability to lower their metabolism (Voges et al., 2024).

The effects of increased temperature and pollutants may affect nestlings and adults differentially. Are there long-term changes from early life (eggs and nestlings) exposure to environmental stressors? A lot of research deals with this question. Recent data indicate that there are, in fact, epigenetic and gut microbiome changes that are induced by both biotic (e.g., food and sociality) and abiotic (e.g., temperature change) factors (Ruuskanen, 2024; Wada and Coutts, 2021). It is not clear yet which or what yields positive or negative welfare states.

How much do we want, or need, to intercede in wild population health? Should we intercede? Is saving nonhuman species enough of a reason to intercede? Or should we only intercede if humans are potentially at risk from zoonoses? There is a precedent for wildlife vaccination programs to stem risk of human disease. Vaccines in bait targeted for raccoons, and coyotes has been used to thwart/slow potential rabies infection in these and other species with the goal of reducing risk to humans (APHIS, USDA). Wild vaccination programs also exist for many other diseases including *Mycobacterium bovis*, amphibian *Batrachochytrium*, *Chlamydia* in koalas, and distemper in pinnipeds. (Gulland et al., 2024; Barnett and Civitello, 2020). These programs are not perfect, and wild vaccination programs have particular challenges. These include waning immunity, partial immunity, the need for frequent boosters, and potential for development of resistance and increased pathogen virulence (Gulland et al., 2024). Many of these challenges are manageable.

Most of the current wild vaccination programs have involved mammals. One program though involves a bird, the endangered Indian yellow-neck albatross (*Thalassarche carteri*). In 2015–2016, young nestlings were vaccinated against avian cholera (Bourret et al., 2018). This resulted in good seroconversion rates and increased survivorship relative to unvaccinated control birds. We know that vaccination of commercial and backyard poultry also works to help decrease spread and spillover of disease. Perhaps we should be discussing increasing vaccination programs for more wild bird species?

We should mention the trade of birds across the world (although we won't be going into any detail about it). Careless or illegal movement of birds across the world for whatever purpose (pets, feathers, etc.) poses a huge risk for pathogen transfer and spread of antimicrobial-resistant bacteria. Some of these pathogens may be zoonotic. Conservation status of these birds and their welfare during their transport are also big issues to contend with. There are insufficient captive breeding programs to support the increasing demand for bird trade across the world, thus animals are still collected from the wild (Davies et al., 2023; Donald et al., 2023). Obviously, these issues apply to avian and non-avian animal trade. More controls and planning are needed to decrease this avenue of disease spread and avian health risks. Educating the public on trade issues is also needed to help manage this issue.

As the environment changes and urbanization pressures increase, we can find brilliant examples of birds adapting to city life! In Sydney, sulfur-crested cockatoos have learned how to activate and drink from water fountains, and the activity is spreading throughout their population (Figure 12.4; Klump et al., 2025). They have also learned how to open

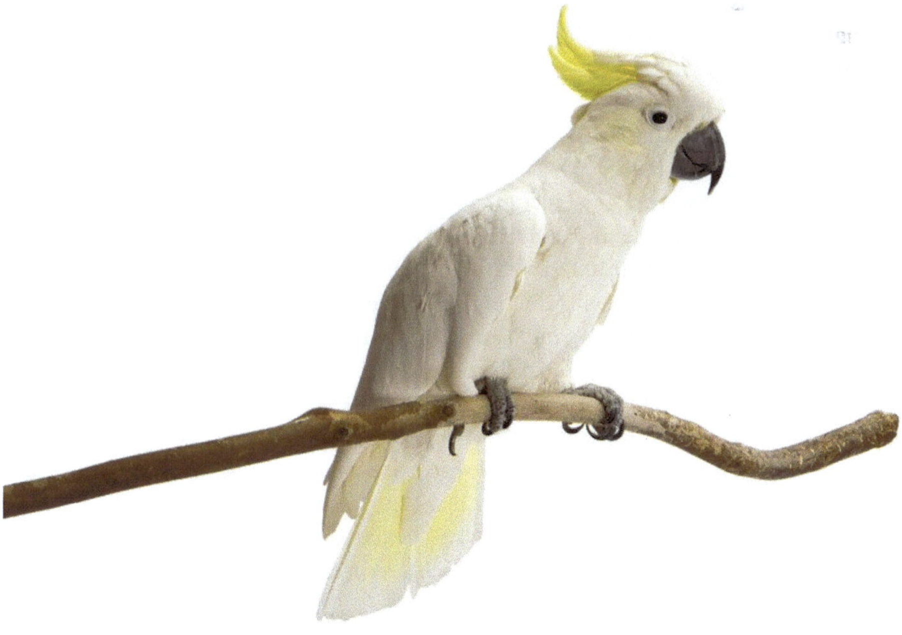

Figure 12.4 Sulfur crested cockatoo! *Source*: andrewburgess / Adobe Stock Photos.

garbage bin lids to access food waste! Not a skill most would brag about! But clearly an activity with a big caloric reward! (Much different from gulls visiting garbage dumps! But I'll give the gulls some props for that, even though it is still embarrassing!) Here is another example of clever adaptation to urban life. A Cooper's hawk learned that when the traffic light turned red, the stopped cars provided cover so the hawk could swoop down and surprise attack birds foraging on the ground (Dinets, 2025)! As mentioned in Chapter 8, seagulls hitch a ride in a garbage truck to a waste dump! (Still gets my goat, but kudos to that bird for figuring that out!) Birds are smart! As smart as some species are, however, we humans still need to act.

I think we know what we need to do to address the health of and protect bird populations in a changing world – be proactive in monitoring for pathogen spread, new diseases, antibiotic resistance changes, etc. Monitor bird species that are good sentinels for their environments such as raptors and other birds of prey for terrestrial environments (Badry et al., 2020) and marine birds as sentinels of the oceans (Burger and Gochfeld, 2004). Maintaining the integrity of habitats likely provides a buffer against disease transmission (Chen et al., 2024). We should especially be monitoring areas of intersection of animals and humans to be aware of emerging (or potential) zoonotic diseases as promulgated in the One Health approach (Chen et al., 2024; D'Elia, 2010). These are the main threats to avian health in the coming years as a result of anthropomorphic and climate-induced environmental changes. At least we know of VARIOUS ways we can approach this task. So, let's get to it! "We can do it. We must do it!" (Sir David Attenborough, 2024).

Literature Cited

Badry, A., Krone, O., Jaspers, V. L. B., et al. (2020). Towards harmonisation of chemical monitoring using avian apex predators: Identification of key species for pan-European biomonitoring. *Science of the Total Environment* 731:139198. https://doi.org/10.1016/j.scitot.2020.139198.

Barnett, K. M. and Civitello, D. J. (2020). Ecological and evolutionary challenges for wildlife vaccination. *Trends in Parasitology* 36(12):970–978. https://doi.org/10.1016/j.pt.2020.08.006.

Biega, A. M., Lamont, M., Mooers, A., et al. (2019). Guiding the prioritization of the most endangered and evolutionary distinct birds for new zoo conservation programs. *Zoo Biology* 38(3):305–315. https://doi.org/10.1002/zoo.21482.

Bourret, V., Gamble, A., Tornos, J., et al. (2018). Vaccination protects endangered albatross chicks against avian cholera. *Conservation Letters* 11(4):e12443.

Burger, J. and Gochfeld, M. (2004). Marine birds as sentinels of environmental pollution. *EcoHealth* 1:263–274. https://doi.org/10.1007/s10393-004-0096-4.

Cayuela, H., Roques, S., Arnaud, A., et al. (2025). Migration shapes senescence in a long- lived bird. *Proceedings of the National Academy of Sciences of the United States of America* 122(36): e2422882122. https://doi.org/10.1073/pnas.2422882122.

Che-Castaldo, J. P., Grow, S. A., and Faust, L. J. (2018). Evaluating the contribution of North American Zoos and aquariums to endangered species recovery. *Scientific Reports* 8:9789. https://doi.org/10.1038/s41598-018-27806-2.

Chen, F., Jiang, F., Ma, J., et al. (2024). Intersecting planetary health: Exploring the impacts of environmental stressors on wildlife and human health. *Ecotoxicology and Environmental Safety* 283:116848. https://doi.org/10.1016/j.ecoenv.2024.116848.

Davies, A., D'Cruze, N., and Martin, R. (2023). A review of commercial captive breeding of parrots as a supply-side intervention to address unsustainable trade. *Conservation Biology* 38:e14338. https://doi.org/10.1111/cobi.14338.

D'Elia, J. (2010). Evolution of avian conservation breeding with insights for addressing the current extinction crisis. *Journal of Fish and Wildlife Management* 1(2):189–210. https://doi.org/10.3996/062010-JFWM-017.

Dinets, V. (2025). Street smarts: A remarkable adaptation in a city-wintering raptor. *Frontiers in Ethology* 4:1539103. https://doi.org/10.3389/fetho.2025.1539103.

Donald, P. F., Fernando, E., Brown, L., et al. (2023). Assessing the global prevalence of wild birds in trade. *Conservation Biology* 38:e14350. https://doi.org/10.1111/cobi.14350.

Flanagan, A. M., Masuda, B., Pribble, J., et al. (2024). Starting from scratch: Husbandry techniques to establish the first population of ʻAkikiki (*Oreomystis bairdi*) in human care using wild caught eggs. *Zoo Biology* 43(6):585–589. https://doi.org/10.1002/zoo.21862.

Fuller, T., Bensch, S., Müller, I., et al. (2012). The ecology of emerging infectious diseases in migratory birds: An assessment of the role of climate change and priorities for future research. *Ecohealth* 9(1):80–88. https://doi.org/10.1007/s10393-012-0750-1.

Gulland, F. M. D., Barbieri, M., Cleaveland, S., et al. (2024). Vaccination of endangered wildlife as a conservation tool: Hindsights and new horizons in the pandemic era. *Biological Conservation* 300:110842. https://doi.org/10.1016/j.biocon.2024.110842.

Hutchins, M., Marra, P. P., Diebold, E., et al. (2017). The evolving role of zoological parks and aquariums in migratory bird conservation. *Zoo Biology* 37:360–368. https://doi.org/10.1002/zoo.21438.

Jennings, M. K., Pairis, A., Walker, A., et al. (2025). Climate transformation and stewardship: Reflections on meaningful collaboration to support indigenous-led research. *Ecology and Evolution* 15(12):e72715. https://doi.org/10.1002/ece3.72715.

Klump, B. C., Walter, D., Martin, J. M., et al. (2025). Emergence of a novel drinking innovation in an urban population of sulphur-crested cockatoos, *Cacatua galerita*. *Biology Letters* 21(6):20250010. https://doi.org/10.1098/rsbl.2025.0010.

Klusener, R., Hurtado, R., Parsons, N. J., et al. (2018). From incubation to release: Hand-rearing as a tool for the conservation of the endangered African penguin. *PLoS One* 13(11):e0205126. https://doi.org/10.1371/journal.pone.0205126.

Mooney, A., Teare, J. A., Staerk, J., et al. (2023). Flock size and structure influence reproductive success in 4 species of flamingo in 540 captive populations worldwide. *Zoo Biology* 42:343–356. https://doi.org/10.1002/zoo.21753.

Ramont, M., Hickman, C., Snyder, T., et al. (2025). From hatch to fledge: Growth and development of Sihek (*Todiramphus cinnamominus*) chicks at Brookfield Zoo Chicago. *Journal of Zoological and Botanical Gardens* 6:16. https://doi.org/10.3390/jzbg6010016.

Rose, P. and Riley, L. (2019). The use of Qualitative Behavioural Assessment to zoo welfare measurement and animal husbandry change. *Journal of Zoo and Aquarium Research* 7(4):150–161. https://hdl.handle.net/10871/39449.

Ruuskanen, S. (2024). Early-life environmental effects on birds: Epigenetic and microbiome as mechanisms underlying long-lasting phenotypic changes. *Journal of Experimental Biology* 227:jeb246024. https://doi.org/10.1242/jeb.246024.

Sherley, R. B., Waller, L. J., Strauss, V., et al. (2014). Hand-rearing, release and survival of African penguin chicks abandoned before independence by moulting parents. *PLoS One* 9(10):e110794. https://doi.org/10.1371/journal.pone.0110794.

Stoyanov, G., Peshev, H. V., Kmetova-Biro, E., et al. (2023). Results of the re-introduction of the Griffon Vulture (*Gypsfulvus*) in Vrachanski Balkan Nature Park, Bulgaria – completion of the establishing phase 2010–2020. *Biodiversity Data Journal* 11:e100834. https://doi.org/10.3897/BDJ.11.e100834.

Theule, J. and Rimlinger, D. (2023). Breeding history and husbandry of the Raggiana Bird of paradise (*Paradisaea raggiana*). *Zoo Biology* 42:162–170. https://doi.org/10.1002/zoo.21714.

Voges, J. J., Freeman, M. T., Wolf, B. O., et al. (2024). Functional role of metabolism suppression in avian thermoregulation in the heat. *Journal of Thermal Biology* 123:103924. https://doi.org/10.1016/j.therbio.2024.103924.

Wada, H. and Coutts, V. (2021). Detrimental or beneficial? Untangling the literature on development stress studies in birds. *Journal of Experimental Biology* 224(19):jeb227363. https://doi.org/10.1242/jeb227363.

Werner, C. S., Chapman, M., Peach, D. A. H., et al. (2026). Use of contaminated habitat and associated selenium uptake mediate Haemosporidian parasite infections in wild passerine birds. *Ecology and Evolution* 16(1):372681. https://doi.org/10.1002/ece3.72681.

Wernery, U., Liu, C., Baskar, V., et al. (2010). Primordial germ cell-mediated chimera technology produces viable pure-line Houbara bustard offspring: Potential for repopulating an endangered species. *PLoS One* 5(12):e15824. https://doi.org/10.1371/journal.pone.0015824.

Whitfort, H. L. and Young, R. J. (2004). Trends in the captive breeding of threatened and endangered birds in British zoos, 1988–1997. *Zoo Biology* 23:85–89. https://doi.org/10.1002/zoo.10122.

Zhang, J., Zhang, D., Zhang, Y., et al. (2026). A method for preparing morphologically preserved wildlife fecal specimens for long-term ecological studies. *Ecology and Evolution* 16:e72931. https://doi.org/10.1002/ece3.72931.

13

Epilogue – Ode to the Chicken

Gallus gallus domesticus. Domesticated descendant of the red jungle fowl (*Gallus gallus*; Figure 13.1). Chickens have been some of the most famous comedic characters in cartoons over the years (Figure 13.2). Foghorn Leghorn, a tall, endearing rooster of the Looney Tunes heyday (Warner Bros.); Chicken Little, the title character and defender of his town from alien invaders (Disney); Heihei, the most recent addition, as Moana's friend and companion on her journeys (Disney); and Torchic, a Pokémon character! (The chicken has made it into the Pokémon genre!) The chicken is an infamous farm resident, but the rooster may be seen as an annoyance when he crows at daybreak. They are frequently raised in backyards, almost as pets, but not allowed inside the home, like a dog or cat. They are a favorite meal of young and old, from chicken nuggets to elegant chicken cuisine.

But do we really know the chicken? Often the term "chicken" is used to refer to someone who is afraid and meek. This is despite the fact that the chicken has a rich history in many cultures around the world as a symbol of fortune, prosperity, longevity, strength, and fertility. It is revered and is considered sacred in India and African nations.

But really, do we/you really *know* the chicken? Its history in biomedical research and science? Its contributions to genetics, immunology, virology, vaccine development, developmental biology, neurology, and carcinogenesis (among other areas)? Or do we only "know" the chicken because it is the most common food item, and the way the poultry industry has managed the chicken raises furor in many people?

The ability to observe embryonic development in an egg, outside of the female, was revolutionary to the field of embryology and development. The discovery of oncogenes (genes that cause cancer/neoplasia) and that viruses can cause cancer was made in a sarcoma tumor of a chicken! The scientist, Dr Rous, discovered the tumor was due to a virus, ultimately named Rous Sarcoma virus. And this discovery led to a multitude of details about the pathogenesis of cancer. The finding of different types of lymphocytes (B and T lymphocytes) in birds led to fundamental discoveries of the different arms of the immune system (Tregaskes and Kaufman, 2021).

The chicken was, and remains, a model for various human diseases. Chickens are easy to raise and manage, making them an attractive model organism. The study of Rous Sarcoma virus revealed it to be an immunosuppressive virus. This led to the chicken as an early model for AIDS and HIV studies. Viruses were cultured (grown) in chicken eggs before *in-vitro*

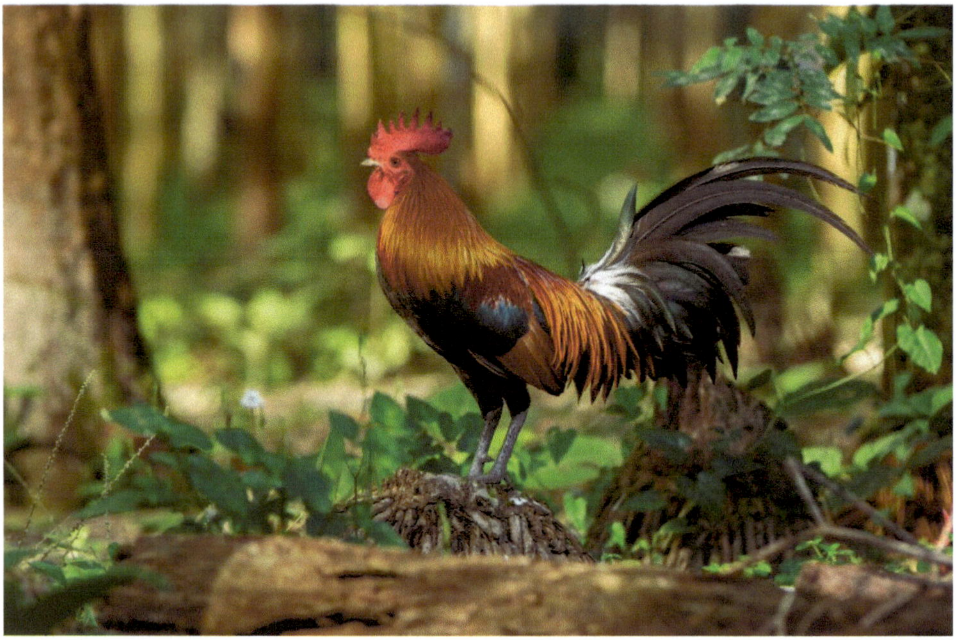

Suksamranpix/Adobe Stock Photos

Figure 13.1 Red jungle fowl (*Gallus gallus*).

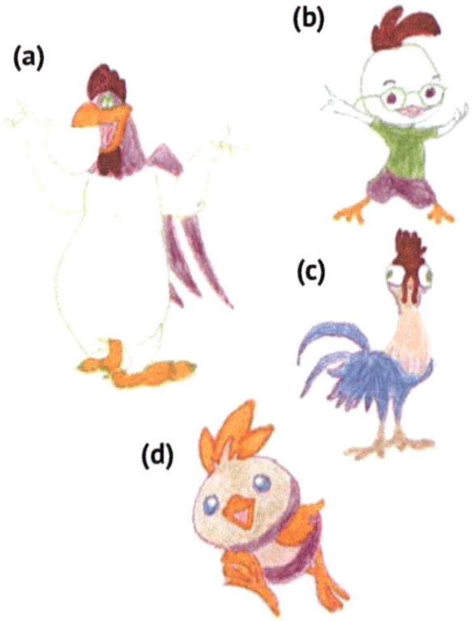

Figure 13.2 Famous chicken cartoon characters. (a) Foghorn Leghorn, (b) Chicken Little, (c) Heihei, (d) Torchic. *Source:* Illustration by author.

methods were developed. Chicken eggs are used in vaccine development. Autoimmune diseases, including rheumatoid arthritis, have been studied in chickens (Tregaskes and Kaufman, 2021). Even though the models of human disease most often used now are mice, the chicken's role in biomedical research, and the discoveries made therein, is solid and impressive.

From a simply a biological viewpoint, one of the most interesting demonstrations of selective breeding and genetics belongs to the chicken (and I guess the poultry geneticists too). The development and selective breeding of chickens raised for meat and egg is impressive! (The business end of poultry production is also impressive, but I am focused on the birds.) Even the undesirable side effects observed in the chickens secondary to the selection for increased muscle mass and continual daily egg laying are medically instructive and largely nutritionally manageable. For example, selection for daily consecutive egg production for over a year straight may lead to brittle bones (decreased bone calcium) as the calcium is used in producing the eggshell. This side effect is relatively infrequent and can be mitigated by supplementation of calcium and other minerals. But this provides a different avenue to study metabolic bone diseases relevant to humans.

My foray into learning about poultry science was while researching this book. The result of that foray is immense respect for the chicken! I have owned a few chickens as pets, and I found them to be quite intelligent! My daughter dislikes chickens because one of the chickens we had as a pet didn't like her and chased her all the time! But I love chickens! Especially the variety in plumage of some strains (Figure 13.3). In Miami where I live, there are many chickens now roaming many neighborhoods. And I drive my daughter crazy by slowing down the car to watch them every time we pass some. On the way home from work every day, I pass a woman who lives on the street, and inevitably, there are a few chickens by her on the sidewalk or with her on her bench. Her friends! And she shares food with them, and they return the favor by being company for her. It is very sweet. So we can add companion as another quality of chickens.

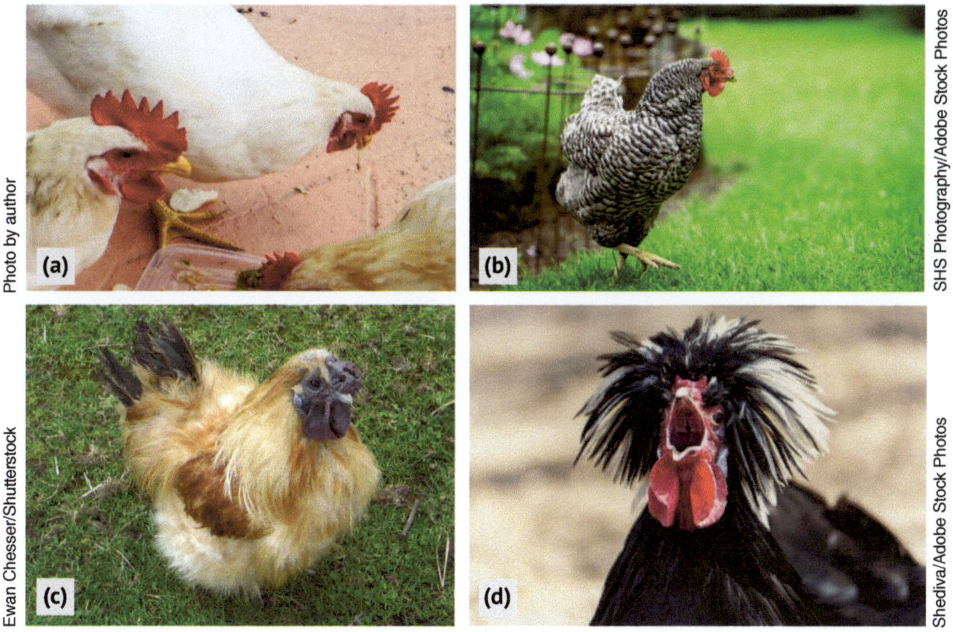

Figure 13.3 Examples of varieties of chickens. (a) Author's pet chickens. (b) Dominique chicken. (c) Silkie chicken. (d) Black polish chicken.

And let us not forget, in Jewish culture, the ultimate contribution from the chicken, the tried-and-true cure for *everything*...chicken soup!

Thank you to all chickens.

Literature Cited

Tregaskes, C. A. and Kaufman, J. (2021). Chickens as a simple system for scientific discovery: The example of the MHC. *Molecular Immunology* 135:12–20. https://doi.org/10.1016/j.molimm.2021.03.019.

Index

Note: Page numbers in *italics* and **bold** refers to figures and tables respectively.